EXAMKRACKERS

16 MINI MCATS

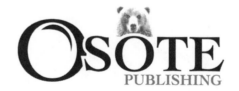

OSOTE
PUBLISHING

ISBN 1-893858-43-X

2004 Edition

Design and production by Saucy Enterprizes, LLC [www.saucyenterprizes.com]

To purchase additional copies of this book, call 1-(888)-572-2536 or fax orders to 1-(201)-797-1644

Examkrackers.com

Osote.com

TABLE OF CONTENTS

INSTRUCTIONS

ExamKrackers 16 Mini-MCATs is designed to provide practice in all topics covered by the MCAT. For best results, the exams can be taken in conjunction with study from the *Examkrackers Complete MCAT Study Package as follows:

After Studying:	Take Exams:
Verbal Introduction: Introduction to MCAT Including MCAT Math Physics Lecture 1: Translational Motion Biology Lecture 1: Molecular Biology; Cellular Respiration Verbal Lecture 1: Strategy and Tactics	1 and 2
Chemistry Lecture 1: Atoms, Molecules, and Quantum Mechanics Physics Lecture 2: Force Biology Lecture 2: Genes Verbal Lecture 2: Answering the Questions	3 and 4
Chemistry Lecture 2: Gases, Kinetics, and Chemical Equilibrium Physics Lecture 3: Equilibrium, Torque, and Energy Biology Lecture 3: Microbiology Verbal Lecture 3: The Main Idea	5 and 6
Chemistry Lecture 3: Thermodynamics Physics Lecture 4: Momentum, Machines, and Radioactive Decay Biology Lecture 4: The Eukaryotic Cell; The Nervous System Organic Chemistry Lecture 1: Molecular Structure Verbal Lecture 4: How to Study for the Verbal Reasoning Section	7 and 8
Chemistry Lecture 4: Solutions Physics Lecture 5: Fluids and Solids Biology Lecture 5: The Endocrine System Organic Chemistry Lecture 2: Hydrocarbons, Alcohols, and Substitutions	9 and 10
Chemistry Lecture 5: Heat Capacity, Phase Change, and Colligative Properties Physics Lecture 6: Waves Biology Lecture 6: The Digestive System; The Excretory System Organic Chemistry Lecture 3: Carbonyls and Amines	11 and 12
Chemistry Lecture 6: Acids and Bases Physics Lecture 7: Electricity and Magnetism Biology Lecture 7: The Cardiovascular System; The Respiratory System Organic Chemistry Lecture 4: Biochemistry and Lab Techniques	13 and 14
Chemistry Lecture 7: Electrochemistry Physics Lecture 8: Light and Optics Biology Lecture 8: Muscle, Bone, and Skin Biology Lecture 9: Populations	15 and 16

*Examkrackers Complete MCAT Study Package is available at www.examkrackers.com.

BIOLOGICAL & PHYSICAL SCIENCES

DIRECTIONS. Most of the questions in 16 MINI MCATS are organized into groups, each preceded by a descriptive passage. After studying the passage, select the one best answer to each question in the group. Some questions are not based on a descriptive passage and are also independent of each other. You must also select the one best answer to these questions. If you are not certain of an answer, eliminate the alternatives that you know to be incorrect and then select an answer from the remaining alternatives. Indicate your selection by blackening the corresponding oval on your answer document. A periodic table is provided for your use.

PERIODIC TABLE OF THE ELEMENTS

1 H 1.0																	2 He 4.0
3 Li 6.9	4 Be 9.0											5 B 10.8	6 C 12.0	7 N 14.0	8 O 16.0	9 F 19.0	10 Ne 20.2
11 Na 23.0	12 Mg 24.3											13 Al 27.0	14 Si 28.1	15 P 31.0	16 S 32.1	17 Cl 35.5	18 Ar 39.9
19 K 39.1	20 Ca 40.1	21 Sc 45.0	22 Ti 47.9	23 V 50.9	24 Cr 52.0	25 Mn 54.9	26 Fe 55.8	27 Co 58.9	28 Ni 58.7	29 Cu 63.5	30 Zn 65.4	31 Ga 69.7	32 Ge 72.6	33 As 74.9	34 Se 79.0	35 Br 79.9	36 Kr 83.8
37 Rb 85.5	38 Sr 87.6	39 Y 88.9	40 Zr 91.2	41 Nb 92.9	42 Mo 95.9	43 Tc (98)	44 Ru 101.1	45 Rh 102.9	46 Pd 106.4	47 Ag 107.9	48 Cd 112.4	49 In 114.8	50 Sn 118.7	51 Sb 121.8	52 Te 127.6	53 I 126.9	54 Xe 131.3
55 Cs 132.9	56 Ba 137.3	57 La* 138.9	72 Hf 178.5	73 Ta 180.9	74 W 183.9	75 Re 186.2	76 Os 190.2	77 Ir 192.2	78 Pt 195.1	79 Au 197.0	80 Hg 200.6	81 Tl 204.4	82 Pb 207.2	83 Bi 209.0	84 Po (209)	85 At (210)	86 Rn (222)
87 Fr (223)	88 Ra 226.0	89 Ac† 227.0	104 Unq (261)	105 Unp (262)	106 Unh (263)	107 Uns (262)	108 Uno (265)	109 Une (267)									

	58 Ce 140.1	59 Pr 140.9	60 Nd 144.2	61 Pm (145)	62 Sm 150.4	63 Eu 152.0	64 Gd 157.3	65 Tb 158.9	66 Dy 162.5	67 Ho 164.9	68 Er 167.3	69 Tm 168.9	70 Yb 173.0	71 Lu 175.0
*														
†	90 Th 232.0	91 Pa (231)	92 U 238.0	93 Np (237)	94 Pu (244)	95 Am (243)	96 Cm (247)	97 Bk (247)	98 Cf (251)	99 Es (252)	100 Fm (257)	101 Md (258)	102 No (259)	103 Lr (260)

16 MINI MCATS

EXAMINATION 01

Questions 1–47

Physical Sciences
Time: 20 Minutes
Questions 1–16

Passage I (Questions 1-7)

Students in a physics lab use a camera with a timer to record the displacement of several objects undergoing accelerated motion. The students record each object's displacement at 0.2 second intervals. The instantaneous velocities of the objects were then approximated from the displacement readings. The students used their data to construct the graphs below, depicting the velocities of the four objects over time.

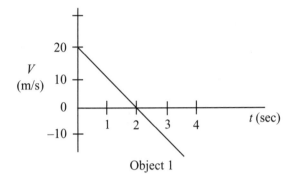

Object 1

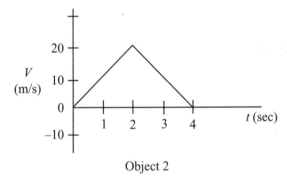

Object 2

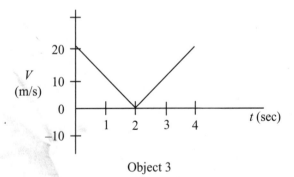

Object 3

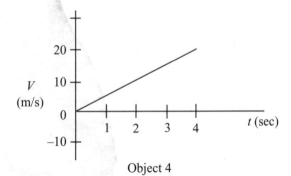

Object 4

Figure 1

1. One of the objects was tossed straight up into the air. A student recorded its motion as the object rose to maximum height and then returned to the starting position. This motion of this object is best represented by the graph of:

   A. Object 1
   B. Object 2
   C. Object 3
   D. Object 4

2. Which of the following is true of the displacement of Object 2 over the course of the 4 seconds shown in the graph?

   A. It is always decreasing.
   B. It is always increasing.
   C. It increases, then decreases.
   D. It decreases, then increases.

3. Which of the following graphs represents the acceleration of Object 3?

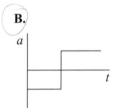
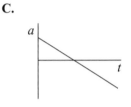
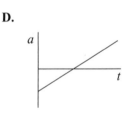

4. Which of the following is true of the speed of Object 1 over the course of its four seconds of recorded motion?

   A. It is always increasing.
   B. It is always decreasing.
   C. It increases, then decreases.
   D. It decreases, then increases.

5. If Object 4 started from rest at a displacement of zero, which of the following is equal to its displacement during the course of its motion?

	1 sec	2 sec	3 sec	4 sec
A	5 m	10 m	15 m	20 m
B	5 m	20 m	45 m	80 m
C	2.5 m	5 m	7.5 m	10 m
D	2.5 m	10 m	22.5 m	40 m

4

6. The displacement measurements taken by the students were used to approximate the instantaneous velocities of the particles. The students' approximations will be most accurate if the time intervals between their measurements are:

   A. short, and the acceleration of each object is small.
   B. short, and the acceleration of each object is large.
   C. long, and the acceleration of each object is small.
   D. long, and the acceleration of each object is large.

7. Which Object(s) will have a displacement of zero at the end of 4 seconds?

   I. Object 1
   II. Object 2
   III. Object 3

   A. I only
   B. II only
   C. I and II only
   D. II and III only

Passage II (Questions 8-13)

A picture of the Red River is shown below. The river's current flows directly from West to East at a rate of 8 meters per second. The banks of the river are parallel to each other and are separated by a distance of 1,800 meters. There is a launching area for boats on the river's South bank.

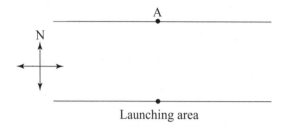

Launching area

Figure 1 River bank diagram

A fisherman who wishes to cross the river can choose to take a motorized canoe which moves at a constant forward velocity of 6 meters per second, or a motorboat which moves at a constant forward velocity of 15 meters per second. In either case, in addition to the velocity due to the boat's motor, a boat crossing the river will be swept down the river by the current with a velocity of 8 meters per second. A person wishing to reach a particular point on the North shore must direct the boat at the angle to the current that will generate the appropriate resultant velocity vector.

8. If the fisherman steers the motorboat due North across the river, what will be the magnitude of the velocity of the boat's actual motion?

   A. 17 m/s
   B. 19 m/s
   C. 23 m/s
   D. 25 m/s

9. If, instead, the fisherman directs the canoe at an angle of 30° to the West of his original Northbound direction, what will be the magnitude of the velocity component that is parallel to the banks of the river?

   A. 2 m/s
   B. 5 m/s
   C. 11 m/s
   D. 14 m/s

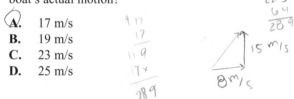

GO ON TO THE NEXT PAGE.

10. The fisherman wishes to cross the river to point A, directly to the North of the launching area. In which direction should he direct the canoe?

    A.   Directly North
    B.   To the West of North
    C.   To the East of North
    D.   The canoe can never land at point A

11. To travel across the river in the least amount of time, the fisherman should direct the boat:

    A.   to the West of North, to minimize the distance traveled.
    B.   to the East of North, to maximize the speed of the boat.
    C.   directly to the North, to maximize the Northward velocity.
    D.   in any direction with a Northward component because the time will always be the same.

12. The fisherman steered the motorboat directly North and reached the far shore at point B, which is 2,040 meters to the East of point A. How long did the trip take?

    A.   1 minute
    B.   2 minutes
    C.   3 minutes
    D.   4 minutes

13. When traveling due North across the river, the fisherman's acceleration is?

    A. 0 m/s^2
    B. 2 m/s^2
    C. 10 m/s^2
    D. 14 m/s^2

Questions 14 through 16 are **NOT** based on a descriptive passage.

14. A series of projectiles were all launched at the same speed, but will different angles of elevation. As the sine of the angle of elevation is increased, the horizontal speed of the projectile:

    A.   increased and the vertical speed decreased.
    B.   increased and the vertical speed increased.
    C.   decreased and the vertical speed decreased.
    D.   decreased and the vertical speed increased.

15. An automobile is traveling eastbound across a flat surface with a velocity of 20 m/s. If the automobile is accelerating westward at 20 m/s^2, which of the following is true of the automobile?

    A.   It is speeding up.
    B.   It is slowing down.
    C.   Its speed is constant.
    D.   Its displacement is constant.

16. Projectile A, with a mass of 10 kg, and Projectile B, with a mass of 20 kg, were launched straight up into the air at the same speed. Compared to Projectile A, Projectile B will experience:

    A.   greater force due to gravity and greater acceleration.
    B.   greater force due to gravity and equal acceleration.
    C.   equal force due to gravity and greater acceleration.
    D.   equal force due to gravity and equal acceleration.

STOP. IF YOU FINISH BEFORE TIME IS CALLED, CHECK YOUR WORK. YOU MAY GO BACK TO ANY QUESTION IN THIS TEST BOOKLET.

Verbal Reasoning
Time: 20 Minutes
Questions 17–31

...In the rush to get their products printed, with time and money frequently being the determining factors, many smaller publishers fail to recognize the differences between the printing companies from which they are choosing. Let
5 me first say, that if you can detect no difference between the full-color look of a *USA Today* and a *Cosmopolitan*, this discussion may not seem very compelling. Loupes have been largely relegated to the stereotypical squinting diamond merchant, and with them, the skills to detect such
10 minor visual variations. Yet the various types of printing presses that these printing companies use do make a difference in the final product.

Outside of the publishing world, the majority of us are familiar with digital style printers. Even very high-end post-
15 script printers and copiers use this technique. We have all had to change toner cartridges. *Digital* printing uses toner that is laid down on the paper and then fused to the paper using extreme heat. This occurs on almost all copiers. In contrast, *offset* printing uses ink, rather than toner, which
20 will penetrate the paper. Where graphic images and text collide the visual differences can be striking. However, there are other notable differences as well.

The warmth we feel when removing fresh copies from our copying machine reminds us of the aforementioned
25 'extreme heat' required in digital printing and copying. This heat has a desiccating effect on the paper. One would notice, for instance, that the 100 pages of paper run through a copying machine—and subjected to heat—take up less room than 100 pages of paper waiting in the feed tray.
30 Normally, the desiccated paper will gradually reabsorb moisture until it reaches ambient humidity conditions without our noticing anything has occurred. But in the rapid-fire printing and book binding process, this reabsorption may not become noticeable until later in the life of the book.

35 In the book binding process, high speed rollers and cutters immediately take the printed pages—whether digital or offset—and assemble them in blocks for binding. Most commonly nowadays—in paperbacks—this is the so-called "perfect binding" process whereby the long edge of the
40 paperback 8 1/2 × 11 book is roughened and then smeared with adhesive. This adhesive effectively seals the bound edge of all of the pieces of paper that make up that book. Remember, however, that the digitally printed pages have become abnormally dry due to the heat of the printing
45 process and are now reabsorbing moisture and resuming their previous size. The problem is that the pages cannot absorb moisture equally on all sides, because the binding has sealed one edge. This may cause the pages of the book to curl, which is not only unsightly and annoying, but will
50 eventually weaken the binding itself with resultant page loss. These problems are exacerbated if the book is smaller than the common 8 1/2 × 11 inches.

Commonly, paper is made from pulp by machines laying down long strands that eventually lie down length-
55 wise along the long axis of the paper. This actually gives the paper a "grain", and can be demonstrated by taking a sheet of common paper and folding it lengthwise, which will result in a smooth and neat fold. Folding that same sheet of paper in half the short way will result in an irregular and
60 rough fold—it goes against the grain. This becomes one of the most significant factors in broken bindings and resultant lost pages when books smaller than 8 1/2 × 11 are printed and bound. For some reason, digital printers are notorious for ignoring paper grain.

65 The newer high-speed digital presses are becoming increasingly prolific due to their ease of use and extremely competitive pricing. But the wary publisher would do well to consider other factors as well. His best bet would be to use an older established printer who has recently acquired a
70 digital printing capability.

GO ON TO THE NEXT PAGE.

17. Suppose that a study found that contrary to popular belief, the majority of people have little or no experience with copiers and printers, but instead patronize commercial printers and copiers for these services. Which of the following statements is an assumption of the author related to this study that would be called into *question*?

   A. Smaller publishers should choose their printing services wisely.
   B. One of the differences between offset and digital printing is visual.
   C. The experience of changing a toner cartridge is common to us all.
   Most people own their own copiers or printers.

18. According to information in the passage, the loss of pages would be likely to occur later in the life of the book, when:

   I. bound with the use of high speed rollers and cutters.
   II. the pages have been dried out and part of the pages are sealed.
   III. the book is smaller than 8 1/2 × 11 inches.

   A. I only
   B. II only
   C. III only
   D. II and III only

19. Which of the following conclusions can most reasonably be drawn from the author's description of printing companies, printers, and his advice to publishers?

   A. Digital printers, though less expensive, are not worth using in the long run.
   B. Older established publishers should seek out printers who use offset presses.
   C. Older establisher printers would be less likely to ignore paper grain, even if they were using digital printers.
   D. A publisher would be well advised to avoid using digital printing altogether.

20. If the hypothesis of the passage is correct, one should find that generally, in the printing business:

   A. a printer who has only used high-speed digital presses has not been in business as long as an offset printer.
   B. the grain of the paper is one of the most important characteristics of the binding process to be aware of.
   C. digital style printers and presses are by far the most prevalent in existence today.
   D. a recently acquired digital printing capability indicates that the printer will be better established in the practice.

21. What is the intended relevance of the comment, "Loupes have been largely relegated to the stereotypical squinting diamond merchant, and with them, the skills to detect such minor visual variations" (lines 8-10), to the rest of the passage?

   A. To explain how difficult it is to acquire the skills necessary to distinguish one style of printing from another.
   B. To provide a framework from which to understand the more arcane areas of offset printing
   C. To express the subtleties in the flaws of diamonds and other gemstones
   D. To indicate that there is less attention paid to minute visual detail than there has been in the past

22. Suppose that the author was unaware of a new adhesive, which is permeable to air and moisture, that had been introduced into the perfect binding process. Which of the following *changes* in the author's advice would be most appropriate?

   A. Since the heat from digital printing would not cause curling, the only difference between offset and digital press would be the almost imperceptible visual differences.
   B. The author's advice to smaller publishers would still be valid, though his reasoning regarding why the paper was curling would have to be changed.
   C. Because curling of the pages later in the life of a book would not be a problem, a publisher would only have to ensure that digital printers were aware of the ramifications of paper grain.
   D. There would no longer be a strong argument supporting the use of offset printers over digital printers.

23. The author's primary purpose in addressing his audience is to:

   A. Consider the effects of newer technology on smaller publishing businesses as a whole.
   B. Clarify the advantages and disadvantages of one form of printing over another.
   C. Question the need for the newer digital presses in the printing industry.
   D. Justify the use of older, well-established businesses and offset printers.

_____

"Wow, that is a *beautiful* dog. Does he have papers?" Papers? Is this Communist East Germany or something?! Hey, we don't need no stinking papers! Yet, anyone who owns a dog understands what this rather cryptic question is
5 referring to. The 'innocent' wishes to know whether your dog has "papers" from the American Kennel Club (AKC) validating that your canine is a pure breed. To most American dog lovers, having papers would also seem to convey something more. That their dog is really something
10 special; beautifully obedient with wonderful conformation, and a striking example of its breed.

What a sad joke. This naïve idea has ruined more than one breed of dog in the United States. Think about it a moment. If you had a purebred (i.e. papered) male and
15 female Lhasa Apso and bred them, then bred their children, then bred their children's children, sooner, rather than later, the inbreeding would begin to show itself through genetic defects, both physical and mental. The puppies might be born blind, three-legged, or inherently vicious. Yet the good
20 old AKC would still be glad to have you, the breeder, adver- tise that these sickened little degenerates had their "papers". This is, in fact, what actually happens again and again throughout the United States at 'puppy farms' and even within the households of well meaning, yet poorly educated
25 self-styled dog 'breeders'. Moreover, other dolts go out and buy these dogs secure in the knowledge that their dog is a purebred with papers!

Far better is what occurs in West Germany with German Shepherds, which are considered a national treas-
30 ure and an icon of the country. I am referring to the nationally sanctioned Schutzhund competitions wherein the dogs are judged in three areas. First is Conformation. The judges look very closely for physically disqualifying char- acteristics, such as floppy ears, missing teeth, poor or
35 discolored eyes, or hip dysplasia. The dog is actually given a rating and ranking based upon how well it physically looks like what a German Shepherd is *supposed* to look like. During this phase, any outward signs of aggression by the dog, either towards the judges, or other dogs and
40 strangers is immediately disqualifying. Next comes the Tracking and Obedience portion of the trials where the dog is ranked on its ability to concentrate and discriminately track on a trail laid earlier by the judges. Further, the dogs are rated on how quickly they obey the commands of their
45 handlers. Finally, comes the Protection phase where the dogs must react appropriately in a given scenario. Usually this involves an aggressive "mugger" attacking the handler. This mugger has a gun that he fires in the air while the dog is attacking him. If the dog fails this courage test by fleeing
50 or not engaging the attacker, he is disqualified.

There are three mandatory Schutzhund trials through- out the life of a dog which increase in difficulty until the animal reaches Schutzhund III. "Mandatory?!" you ask. That's right. If the animal fails its Schutzhund trials it is
55 *illegal* to breed that German Shepherd. Puppies which the breeders believe lack the proper conformation, are destroyed in order that they don't breed.

It is this exacting competition and the rules behind the competition that allow the preservation and perpetuation of
60 the German Shepherd breed; at least, those German Shepherds which are bred in Germany. While all the while, because of the AKC, a German Shepherd in the U.S. can exhibit crippling hips, floppy ears, and poor temperament, while still touting its "papered" "purebred" status.

24. Which of the following statements, if true, would most directly *challenge* the ideas of the author?

   A. Canine identificationIdentification is actually not required in East Germany.
   B. Puppies that don't pass their Schutzhund trials are neutered.
   C. Most American 'dog lovers' have a good under- standing of the conformation characteristics of their particular breed.
   D. The Schutzhund competitions have become increas- ingly lax in their standards.

25. Elsewhere, the author of the passage states that far too many people in so-called 'free societies' place more trust in well-known organizations thatthan is unwarranted by the tangible results of these organizations' performance. This statement most directly supports the passage asser- tion that:

   A. The the West German Schutzhund trials are a model which the United States should be following.
   B. Itit should be illegal to breed dogs within the United States unless they have passed a Schutzhund trial.
   C. Purebred purebred breeding within the United States has proven disastrous for dogs.
   D. Reliancereliance upon a purebred status from the AKC has resulted in inbreeding.

26. For which of the following conclusions does the passage offer the *most* support?

   A. In West Germany, the German Shepherd breed benefits from the Schutzhund trials.
   B. It is the desire of the AKC that as many dog owners as possible register their dogs as purebreds.
   C. It is the goal of the AKC to ruin breeds of dogs within the United States.
   D. The goals of the Schutzhund trials and the AKC are diametrically opposed to one another.

27. On the basis of the passage, one can most reasonably infer that careful judging has the capacity to distinguish:

   A. between who should and who should not be breeding dogs.
   B. which animals will contribute most to the future of a given breed.
   C. whether or not 'papers' should be conferred upon a given dog.
   D. why a certain dog might or might not be able to pass a Schutzhund competition.

28. Implicit in the passage is the assumption that:

   A. most people love dogs.
   B. whoever is reading the passage must love dogs as much as the author.
   C. anyone who doesn't agree with the author is stupid.
   D. an animal's purebred status means nothing.

29. According to the passage, the Conformation area of Schutzhund (lines 34-53) focuses primarily on which of the following aspects of a German Shepherd?

   A. Will the dog be able to perpetuate the breed?
   B. Should the dog be disqualified for hip displasia?
   C. Can the dog obey the rules of the Schutzhund competition?
   D. Does the dog meet the standards for physical perfection?

30. In the past, some breakaway chapters of the AKC have placed stricter limits on their certification of an animal for breeding purposes than those now used by the parent association. Given this information, the author could best clarify his argument withAn appropriate clarification of the passage would be the stipulation that:

   his the author's argument applies only to both :

   A. the present and future.
   B. the passage addresses only certain parts of the AKC.
   C. the passage addresses only these breakaway chapters.
   D. his argument applies to certifications in West Germany.

31. If the following statements are true, which would most weaken the purpose argument of the proponents of the Schutzhund trials?

   A. Strict adherents to AKC breeding guidelines produce dogs that are very sound, both structurally, and temperamentally.
   B. The Schutzhund trials invariably produce the soundest animals for perpetuation of the breed.
   C. Euthanizing dogs who have failed the trials is inhumane.
   D. National sanctioning of the trials results in bribery and unfair judging.

STOP. IF YOU FINISH BEFORE TIME IS CALLED, CHECK YOUR WORK. YOU MAY GO BACK TO ANY QUESTION IN THIS TEST BOOKLET.

STOP.

Biological Sciences
Time: 20 Minutes
Questions 32-47

The human digestive system orchestrates highly coordinated and specific mechanisms for digestion and absorption of nutrients. Digestion is a progressive process that begins in the mouth and continues in the stomach and small intestine. In general, macromolecules are digested by enzymes into their component molecules before absorption. Nutrients from digested macromolecules, such as water, monosaccharides, amino acids, and lipids are absorbed via passive, facilitated, and active transport mechanisms. These transport mechanisms may occur with or without mineral co-transport.

Digestive enzymes, at the intestinal brush border, work together with those secreted by salivary glands and pancreas to facilitate nutrient absorption. The digestion of complex carbohydrates provides a good example of this synchrony. Alpha-amylases, both salivary and pancreatic, hydrolyze 1,4-glycosidic bonds in starch, yielding maltose, maltotriose, and alpha-limit dextrins. Maltase, α-dextrinase, and sucrase in the intestinal brush border hydrolyze these oligosaccharides to their final monosaccharide products: glucose, galactose, and fructose. Other brush border enzymes, Lactase, trehalase, and sucrase degrade their respective dissacharides to monosaccharides.

Acarbose is a commonly used diabetic medication which directly inhibits α-1,4-glucosidases, with a 10^5-fold higher affinity than typical substrates. The graph below demonstrates α-glucosidase kinetics in the absence and presence of acarbose.

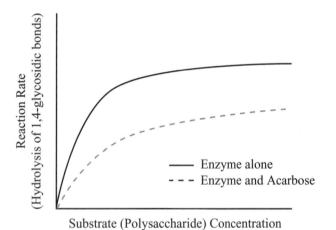

32. Which of the following molecules is NOT transported via Na$^+$ dependent transport?

   A. Bile Acids
   B. Galactose
   C. Proteins
   D. Fatty Acids

33. Pancreatic peptidases do not demonstrate discretion between ingested proteins and self-proteins. For this reason, they are closely regulated. Pancreatic peptidases are activated by which of the following mechanisms?

   A. proteolytic cleavage
   B. temperature change
   C. pH change
   D. cofactor binding

34. Micelle formation is necessary for the intestinal absorption of all of the following molecules, EXCEPT:

   A. cholesterol
   B. triglycerides
   C. bile acids
   D. vitamin D

35. Which of the following products of digestion is NOT absorbed by a specific carrier in intestinal cell wall?

   A. fructose
   B. sucrose
   C. alanine
   D. tripeptides

36. From the graph above, Acarbose most closely demonstrates which type of inhibition on α-1,4-glucosidase?

   A. allosteric
   B. reversible covalent modification
   C. negative cooperativity
   D. competitive

37. According to the graph, acarbose affects α-1, 4-glucosidase enzyme kinetics by:

   A. altering enzyme specificity
   B. irreversible inactivating the enzyme's active site residue(s)
   C. changing the enzyme's affinity for its normal substrate
   D. decreasing the concentration of available enzyme

38. By inhibiting α-1,4-glucosidases, acarbose induces a clinical syndrome that most closely resembles :

   A. lactase deficiency
   B. *Vibrio cholera* infection
   C. Bile acid deficiency
   D. Intrinsic factor deficiency

39. Glucosidase can be best described as a:

   A. lyase
   B. hydrolase
   C. oxidoreductase
   D. kinase

GO ON TO THE NEXT PAGE.

Glycolysis is one of the oldest metabolic pathways in evolution. In this ten-step process, glucose is converted to 2 molecules of pyruvate, yielding a net 2 molecules of ATP. In the presence of oxygen, pyruvate is decarboxylated and esterified with coenzyme A in the mitochondria to enter the Krebs cycle. Ostensibly, when glucose levels exceed energy demand, the body stores the sugar for future oxidation. When glucose levels are insufficient, the body will synthesize the carbohydrate from metabolites such as pyruvate or certain amino acids. In fasting conditions, for instance, the liver and kidney convert pyruvate and glucogenic amino acids into glucose for export to the bloodstream. This process of gluconeogenesis occurs in an opposite pathway to glycolysis. Thus, where glycolysis provides a net gain of ATP, gluconeogenesis requires a net input of energy. Understandably, operating both pathways simultaneously would be an inefficient use of cell resources. As a result, these pathways are tightly regulated according to the changing needs of the cell. Coordination of glucose metabolism is also important at tissue, organ, and system levels. For example, at low blood sugar levels, glucose will be preferentially supplied to the brain.

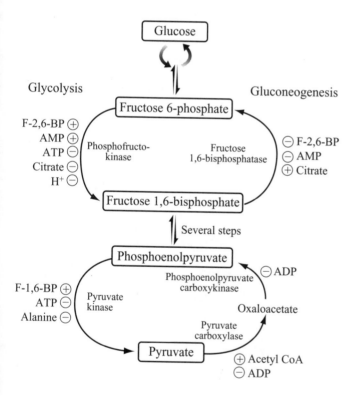

Figure 1 Glycolysis/Gluconeogenesis

40. Feedback regulation, a method of controlling different pathways in the body, is of paramount importance in glucose metabolism. In glycolysis, under aerobic conditions:

    A. citrate is involved in negative feedback regulation
    B. The synthesis of ATP results in positive feedback
    C. Fructose-1,6-bisphosphate functions in endpoint regulation
    D. AMP is involved in positive feedback regulation

41. A student in a biology lab simulates *in vitro* glycolysis. In order for the reaction to proceed in the forward direction, her experiment vessel, along with glucose and glycolytic enzymes, must contain:

    A. NADH, ADP, Pi, CoA
    B. FAD$^+$, ATP, ADP
    C. NAD$^+$, ATP, ADP, Pi
    D. NAD$^+$, ADP, Pi,

42. Which of the following statements regarding glycolysis is FALSE:

    A. glycolysis only occurs in the cytosol
    B. the reactions only takes place in the presence of oxygen
    C. it involves the oxidation of glucose
    D. it provides less ATP than oxidative phosphorylation

43. Once glucose enters the cell, it is promptly phosphorylated by the enzyme glucokinase. The purpose of this reaction is to:

    A. allow glucose to enter the mitochondria
    B. prevent glucose from leaving the cell
    C. convert glucose to CoA
    D. reduce the sugar

44. After a three day period of starvation, the body will participate in which of the following conditions:

    I. upregulated glucagon levels
    II. the upregulation of glycolysis
    III. the downregulation of gluconeogenesis

    A. I only
    B. I and III only
    C. II and III only
    D. I, II, and III only

Question 47 is **NOT** based on a descriptive passage.

45. AMP is an allosteric regulator of phosphofructokinase. In this scenario, enzyme activation is achieved by:

  A. covalent modification of the enzyme
  B. converting the zymogen to an active form
  C. binding of the active site
  D. changing the conformation of the enzyme

46. The Gibbs free energy change, ΔG, is negative for all of the following reactions, EXCEPT:

  A. Diffusion of a solute down its concentration gradient.
  B. ATP hydrolysis.
  C. Diffusion of a solute up its concentration gradient.
  D. Proton entry into the mitochondrial matrix via ATP synthase.

47. The primary function of an erythrocyte is to serve as a carrier of oxygen to the other tissues in the body. In a mature erythrocyte, glucose metabolism :

  A. occurs along with aerobic respiration
  B. occurs without aerobic respiration
  C. occurs only if the RBC is not oxygen bound
  D. does not occur at all

STOP. IF YOU FINISH BEFORE TIME IS CALLED, CHECK YOUR WORK. YOU MAY GO BACK TO ANY QUESTION IN THIS TEST BOOKLET.

STOP.

16 MINI MCATS

EXAMINATION 02

Questions 48–94

Physical Sciences
Time: 20 Minutes
Questions 48-63

Passage I (Questions 48-55)

A projectile's horizontal distance and maximum height are both functions of the projectiles launch speed and angle of elevation. The maximum height of a projectile can be predicted using the equation,

$$h = \frac{(v \sin x)^2}{2g}$$

In this formula, h represents the maxiumum height, v the initial speed of the projectile, x the angle of elevation, and g the acceleration due to gravity. The horizontal distance traveled by a projectile may also be calculated using the following formula:

$$d = \frac{2v^2}{g} \sin(90 - x) \sin x$$

d, the horizontal distance, is presented as a function of three variables: v, the initial speed of the projectile; x, the angle of elevation; and g, the acceleration due to gravity.

A launching device is able to consistently launch smooth, spherical projectiles at a speed of 50 m/s. Three projectiles are launched by the device at varying angles of elevation. The graph below depicts the height of three projectiles over the course of their flight. For the purposes of this passage, air resistance may be ignored and the acceleration due to gravity is 10 m/s^2.

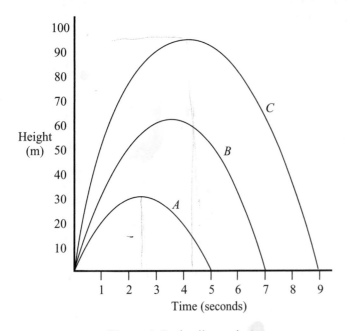

Figure 1 Projectile graph

48. According to the graph, which of the projectiles is launched with the greatest angle of elevation?

   A. Projectile A
   B. Projectile B
   C. Projectile C
   D. The angle of elevation cannot be determined without further information.

49. As the launching device increases the angle of elevation from 0° to 90°, the horizontal distance traveled by a projectile will:

   A. increase only.
   B. decrease only.
   C. increase, then decrease.
   D. decrease, then increase.

50. If the launching device is set at an angle of 45°, what will be the horizontal distance traveled by the projectile? (sin 45° = 0.707)

   A. 60 m
   B. 125 m
   C. 200 m
   D. 250 m

51. At what point in its trajectory does projectile A have the least amount of speed?

   A. 1.5 seconds
   B. 2.5 seconds
   C. 3.5 seconds
   D. 4.5 seconds

52. What is the value of sin x for projectile C?

   A. $\sin x = \dfrac{5}{19}$

   B. $\sin x = \dfrac{19}{25}$

   C. $\sin x = \sqrt{\dfrac{5}{19}}$

   D. $\sin x = \sqrt{\dfrac{19}{25}}$

53. When the horizontal distances for the three projectiles were measured, it was found that projectile A and projectile C traveled the same distance. If the angle of elevation for projectile A is given by y and the angle of elevation for projectile C is given by z, which of the following is true of y and z?

A. $y = z$
B. $y + z = 45°$
C. $y + z = 90°$
D. $y + z = 180°$

54. The horizontal distance traveled by projectile A is 125 meters. What was the horizontal speed of the projectile?

A. 5 m/s
B. 10 m/s
C. 20 m/s
D. 25 m/s

55. Which of the projectiles demonstrates the greatest acceleration?

A. Projectile A
B. Projectile B
C. Projectile C
D. The acceleration is the same for all three projectiles.

Passage II (Questions 56-60)

During the busiest hours at Center City Airport, planes take off from the principal runway every 3 minutes. Each plane starts from rest and accelerates down the runway at a rate of 3.0 m/s². The planes become airborne when their horizontal speeds reach 60 m/s. Each plane leaves the runway pointed due north, and gains altitude at a rate of 9 m/s until it reaches a cruising altitude of 2.25 km. Most commercial airplanes have a mass of approximately 4500 kg.

After becoming airborne, Airplane A flew due north for a distance of 12 km while accelerating at a rate of 0.01 m/s². The plane then turned due east and flew at constant horizontal speed for another 16 km. At this point, the plane turned south.

Airplane B flew north for two minutes with a horizontal acceleration of 0.02 m/s², then turned west and continued at a constant horizontal speed.

Airplane C flew north with constant horizontal acceleration for a distance of 20 km. At this point, the plane had reached a horizontal speed of 200 m/s, which it maintained in the same direction.

(For the purposes of the passage, assume that the time spent changing direction is insignificant. Please ignore the curvature of the Earth in all calculations due to the short nature of the distances traveled.)

56. Which of the following expressions is equal to the horizontal speed of an airplane at takeoff?

A. $(60)(3600)\left(\dfrac{1}{1000}\right)$ km / hr

B. $(60)\left(\dfrac{1}{3600}\right)(1000)$ km / hr

C. $(60)\left(\dfrac{1}{3600}\right)\left(\dfrac{1}{1000}\right)$ km / hr

D. $(60)(3600)(1000)$ km / hr

GO ON TO THE NEXT PAGE.

57. The Center City airport has nearly doubled in air traffic over the last few years. In order to accommodate this increased volume of air traffic, the city must maximize the amount of runways, by making the runways as small as possible. What is the shortest possible length for the Center City principal runway?

    A.   400 m
    B.   600 m
    C.   900 m
    D.   1200 m

58. What is the horizontal displacement of Airplane A at the end of its Eastward leg?

    A.   0 m
    B.   4 m
    C.   20 m
    D.   28 m

59. How long does it take for a plane to achieve cruising altitude from rest?

    A.   250 sec
    B.   260 sec
    C.   270 sec
    D.   280 sec

60. As Airplane B climbs towards its cruising altitude, its acceleration vector is directed:

    A.   horizontally.
    B.   slightly above the horizontal.
    C.   slightly below the horizontal.
    D.   straight downward.

Questions 61 through 63 are **NOT** based on a descriptive passage.

61. A gust of wind blows a small potted plant off a windowsill. If the windowsill is 3 meters high, what is the approximate vertical speed of the plant when it hits the ground?

    A.   5 m/s
    B.   8 m/s
    C.   10 m/s
    D.   20 m/s

62. It takes about 8 minutes and 20 seconds for light from the Sun to reach the Earth. If the Earth orbits the Sun in a circular path and the speed of light is 3×10^8 m/s, what is the approximate distance traveled by the Earth in one year?

    A. 3×10^8 m
    B. 9×10^8 m
    C. 3×10^{11} m
    D. 9×10^{11} m

63. A 10 kg cardboard box is pushed up a 60° incline at a constant velocity against a frictional force of 60 N. Which of the following is equal to the acceleration of the box?

    A. 0 m/s^2
    B. $6 \cos 60°$ m/s^2
    C. $6 \sin 60°$ m/s^2
    B. $6 \tan 60°$ m/s^2

STOP. IF YOU FINISH BEFORE TIME IS CALLED, CHECK YOUR WORK. YOU MAY GO BACK TO ANY QUESTION IN THIS TEST BOOKLET.

STOP.

Verbal Reasoning
Time: 20 Minutes
Questions 64-78

Through a battery of magazine, radio, and television advertisements, consumers are repeatedly urged to create an almost surgically clean environment in which to live. We *must* strive to eliminate not only the execrable bacteria in,
5 on, and around our toilets, but also on the doorknobs, kitchen floors, in our air ducts, and in our yards. It is now more common than not when viewing news footage from many countries to see the business-attired local populace nonchalantly sporting surgical facemasks! Yet, assumed
10 amid the increasing prevalence of anti-bacterial soaps, disinfecting bathroom cleaners, and other household super-cleaners, is the idea that the elimination of as much bacteria and germs on and around the body is a good idea. Dirt, and accompanying bacteria and germs, makes us sick so let's
15 get rid of as many of them as we can, right? Maybe. Maybe not.

Beyond the well-known fact that many of these organisms are actually helpful and necessary to human life, lie the less intuitive ideas that a little dirt and grunge may be a
20 good thing. The first suggestion of this came about as a result of a rather bland study regarding the household living environments of children with allergies; or more accurately the *control group* of children for the study who did *not* have allergies. A young graduate student attempting to analyze
25 the data from a different perspective began looking more closely at this control group and realized that a commonality among most of them was the presence of a household pet; either an 'inside' cat or a dog. This coincidence was regarded with little interest and the student quickly chose
30 another subject for his dissertation. It was not until several years later that further studies, which were actually attempting to prove that these same types of 'indoor' pets were very 'clean', instead pointed toward the seemingly obvious conclusion that these animals in fact brought additional dirt,
35 bacteria and germs into a household and into contact with the inhabitants of that household. The domiciles with pets were not nearly so clean as those without, despite the best efforts of the person responsible for cleaning the home. Though the 'animals-r-cleaner-than-us' group who had
40 commissioned the study was disappointed, these results were noticed by the grad-student-now-associate-professor who began to once again take a look at his previous findings. It was his eventual conclusion that the control group of children from the previous studies was without allergies
    precisely because they had been exposed to their pets for a prolonged period during their youth. The fact that they had
45 grown up in a less than aseptic environment had benefited them.

More recently, though it is reported that "no one is sure why", incidences of eczema—as well as other atopic disorders such as asthma, hay fever and peanut allergy—
50 appear to be rising. According to recent studies from Denmark, Germany, Sweden and the United States, up to 17 percent of schoolchildren have eczema—about three times as many as in earlier generations. "There's better data for the asthma, but [eczema is] following the same direction,
55 with a significant increase over the last few years," said Alan Moshka, a skin diseases specialist with the National Institute of Arthritis and Musculoskeletal and Skin Diseases. Dr. Moshka went on to explain "possible explanations for the increase range from too little exposure to
60 antigens (because our houses are too clean) to too much exposure to dust mites (because our houses are too warm and well-insulated)."

64. Which of the following assertions did the author NOT provide support for in the passage?

   A. Some people in Denmark, Germany, Sweden, and the U.S are wearing surgical facemasks.
   B. It is a fact that many bacteria and germs are actually helpful to human life.
   C. Having pets that bring dirt into your home might make you healthier.
   D. Anti-bacterial soaps, in particular, are not good for us.

65. Which of the following conclusions can justifiably be drawn from the experience of the "grad-student-now-associate-professor" (lines 42-43) mentioned in the passage?

   A. Frequently, a seemingly failed study can provide valuable insights when analyzed from a different perspective.
   B. A researcher who does not have preconceived notions of what he will find from the data may do a better job.
   C. Important information may be gained from a study that does not support its initial hypothesis.
   D. It is possible that the "grad student" got his associate professor position because of his findings from the first study.

24

66. The author's referral to the *first* "rather bland study" in lines 20-31 contains the unstated assumption that:

   A. all of the children in the control group had indoor pets.
   B. the children with allergies did not have household pets.
   C. the homes were not as clean as the owners might have wanted them to be.
   D. the young graduate student had been one of the children in the control group.

67. The statement that pets were bringing "dirt, bacteria and germs into a household" (line 36), is NOT supported by information in the passage regarding:

   A. the types of owners of these pets.
   B. the fact that the pets were 'inside' cats and dogs.
   C. the original goals of the study.
   D. the cleanliness of the children themselves.

68. A critic asks the author, "Suppose it were possible to raise a child in an absolutely germ-free environment, and this resulted in an adult who was free of allergies and relatively impervious to infectious diseases. How would this affect your recommendations to parents?" Which of the following responses would best allow the author to maintain his thesis:

   A. "Though this might be physically healthy, it would pose serious social and developmental problems for the child."
   B. "The supposition is flawed and I stand by my thesis."
   C. "It is important to find options that are available to people from all walks of life all over the world."
   D. "Since the supposition is not feasible at present, it is currently the best practice to allow child some exposure to germs and bacteria."

69. The author would most likely agree with which of the following statements?

   A. If the trend towards using 'anti-bacterials' continues, we will all soon be forced to wear surgical masks.
   B. Being exposed to antigens at an early age can only be beneficial to children.
   C. Advertisements are not usually meant to be accurate health advisements.
   D. Increasing incidences of atopic disorders are probably the result of our houses being too clean.

70. The author's purpose in referencing the "business-attired local populace nonchalantly sporting surgical facemasks" (lines 8-10), is to suggest that:

   A. wearing these facemasks has become fashionable in certain parts of the world.
   B. the 'better-educated' are not taking chances with their health.
   C. people have begun acting in an unreasonable manner.
   D. surgical facemasks alone will not protect you from germs and bacteria.

GO ON TO THE NEXT PAGE.

The work of L.&J.G. Stickley can often be identified by the most obvious details of joinery. The loose wedge pins are usually shaped with a faceted rather than curved outline, the latter being more typical of Craftsman furniture.
5 The tabletop spline is more precise than those found on Limbert Arts and Crafts furniture, though the designs of the L.&J.G. Stickley factory seldom approached the degree of European sophistication that was evident in Limbert's production ...

10 The catalog's claim that this was "entirely American" furniture may have been an overstatement. Many ideas used by L.&J.G. Stickley were "second generation" having been interpreted earlier by Gustav Stickley from such British designers as C.F.A. Voysey and H.M. Baillie Scott. The
15 concept of "honest construction through handwork" was no longer revolutionary. However, it was, in fact, so firmly established that the Stickleys were free to use machines to state the idea symbolically.

Construction technique at the L.&J.G. Stickley facto-
20 ries during the years it was evolving from the Onondaga Shops does not seem to have been standardized. As in the early perhaps experimental production of the Gustav Stickley factory details of construction often varied from one piece to the next for any given design. Drawer pulls on
25 early case pieces took the form of crisply faceted rectangular wooden knobs. Metal escutcheons were sometimes fastened with square headed screws and hardware in general could be found in brass as well as the copper that later became standard. Legs on early furniture were some-
30 times of solid wood and sometimes built up with a sandwich-like lamination. The sides of drawers were sometimes held together with dovetails hand shaped in the English tradition while others were fastened without dovetails. A range of stains, from almost black to natural, was
35 more frequently used and the later preference for "quarter sawed" oak was less evident.

By the time the circa 1905 catalog appeared, the company was willing to forego any pretense toward Arts and Crafts adherence to a medieval kind of handcraft and
40 opted for "a scientific manner [that] does not attempt to follow the traditions of a bygone day." This approach may well have contributed to the company's longevity and it certainly removed their production from the restricted and ephemeral realm of a philosophical trend to allow them to
45 continue making "mission oak" well into the 20's. Though many designs still carried appendix-like vestiges of Arts and Crafts theory such as loose wedge pinned mortise and tenon joints that appeared in non-functional situations on case pieces, the company's directors were sensitive enough
50 to realize the advantages of adapting to machine production. The almost trademark use of four interlocking pieces of wood around a central core for furniture legs became

standard. The claim was that this joinery was superior in strength and durability because it circumscribed the use of
55 veneers and was made of solid wood. More practically, it allowed smaller sections of wood to be utilized and the precision machine cuts eliminated the time consuming dual process of laminating and veneering.

Examination of labeled L.&J.G. Stickley furniture
60 reveals that quarter-sawn oak was not used consistently even after production became more standardized. The "fine silver flake of the quartering" was certainly appreciated by the manufacturers but they obviously did not see this elaborate grain pattern as essential to the enrichment of their
65 designs. The oak was generally fumed and the customer was encouraged to select a color for the finish most suited to his individual taste, but with the majority of extant L.&J.G. Stickley pieces retaining original finish in the standard medium brown factory finish. As previously noted,
70 dark finishes do appear on some early pieces and some custom stains such as the then popular green are known.

71. According to the passage, handmade details with respect to furniture is characteristic of:

   I.   Arts and Crafts
  II.   L.&J.G. Stickley
III.   European sophistication.

  A.   I only
  B.   II only
  C.   III only
  D.   I and III only

72. In line 12, the use of the phrase *second geneneration* indicates which of the following characteristics of L.&J.G Stickley's ideas:

  A.   European.
  B.   poorly crafted.
  C.   finely crafted.
  D.   unoriginal.

73. On the basis of the passage, it is reasonable to conclude that:

A.   the Stickleys were the forefathers of the Arts and Crafts furniture movement.
B.   the Stickleys were not interested in producing consistently high-quality furniture.
C.   the Stickley's catalog claims were often self-serving.
D.   the Stickleys usually used fumed quarter sawn oak.

74. The author implies that, for a furniture company, production of strictly hand-made furniture is NOT:

A.   an antique vestige.
B.   possible.
C.   without risks.
D.   practical.

75. According to the author, L.&J.G. Stickley was not only able to evolve to changing production methods, but also a relatively successful company. If both of these assertions are true, which of the following statements is true?

A.   If a company was able to evolve to changing production methods, then it would probably be successful.
B.   If the Stickley company had not evolved to changing production methods then it would not have been successful.
C.   If a company was not able to evolve to changing production methods, then it was not the Stickley company.
D.   If a company was not able to evolve to changing production methods, then it was probably not successful.

76. The passage states that Stickley furniture could often be identified by the most obvious details of joinery. Which of the following assertions is NOT clearly consistent with above statement?

A.   "loose wedge pinned mortise and tenon joints… appeared in non-functional situations"
B.   L&J.G. Stickley began a philosophical evolution in Arts and Crafts beginning in Britain.
C.   the Stickley's employed trademark use of four interlocking pieces of wood for furniture legs.
D.   "details of construction often varied from one piece to the next"

77. The author of the passage would be most likely to agree with which of the following ideas expressed by other furniture craft historians?

A.   The Stickleys were the originators of using four interlocking pieces for furniture legs.
B.   Many of the claims made by the Stickley company have been embellished.
C.   The Stickley company was driven to make money and succeed at all costs.
D.   Limbert and Stickley were on par with one another regarding their level of craftsmanship.

78. Elsewhere, the author of the passage states that the Stickley's name became synonymous with the finest of painstakingly handmade furniture. This statement most directly supports the passage assertion that:

A.   the Stickley's name became almost a trademark for the Arts and Crafts movement's emphasis on hand-crafted quality.
B.   Stickley furniture can be identified by the more obvious handmade details of its joinery.
C.   the Stickleys were later able to make furniture by more modern machine methods, yet fool the consumer into thinking the furniture was actually hand-made.
D.   the Stickleys were later able to make furniture by more modern machine methods, yet still have it perceived as having the original handmade quality.

STOP. IF YOU FINISH BEFORE TIME IS CALLED, CHECK YOUR WORK. YOU MAY GO BACK TO ANY QUESTION IN THIS TEST BOOKLET.

Biological Sciences
Time: 20 Minutes
Questions 79-94

Passage V (Questions 79-84)

Many bacteria achieve glycerol metabolism via conversion to dihydroxyacetone phosphate (DHAP), an intermediate in the glycolytic pathway. This cytoplasmic reaction requires the hydrolysis of one molecule of adenosine triphosphate, as well as the reduction of one molecule of NAD^+. The carbons adjacent to DHAP's carbonyl carbon contain a hydroxyl group and a phosphate group. In the absence of oxygen, many bacteria, like the human body, will utilize fermentation to produce lactic acid.

A hypothetical bacteria known as *M. evanisa* possesses the required enzymes for the conversion of glycerol to DHAP. A microbiologist runs the following experiments in an attempt to identify the optimal conditions for energy production.

Experiment One:

The bacteria is grown aerobically on a glucose medium.

Experiment Two:

The bacteria is grown anaerobically on a glucose medium.

Experiment Three:

The bacteria is grown anaerobically on a glycerol medium.

Experiment Four:

The bacteria is grown aerobically on a glycerol medium.

Partial Results of the scientist's finding are listed below in Table 1. A diagram of the Kreb's cycle and glycolysis are provided as well.

Experiment Number	Net ATP Produced	Other byproducts
1	36	CO_2, H_2O
2	2	???
3	???	CO_2, lactic acid
4	???	CO_2, H_2O

Table 1 Products of Experimental Trials 1-4.

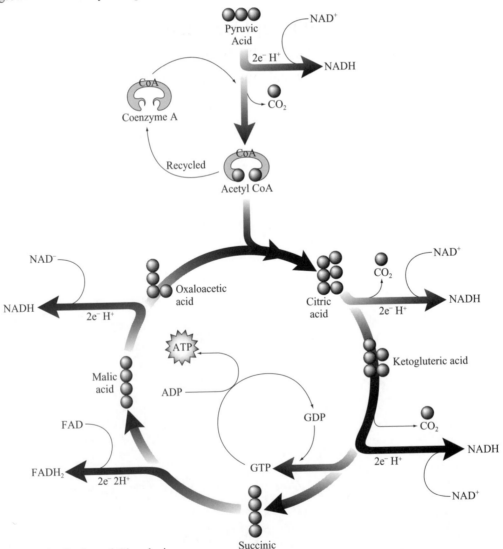

Figure 1 The Krebs Cycle and Glycolysis

30

GO ON TO THE NEXT PAGE.

79. In experiment 3, how many moles of ATP are produced per mole of glycerol, and why?

    A. 0 moles; A shortage of NAD^+ will stall the glycolytic pathway.

    B. 1 mole; Two moles of ATP are produced per molecule of glycerol, however, one mole of ATP is consumed in the conversion of glycerol to DHAP.

    C. 2 moles; Anaerobic respiration produces two moles of ATP.

    D. 3 moles; Though two moles of ATP are produced per molecule of glucose, one less ATP is used to convert glycerol to DHAP than is used to convert glucose to DHAP.

80. Which of the following are byproducts of experiment 2?

    I. Lactic acid
    II. Heat
    III. H_2O

    A. I only
    B. I and III only
    C. II only
    D. I, II, and III

81. In experiment 4, how many moles of ATP are produced per mole of glycerol?

    A. 22 moles
    B. 20 moles
    C. 37 moles
    D. 40 moles

82. Enzyme X is required for the conversion of Succinic acid to Fumaric acid. The enzyme is irreversibly bound by inhibitor Y. If in experiment 1, the scientist adds an excess of inhibitor Y to the medium, levels of which of the following molecules will show the greatest increase?

    I. Succinic Acid
    II. Pyruvic Acid
    III. FAD
    IV. Lactic Acid

    A. I only
    B. II only
    C. IV only
    D. I an III only

83. Inhibitor W works by binding to enzyme X at a site adjacent to the active site for Succinic acid. In the case of such an inhibitor, which of the following best describes the effect on the apparent maximum rate (V_{max}) of the reaction and on the apparent Michaelis constant (K_m)?

    A. V_{max} remains the same and K_m remains the same.
    B. V_{max} remains the same and K_m increases.
    C. V_{max} increases and K_m decreases.
    D. V_{max} decreases and K_m remains the same.

84. Which of the following values could represent the equilibrium constant for the isomerization of DHAP as shown below?

$$DHAP \leftrightarrow GAP$$

    A. 1
    B. .8
    C. 4.73×10^2
    D. 4.73×10^{-2}

GO ON TO THE NEXT PAGE.

Passage VI (Questions 85-91)

In fermentation, ATP is produced in the absence of oxygen. There are 2 major subtypes of the process: lactic acid and alcohol fermentation. Both serve similar purposes, though each has evolved separately.

In yeast, and certain bacteria, one molecule of pyruvate is reduced and decarboxylated (generates CO_2) to ethanol with concomitant oxidation of NADH to NAD^+. This process has been utilized for thousands of years by people to make beer and wine.

Human muscle cells engage in lactic acid fermentation when the oxygen supply is insufficient. The reaction converting pyruvate, the end product of glycolysis, into lactic acid is catalyzed by lactate dehydrogenase. Along with the production lactic acid, NAD^+ is regenerated from NADH. Anaerobic metabolism allows the muscle cells to produce ATP and continue functioning in the absence of oxygen.

To better understand the structure and mechanism of the lactate dehydrogenase enzyme, researchers have synthesized a novel drug that modulates lactic acid fermentation. The researchers perform a series of experiments in order to determine the drug's mechanism of action; The drug is included in the cell mileu of cell groups 1-3, while groups 4-6 receive only saline. The cells are then placed either in a normal solution, a low NADH solution, or a low ATP solution. The researchers measure the rates of fermentation in all 6 groups under anaerobic conditions. Their data is presented in the table below.

Group	Normal	Low NADH	Low ATP
1	4	7	4
2	3	4	3
3	2	5	4
4	3	1	3
5	2	2	4
6	3	2	2

Table 1 Relative rates of lactic acid fermentation

85. According to the passage, muscle cells are limited in their energy production when there is insufficient oxygen for aerobic metabolism. Which of the following processes will be most affected by a defect in the enzyme responsible for the conversion of pyruvate to lactic acid?

   A. Electron-transport chain
   B. Kreb's cycle
   C. Glycolysis
   D. Fatty acid synthesis

86. According the to the researchers' data from the table, what is the most likely mechanism of action for the drug?

   A. Inhibits pyruvate dehydrogenase
   B. Stimulates glycolysis
   C. Produces ATP
   D. Acts similarly to NADH

87. The passage states that lactic acid fermentation regenerates NAD^+ in the absence of oxygen. Which process regenerates NAD^+ when oxygen is present?

   A. Electron-transport chain
   B. Kreb's cycle
   C. Amino acid synthesis
   D. Glycogenolysis

88. Muscles produce lactic acid when they are contracting under anaerobic conditions. The build-up of lactic acid in muscles is responsible for the sensation of aching and stiffness after strenuous activity. Lactic acid is eventually cleared from the body by conversion back to pyruvate by which of the following?

   A. Muscle cells
   B. Liver cells
   C. Kidney parenchymal cells
   D. Enzymes ubiquitous in the bloodstream

89. Certain bacteria only utilize alcohol fermentation. According to the information in the passage, how many net molecules of ATP do these bacteria produce per molecule of glucose?

   A. 4
   B. 2
   C. 36
   D. 38

90. During a 200m sprint, the heart is unable increase peripheral blood flow at a rate that would provide additional oxygen to muscles during the race. By the time the circulatory system is able to respond, the sprint is over. In this situation, what is the primary source of fuel for the muscles?

- **A.** Glucose
- **B.** Lactic acid
- **C.** Fatty acids
- **D.** pyruvate

91. The researchers discovered that there were no significant differences, for any of the cell groups, in fermentation rates between normal saline and low ATP solutions. Which of the following statements best explains these results?

- **A.** Normal Saline does not contain ATP, and thus the two solutions were really the same.
- **B.** Fermentation does not produce ATP, and thus low ATP is not a driver for the reaction.
- **C.** The results may be attributed to experimental error.
- **D.** ATP production is completely unrelated to fermentation rates.

Questions 92 through 94 are **NOT** based on a descriptive passage.

92. Excess lactic acid production from working muscles can induce acidosis, in which the pH of the blood is reduced. The lungs compensate for this drop in pH by altering the ratio of carbon dioxide to bicarbonate in the blood. The reaction is:

$$CO_2 + H_2O \Leftrightarrow H^+ + HCO_3^-$$

Which of the following statements best describes the compensatory action of the lungs?

- **A.** CO_2 conversion to H^+ and CO_3^- is increased
- **B.** O_2 production is increased
- **C.** CO_2 exhalation is increased
- **D.** The ventilation rate is decreased

93. Many amino acids are metabolized in the human body by conversion to Kreb Cycle intermediates. Only certain amino acids may be directly deaminated, the rest must first undergo transamination. A product of deaminization is ammonia, which is toxic to many cells. Which of the following most accurately describes how the body best deals with the NH_3 waste?

- **A.** NH_3 is broken down by a special set of enzymes to elemental Nitrogen and Hydrogen, which enter the blood system and are breathed out of the lungs.
- **B.** NH_3 enters the blood stream and is filtered out by the kidneys. It is excreted by the body as a component of urine.
- **C.** NH_3 is combined with CO_2 to form urea, which enters the blood stream and is later excreted.
- **D.** The NH_3 is primarily utilized in the formation of new amino acids for protein synthesis throughout the body.

94. Which of the following gradients is essential for the formation of ATP in cellular respiration?

- **A.** A pH gradient between the two sides of the outer mitochondrial membrane.
- **B.** A pH gradient between the mitochondrial matrix and the mitochondrial intermembrane space.
- **C.** An electric gradient between the organelles and the cytoplasm.
- **D.** An electric gradient between the mitochondrial matrix and the mitochondrial intermembrane space.

STOP. IF YOU FINISH BEFORE TIME IS CALLED, CHECK YOUR WORK. YOU MAY GO BACK TO ANY QUESTION IN THIS TEST BOOKLET.

33

STOP.

16 MINI MCATS

EXAMINATION 03

Questions 95–141

Physical Sciences

Time: 20 Minutes
Questions 95–110

Passage I (Questions 95-101)

As part of his landmark theory on the emission spectrum of hydrogen, Neils Bohr presented the following formula for the energy of an electron in any single-electron atom or ion:

$$E_a = -R_H \left(\frac{Z^2}{n^2} \right)$$

E_n represents the energy of an electron in a given energy level n, while R_H symbolizes the Rydberg constant, 2.18×10^{-18} J. Z stands for nuclear charge. For atoms or ions with a single electron, the energy of the electron is determined only by the principal quantum number n.

Later atomic research revealed quantized energy levels for multi-electron atoms and ions as well. For multielectronic atoms or ions, the azimuthal quantum number, or subshell, is also important in determining the energy of a given electron.

For atoms or ions with electrons in more than one shell, the effect of the nuclear charge on the outer electrons is diminished in a phenomenon know as shielding. A very rough estimate of the effective nuclear charge on an outer electron is calculated by subtracting the number of electrons in lower numbered shells from the overall nuclear charge.

When an electron jumps from one atomic orbital to another, the change in energy level is reflected via the absorption or emission of a photon. The photon must have a frequency which corresponds to the change in energy of the electron. For single-electron atoms and ions, the energy change represented by the photon is found using the equation below.

$$\Delta E = hf = Z^2 R_H \left(\frac{1}{n_i^2} - \frac{1}{n_f^2} \right)$$

In this formula, h stands for Planck's constant, which is 6.63×10^{-34} J-s. The frequency of the photon is represented by f, while the initial and final energy levels are depicted by n_i and n_f, respectively. The photons released as electrons transverse various electron shells are delineated in the table below.

Series	n_f	n_i	Spectrum
Lyman	1	2, 3...	Ultraviolet
Balmer	2	3, 4...	Ultraviolet and visible
Paschen	3	4, 5...	Infrared
Brackett	4	5, 6...	Infrared

95. Using the expression given in the passage, what is a very rough estimate of the effective nuclear charge on an aluminum atom?

- **A.** 0
- **B.** 1
- **C.** 3
- **D.** 5

96. Which of the following will be true of the energy of a hydrogen atom when an electron moves from the 2s subshell to the 2p subshell?

- **A.** It will be halved.
- **B.** It will not be changed.
- **C.** It will be doubled.
- **D.** It will be quadrupled.

97. The changes in energy caused by electron movement from the third to the first principal energy levels were compared among H atoms and He+ ions. Compared to the energy change for H, the energy change for He+ will be:

- **A.** greater because He+ has a greater nuclear charge.
- **B.** greater because He+ has a smaller nuclear charge.
- **C.** smaller because He+ has a greater nuclear charge.
- **D.** smaller because He+ has a smaller nuclear charge.

98. An energy change in a hydrogen atom caused by a change in the electron's energy level causes a red band to appear in the atom's emission spectrum. Which of the following could be the jump made by the electron?

- **A.** From $n = 5$ to $n = 3$
- **B.** From $n = 4$ to $n = 3$
- **C.** From $n = 3$ to $n = 2$
- **D.** From $n = 3$ to $n = 1$

38

99. Which of the following statements best describes the process that occurs when a photon is emitted by a hydrogen atom?

   A. The atom absorbs energy when an electron moves to a higher energy level.

   B. The atom absorbs energy when an electron moves to a lower energy level.

   C. The atom releases energy when an electron moves to a higher energy level.

   D. The atom releases energy when an electron moves to a lower energy level.

100. What is the energy of an electron in the second principal energy level of a He^+ ion?

   A. -1.09×10^{-18} J

   B. -2.18×10^{-18} J

   C. -4.36×10^{-18} J

   D. -8.72×10^{-18} J

101. Compared to a He^+ ion, a hydrogen atom has:

   A. smaller radius and smaller ionization energy.

   B. smaller radius and greater ionization energy.

   C. larger radius and smaller ionization energy.

   D. larger radius and greater ionization energy.

Passage II (Questions 102-107)

A farmer drives a tractor across a field, towing a crate full of irrigation machinery. The crate has a mass of 500 kg, and the tractor, a mass of 1200 kg. The farmer attaches the crate with a massless 8m chain. The tractor tows the crate with the chain between them parallel to the ground. The driving force for the tractor originates in the rear wheels, which have diameters of 2.0 meters each.

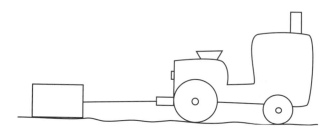

Figure 1

The frictional forces between the ground, the tractor, and crate can have conflicting effects in determining whether the tractor will be able to drag the crate without slipping. If the ground provides a great deal of friction, then the tractor tires will be able to maintain their grip without slipping, however the frictional force impeding the motion of the crate will also increase. If the ground is slippery and provides less friction, then the frictional force impeding the motion of the crate will be smaller, and the tractor will encounter greater difficulty in gaining traction.

The tractor starts from rest and gradually accelerates until it reaches a constant speed. The farmer continues at the constant speed across the field until her nears his destination, at which point he decelerates the tractor and comes to a stop.

102. In order for the tractor to move the crate forward from rest, the:

   A. maximum value of the force of static friction on the tractor must be greater than the maximum value of the force of static friction on the crate.

   B. maximum value of the force of static friction on the tractor must be less than the maximum value of the force of static friction on the crate.

   C. minimum value of the force of static friction on the tractor must be greater than the minimum value of the force of static friction on the crate.

   D. minimum value of the force of static friction on the tractor must be less than the minimum value of the force of static friction on the crate.

GO ON TO THE NEXT PAGE.

103. Which coefficients of friction should be used to calculate the frictional forces on the tractor and crate while the tractor is towing (without tire slippage) the crate across the field at constant speed?

	Tractor	Crate
A.	static	static
B.	static	kinetic
C.	kinetic	kinetic
D.	kinetic	static

104. If the frictional force between the crate and the ground is 500 N, and the tractor and crate accelerate at the rate of 0.6 m/s^2, what is the tension in the chain?

A.   200 N
B.   500 N
C.   700 N
D.   800 N

105. As the tractor tows the crate at constant speed, its back wheels turn at a rate of 30 revolutions per minute. What is the approximate speed of the tractor?

A.   2 m/s
B.   3 m/s
C.   5 m/s
D.   6 m/s

106. As the tractor drags the crate across the field, the force exerted on the tractor by the crate is:

A.   greater than the force exerted on the crate by the tractor.
B.   less than the force exerted on the crate by the tractor.
C.   equal to the force exerted on the crate by the tractor.
D.   equal to zero.

107. If the tractor must exert a force of 1000 N on the crate in order to set it in motion, what is the coefficient of static friction between the crate and the ground?

A.   0.1
B.   0.2
C.   0.4
D.   0.5

Questions 108 through 110 are **NOT** based on a descriptive passage.

108. Which forms of atomic bonding are present in sodium nitrate?

A.   Ionic only
B.   Covalent only
C.   Ionic and covalent
D.   Neither ionic nor covalent

109. A block sits on the slope of an inclined plane as shown below. As the angle of inclination, x, is increased, which of the following will occur?

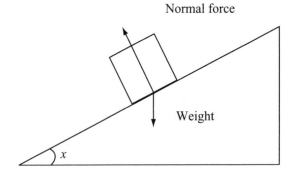

Normal force

Weight

x

A.   The weight of the block will remain the same and the normal force will decrease.
B.   The weight of the block will decrease and the normal force will remain the same.
C.   The weight of the block and the normal force will decrease.
D.   The weight of the block and the normal force will remain the same.

110. The force created by a magnetic field acts on an electron by moving it in a circular path. If the path traveled by the electron remains the same, and the electron's speed is doubled, the magnitude of the force must:

A.   be halved.
B.   remain the same.
C.   be doubled.
D.   be quadrupled.

STOP. IF YOU FINISH BEFORE TIME IS CALLED, CHECK YOUR WORK. YOU MAY GO BACK TO ANY QUESTION IN THIS TEST BOOKLET.

STOP.

Verbal Reasoning

Time: 20 Minutes
Questions 111–125

In comparing himself with his contemporaries, the adolescent often focuses on his external appearance. Good looks, however defined, are valued virtually everywhere—so the adolescent measures his worth as a person, and his
5 chances of success, by the degree to which he meets society's standards of attractiveness. If the adolescent feels inadequate on this scale, he worries. A physician who studied a group of American adolescents over an eight-year period discovered that a third of the boys, and nearly half
10 the girls, were concerned about their appearance. Boys fretted because they were short or fat, did not have athletic frames, because they had bad skin—or simply felt ugly. Girls worried because they were too tall, fat, or generally homely, or because their breasts were small or their figures
15 unformed. Not surprisingly, the 'late-bloomers' were most self-critical. They were, after all, at an obvious disadvantage when they compared themselves to others of the same age.

This disadvantage seems to be more acute among
20 boys than among girls. Late-maturing boys' dissatisfactions with themselves are reflected both in the opinions of their classmates, and in their own responses to psychological tests. Questionnaires circulated among adolescents reveal that late-maturing boys are more often described as 'show-
25 offs' than those who are mature early. Late-blooming males are also considered more restless, bossier, less grown-up, less good-looking. And tests of the late maturers indicate that they are more likely to feel rejected, rebellious, and aggressive. At the same time, they are much more depend-
30 ent, with a much greater need for psychological support from friends and family. In other words, they tend to be both angry and afraid, a combination that obviously makes for conflict, between the boys and their environment as well as within the boys themselves.

35 The slow-growing boy's difficulties are heaped on top of the problems that affect both boys and girls in the early years of adolescence. Social customs in our society ignore an elementary biological fact: until quite late in the teens: girls outpace boys in development. They reach puberty at a
40 younger age, and they experience psychological changes before their male contemporaries. Surveys of junior high school students show that girls are at least two years ahead of their male classmates in physical development. Many have reached puberty by the time they enter junior high, while many boys have not yet reached puberty when they enter senior high. As a result, during these crucial years boys and girls alike have little opportunity to know
45 members of the opposite sex who are on the same level of development as themselves. At the same time, as anthropologist Margaret Mead points out, many American parents press their preadolescent children to "go steady." As a result, the teenagers are not given enough time to learn the
50 meaning of friendship with members of the same sex. This

development Miss Mead finds disturbing. She believes that the capacity to form and keep close friendships with one's own sex can best be developed in childhood and that it is closely related to the ability to achieve mature love rela-
55 tionships in later life.

Are the tensions and anxieties of adolescence dictated by nature or imposed by society? The answer seems to be that they are imposed by society in advanced countries, because society's timetables are not synchronized with
60 man's natural growth timetable.

Almost all human behavior is learned rather than inherited. Man is much less a creature of instinct than any other animal. Indeed, the capacity to learn, to substitute flexible thinking for the rigidities of instinct, is a basic
65 measure of intelligence in man or any other species. Nevertheless, learning is a time-consuming business. Hence, man's protracted childhood is a necessity to give him time to acquire the mass of information and skills without which he could not survive as an adult, even on a
70 primitive level.

111. The contention that the tensions and anxieties of adolescence "are imposed by society in advanced countries, because society's timetables are not synchronized with man's natural growth timetable" (lines 61-63) can most justifiably be interpreted as support for the idea that:

A. in most other countries, adolescents experience less tension and anxiety.
B. a long childhood is necessary to acquire information and skills.
C. in less advanced countries, these timetables are better synchronized.
D. in less advanced countries, society is less concerned about adolescent appearances.

GO ON TO THE NEXT PAGE.

112. The author most likely mentions, "The slow-growing boy's difficulties are heaped on top of the problems that affect both boys and girls in the early years of adolescence. " (lines 35-37) in order to:

 A. demonstrate the strength of his theories regarding a girl's difficulties.

 B. support the claim that a boy's problems are more acute than a girl's.

 C. illustrate the persistence of beliefs that conflict with the author's theories.

 D. provide an example of a girl's problems and to maintain parity in the passage.

113. Which of the following statements would most likely be supported by the author of the passage?

 A. A late-maturing girl would be more self-critical of herself than a normally maturing boy.

 B. Both late-maturing and normally maturing adolescents perceive the former as dissatisfied with themselves.

 C. Boys are much more concerned about their appearances than are girls.

 D. In other societies adolescence does not present much of a problem.

114. What is the author's most likely response to the argument that adolescents focus too much on how they look instead of whom they are?

 A. Acceptance: adolescents prize physical beauty too highly.

 B. Neutral: physical beauty is valued almost everywhere.

 C. Revisionist: this focus is not a cause of concern for the average adolescent.

 D. Skepticism: it is who a person is that is most important.

115. If the author's primary criterion for judging the "intelligence" were applied to different animals in a given situation, which of the following animals would be most intelligent?

 A. A chimpanzee that moves next to its food dish because it knows the exact time it will be fed by its keeper

 B. A mother cat that quickly adapts to nursing orphaned baby skunks

 C. A dog that learns to whine in order to be let outside its master's home

 D. A rat that learns to use a can for a raft in order to obtain food

116. The main idea of the passage is that, in advanced countries:

 A. adolescents are not advancing at a satisfactory rate.

 B. adolescence, particularly in boys, is a difficult time.

 C. adolescents deserve more nurturing societies.

 D. adolescence is a difficult period for both boys and girls.

117. Suppose later child development research reveals that the problems encountered by adolescent boys, as presented in the passage, are unique from those encountered by their female counterparts. Which of the following changes in the passage would be most appropriate?

 A. A distinction regarding which gender was concerned about appearance.

 B. The beliefs of Margaret Mead should be expunged.

 C. There should be more emphasis placed on the adolescence of girls.

 D. Late-maturing girls should no longer be viewed as more self-critical.

118. Which of the following statements is NOT supported by the passage?

 A. Boys are concerned with being too short or ugly.

 B. Boys and girls worry about their height.

 C. Boys and girls worry about being overweight.

 D. Girls worry about having bad skin.

Sub-Saharan Africa comprises a politically and socially complex region of the world that has largely gone unnoticed, especially by inhabitants of the Western world. This region has a human, geographic, and cultural history
5 nearly as old as man himself.

As recent as the beginning of the twentieth century, a layer of mystery shrouded much of the "Dark Continent." Though slave trade has been extant in this region for over a thousand years, much of this commerce was conducted ei-
10 ther from the coastal regions of West and East Africa or from the areas just subjacent the Sahara desert. European penetration of inland areas did not begin until 1850, as missionaries, entrepreneurs, scientists, and explorers broke into the hitherto uncharted sub-Saharan interior. This entry,
15 however, brought its own untoward effects.

Within a few decades, all but two sub-Saharan nations had been colonized by European powers. Subsistence farmers were marginalized and displaced by foreign commercialists intent upon growing cash crops. The indigenous
20 population was used as a repository for cheap labor. To maintain power, preexisting governance and power systems were disrupted and the seeds of civil rivalry were sown as a part of the all too famous "divide and conquer" strategy. Some argue, notwithstanding the immorality of exploita-
25 tion, that colonialism served the positive purpose of creating a vital infrastructure of transportation, medical and education facilities, city planning, governance, and industry, an infrastructure that was inherited by the same African nations following their independence in the latter part of the
30 twentieth century. Such a proposition is tenuous, at best. The transportation links had mostly decayed by the time the nations gained independence or soon after. The state of political instability, elitism, and illiteracy that followed in wake the colonial era perhaps partly due to the abrupt with-
35 drawal of colonizing nations left these facilities existing but useless. Furthermore, colonialism did not end with the departure of European governing bodies from the sub-Sahara. In fact, the legacy of colonialism continues today in the forms of disparate and unjustifiable corporate and political
40 influence in the area.

Importantly, an African identity has endured and survived the mental slavery that colonialist rule many times entails. Most inhabitants of sub-Saharan Africa are subsistence farmers. Africans in this region still share an intimate
45 connection with the earth. For them the divine and spiritual continue to be best embodied by their natural surroundings. In addition, African self-identity still incorporates a sense that life is a continuous chain, and so, ancestry and childbearing continue to be valued. The concept of an extended
50 family persists even today in this region. Also, African of the sub-Sahara share a common feeling of having being vi-

olated by the foreign colonial rule that most in this region have endured.

Sub-Saharan Africa today is in a precarious state of af-
55 fairs. Eighteen of the world's poorest nations lie in this geographic region. Though the overall population density of the area is lower than that of the United States, most Africans are concentrated in specific rural areas. Furthermore, with a population growth rate that is four
60 times that of the U.S., there exists a "1%-gap" between population growth and food production. Recurrent drought, widespread illiteracy, and poor transportation present further obstacles to growth. These industrial-poor nations rely mainly on the export of raw materials to generate income.
65 In contrast, most imports into these countries are manufactured items whose value exceeds that of the raw materials exported. There is no local technocratic class to support the industrialization that would be required to compete in world markets and close this import-export gap. With mounting
70 debt and interest dues to international financial entities like the IMF, governments often place their constituency of subsistence farmers on the wayside by diverting resources toward cash crops in order to make payments. Superimposed on a background of donor fatigue, public health in sub-
75 Saharan Africa presents a striking crisis. Though the knowledge and resources required to surmount this problem are modest, as are those required to industrialize these nations, present access to such ameliorating measures are modest as well.

119. Assume that the United Nations was interested in implementing a program to subsidize sub-Saharan nations in an effort to strengthen their economic standing in the world market. Based on the information provided in the passage, which of the following programs would the author consider most helpful?

   A. A program designed to decrease urban unemployment rates by creating farming jobs for metropolitan youth
   B. A program designed to increase literacy and provide technical training to villagers
   C. A program designed to increase agricultural production, especially cash crops
   D. A program designed to promote family planning and close the "1% gap" (line 60)

44

120. Which of the following statements regarding foreign familiarity with sub-Saharan lands is most consistent with the information in the passage?

  A. The Western world was completely oblivious to sub-Saharan Africa until the twentieth century.
  B. European familiarity with African lands was based only on commercial interests.
  C. Though the lowland coastal areas of sub-Saharan were known to traders, highland, tropic areas of the interior remained unfamiliar territory for some time.
  D. Familiarity with sub-Saharan Africa increased in the Western world after colonial independence, due to an increase of raw materials from African countries.

121. "The lack of utilization of resources developed during the colonial era, resources that became available to African nations post-colonially, was due to none other than the mismanagement of those resources by African aristocracy. Therefore, the post-colonial dilapidation of sub-Saharan nations can be blamed on none but the African people themselves." This statement would most likely elicit which of the following responses from the author?

  A. Strong agreement because the author feels that elitism was a true obstacle to accessing and utilizing the infrastructure left by colonial nations
  B. Partial disagreement because the author feels that colonizing nations are also partly responsible for the post-colonial state of affairs
  C. Strong opposition because the author feels that the colonizing nations were entirely responsible for the post-colonial decline of sub-Saharan nations.
  D. Partial agreement because the author agrees that sub-Saharan nations are in a dilapidated state post-colonially

122. The author would most likely agree with which of the following statements?

  A. Inhabitants of sub-Saharan Africa are, for the most part, very much alike.
  B. The origins of sub-Saharan culture and history antedate the discovery of the New World in the fifteenth century.
  C. Sub-Saharan countries are only now steadily developing into industrialized nations.
  D. If there were better transportation links available, sub-Saharan nations would very easily modernize.

123. According to the passage, which of the following scenarios is NOT characteristic of sub-Saharan inhabitants or sub-Saharan living

  A. A large joint family engaged in growing corn
  B. A group of village people offering devotional services to a tree
  C. An illiterate group of people living in crowded city quarters with poor sanitary conditions
  D. A group of farm workers that are severely emaciated and have several health problems

124. Which of the following statements best conveys the main idea of the passage?

  A. There is a need for greater awareness of the history and current state affairs of sub-Saharan nations in the West.
  B. The subsistence farmers of sub-Saharan African have been repeatedly marginalized due to various political and historical factors.
  C. Colonialism has grossly retarded the growth of sub-Saharan nations.
  D. The sub-Saharan region has historically been wrought with problems and faces many challenges today.

125. The author would be most likely present which of the following statements in an address to the United Nations Hearing Committee?

  A. We must implement controls and policies to remove the remnants of colonial control in the region.
  B. Stiffer tariff regulations need to be in place to close the import-export gap.
  C. There is an undeniable need to create better health care facilities to stave off a pandemic public health crisis.
  D. We must overcome donor fatigue and pump heavy aid into African nations.

STOP. IF YOU FINISH BEFORE TIME IS CALLED, CHECK YOUR WORK. YOU MAY GO BACK TO ANY QUESTION IN THIS TEST BOOKLET.

STOP.

Biological Sciences

Time: 20 Minutes
Questions 126–141

Passage V (Questions 126-132)

All cells of the human body, except mature erythrocytes and gametes, contain the same DNA, yet functions of individual cells are incredibly diverse and specialized. This diversity in cellular function arises primarily from cell to cell variation in protein expression. Most protein expression is in turn regulated at the transcriptional level; which genes are activated, and to what degree, determines cellular function and growth.

More specifically, the transcription of a gene is governed by upstream regulatory sequences, such as regulatory genes and promoters. Regulators and promoters may, in turn, be controlled by extracellular signals such as hormones, or by intracellular signals such as calcium or glucose. Regulators may stimulate or inhibit transcription of a gene, while activated promoters will only increase transcription.

An important cause of cancer is the inability of a cell to regulate its own growth. Genetic mutation can occur at any level in the complex system of cellular growth regulation. There are two categories of genes that when mutated, often lead to cancer: oncogenes and tumor-suppressor genes. Oncogenes regulate cell growth and division; mutation of oncogenes or their promoters can result in uncontrolled cell growth and division. Tumor-suppressor genes regulate the cell cycle and may induce cell death when a cell has aberrant function. Mutations of tumor-suppressor genes result in a lack of this regulation, and thus dysfunctional cells are allowed to proliferate.

If regulators or promoter sequences for genes involved in oncogenesis are elucidated, drugs that regulate transcription of these genes may be used in cancer therapy. One such drug, ZX2, is effective at curtailing the growth of cancerous cells, however has a significant side effect profile, including: decreased immune response, diarrhea, hair loss, and kidney damage.

126. According to the passage, which of the following is the most likely mechanism of action of ZX2?

A. Upregulation of tumor-suppressor gene expression
B. Mutation of an oncogene
C. Inhibition of a tumor-suppressor promoter
D. Upregulation of an oncogene activator

127. Cancers are most often found in tissues that undergo significant cellular division. According to this relationship, which of the following tissues is LEAST likely to develop a cancerous tumor?

A. Intestinal mucosa
B. Thymus
C. Epithelial tissue of the skin
D. Skeletal muscle

128. Promoter sequences may be transcribed along with their associated gene in a single mRNA transcript. In order to make translation possible, the mRNA sequence containing the transcribed promoter must be cleaved. This cleavage most likely takes place in which of the following cellular structures?

A. Endoplasmic reticulum
B. Lysosome
C. Mitochondria
D. Nucleus

129. Oncogene and Tumor-suppressor gene mutations commonly arise during DNA duplication. DNA polymerase has a significant error rate. In which phase of the cell cycle, are cancerous mutations most likely to occur?

A. M
B. S
C. G1
D. G2

130. A novel approach to fighting cancer involves the use of modified tRNA molecules. The modified tRNA carries inappropriate combinations of amino acids and anti-codons. In other words, the nucleotide triplets on one end of the molecule are assigned to incorrect amino acids on the other end of the tRNA molecule. What is the most likely basis for the anticancer activity of these modified RNA molecules?

A. Failure of cancer cells to transcribe protein
B. Altered activity of the translated protein
C. Failure of cancer cells to translate protein
D. Failure of mRNA association with ribosomes

131. A new drug, Colchicine is currently being investigated for anticancer applications. The drug prevents cell division by inhibiting microtubule formation. In which stage of mitosis is Colchicine most effective?

A. Prophase
B. Metaphase
C. Anaphase
D. Telophase

132. A toxin isolated from a rare plant is found to interfere with normal cell division. Which of the following is the LEAST likely mechanism for its action?

A. Substitution of adenine in DNA
B. Destruction of histone proteins
C. Irreversible binding to ribose
D. Prevention of Beta oxidation

GO ON TO THE NEXT PAGE.

Northern blot analysis is a technique employed in the examination of cellular mRNA levels. As mRNA is gene specific, the technique allows one to compare levels of expression of a given gene among different tissues. In the same vein, it may also be used to test candidate genes in patients for certain types of mutations. The technique involves isolation of RNA from blood of the affected and unaffected (control) individuals. For each sample, 15-20 ug of RNA is size fractionated using gel electrophoresis. Similar to DNA gels, the RNA is size fractionated on a porous gel (usually made of agarose) within an electric field that forces the nucleic acids to diffuse from the negative pole to the positive. Smaller fragments pass more easily through gel pores and thus travel further along the gel in a given amount of time. In the case of RNA, formaldehyde is added to the agarose gel in order to maintain the RNA in a denatured state. Following electrophoresis, the gel is rinsed well with water to remove the toxic formaldehyde and soaked in a transfer buffer. The RNA is then transferred via capillary elution onto a nylon or nitrocellulose membrane and cross-linked by UV light. The membrane containing the immobilized RNA, called a Northern blot, can now be evaluated for the presence of specific gene transcripts. This is done by using a radioactively-labeled DNA probe, that contains a fragment of the gene being tested. Before adding the probe, the blot is first prehybridized with a blocking agent, such as denatured salmon sperm, which will prevent nonspecific binding of the DNA probe. Finally, the DNA probe is hybridized to the blot under appropriate conditions, washed, and exposed to film. The film reveals the presence of radioactive bands, which correspond to hybridization of the immobilized RNA with the labeled probe. The level of gene expression is proportional to the intensity of the radioactive band.

133. Northern blot may be employed to identify which of the following mutations in a gene that encodes an intracellular enzyme?

A. A mutation which affects phosphorylation site.
B. A mutation which results in a truncated protein.
C. A mutation which affects exon/intron splice junction.
D. A mutation which results in a large intronic deletion.

134. The Northern Blot protocol is particularly useful in lymphoma and leukemia research. This utility is in part due to the ease of obtaining white blood cells from patients. Which of the following statements best explains the importance of isolating lymphocytes for Northern Blot testing?

A. mRNA is specific to cells which express the gene of interest.
B. Lymphocytes express the greatest variety of genes.
C. Lymphocytes are the only cell type that may be examined by Northern Blot.
D. The mRNA is most stable in lymphocytes and thus easier to examine.

135. Which one of the following mutations will result in a less intense Northern Blot band?

A. Missense mutations
B. Nonsense mutations
C. Small deletions/insertions in the coding region.
D. Small deletions/insertions in a noncoding region.

136. RNA is maintained in a denatured state by formaldehyde in order to prevent formation of secondary structure. Why is this important for the success of Northern Blot analysis?

A. The secondary structure would prevent binding of RNA to the labeled probe.
B. The secondary structure would affect RNA migration through the gel.
C. The secondary structure would prevent transfer of RNA from the gel to the membrane.
D. The secondary structure would prevent the cross-linking of RNA to the membrane.

137. Desmosomes provide flexible yet robust intercellular adhesion for epithelial tissues which are exposed to high levels of stress. A researcher uses Northern Blot Analysis to examine the distribution of a desmosomal plaque protein, Desmoglein 2, in different human tissues. For which of the following sample sets is the researcher most likely to observe the following pattern: a strong band, no band, weak band?

A. Heart, oral mucosa, skin.
B. Skin, skeletal muscle, bladder.
C. Skin, heart, bladder.
D. Brain, skeletal muscle, skin.

GO ON TO THE NEXT PAGE.

138. Family Y is being tested for potential mutations in gene X. A graduate student performs a Northern Blot analysis and does not detect any bands in the patient lanes. All of the following explanations are feasible EXCEPT:

A. There is a deletion upstream of gene X in the Y family.
B. The entire gene X is deleted in the Y family.
C. The patient's DNA contains a chromosomal re-arrangement.
D. The Northern Blot analysis did not work.

139. Which of the following mutations in gene X will NOT result in a longer/further migration of a band on a Northern Blot?

A. A small intragenic deletion that encompasses one exon and the two flanking introns.
B. A large intragenic deletion that encompasses one intron and the two flanking exons.
C. A single point mutation that would alter the splicing junction.
D. A single point mutation that would affect ribosome binding site.

Questions 140 and 141 are **NOT** based on a descriptive passage.

140. "One of the greatest hindrances in battling HIV infection is the high rate of viral genomic mutation. Which of the following reasons best explains the rationale behind the use of triple medication combinations, also known as "triple drug cocktails"?

A. Three medications must be used in order to simultaneously combat opportunistic infection.
B. Using three medications increases the chance that one will work, as therapy is urgent.
C. The likelihood of the virus mutating to become resistant to all three medications is low.
D. Two of the medications decrease the mutation rate so that the virus remains sensitive to the third.

141. Interestingly, an infectious diseases researcher notices that a previously resistant HIV strain isolated from a patient now shows sensitivity to the same antiretroviral medication. What is the most likely explanation for the researcher's observation?

A. backward mutation
B. forward mutation
C. nonsense mutation
D. missense mutation

STOP. IF YOU FINISH BEFORE TIME IS CALLED, CHECK YOUR WORK. YOU MAY GO BACK TO ANY QUESTION IN THIS TEST BOOKLET.

EXAMINATION 04

Questions 142–188

Physical Sciences

Time: 20 Minutes

Questions 142–158

In 1798, Henry Cavendish designed an experiment to measure the force of gravitational attraction between two objects that are separated by a small distance. The diagram below represents a modern version of Cavendish's experiment.

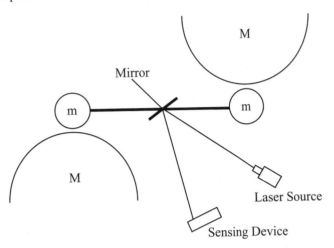

Figure 1 Cavendish diagram

Two small spherical balls of mass m are attached to a light horizontal bar. The bar is suspended at its midpoint by a wire. Two large spheres, each of mass M, are placed in proximity of the smaller spheres as shown in the diagram. The gravitational attraction between the spheres creates a torque on the bar, causing it to rotate about its axis. When the wire is twisted, it acts in a manner that corresponds to a Hooke's law spring, resisting the rotation of the bar.

A mirror is attached to the the wire supporting the bar, and a beam of light from the laser source is directed at the mirror so that the rotation of the reflected beam can be measured by the sensing device. In this way the angle of rotation caused by the gravitational force between the spheres can be measured.

Cavendish repeated the experiment using spheres of different masses and varying the distance between the masses. The spheres are all of uniform density. Through his experiments he was able to determine that the interspherical gravitational force is attractive, that it varies in direct proportion to the mass of each object, and that it varies in inverse proportion to the square of the distance between the centers of mass of the two objects. Thus, he was also able to determine the value of the gravitational constant. The results of Cavendish's experiment, when considered in tandem, are expressed by Newton's law of universal gravitation:

$$F = \frac{GMm}{r^2}$$

F, the interobject gravitational force, is expressed above as the function of the object masses, M and m, and the interobject distance, r. G is the gravitational constant, 6.67×10^{-11} N-m^2/kg^2.

142. If the length of the bar in the Cavendish apparatus is 40 cm and the force exerted by a large sphere on a small sphere is 1×10^{-7} N, what is the total torque on the bar due to gravitational forces?

A. 2×10^{-8} Nm
B. 4×10^{-8} Nm
C. 2×10^{-7} Nm
D. 4×10^{-7} Nm

143. Newton's law of universal gravitation is used to predict the results of an experimental trial using Cavendish's apprraratus. If the spheres used in the experiment are not of uniform density, which of the following variables would be inaccurate?

I. G
II. M
III. r

A. I only
B. III only
C. I and II only
D. II and III only

144. Which of the following is true regarding the wire supporting the rod as the rod rotates in response to the gravitational attraction of the spheres?

A. The wire exerts a constant torque on the bar as the angle of rotation increases.
B. The torque caused by the wire changes direction as the angle of rotation increases.
C. The torque caused by the wire increases as the angle of rotation increases
D. The torque caused by the wire decreases as the angle of rotation increases.

145. If the experiment is repeated with each mass M replaced by a mass of $3M$, how would the torque due to gravity in the second trial compare with the torque in the first trial?

A. It would be the same.
B. It would be three times as large.
C. It would be six times as large.
D. It would be nine times as large.

146. Which of the graphs below depicts the relationship between gravitational force F and distance r?

A.

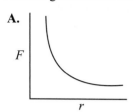

C.

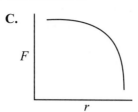

B.

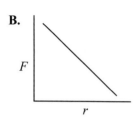

D.

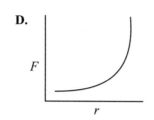

147. The experiment is run using large 24cm diameter spheres and small 6cm diameter spheres. The spheres are placed exactly 1 cm apart. If a student wishes to use Newton's law of universal gravitation to check the results, what value of r should she use?

A. 0.01 m
B. 0.07 m
C. 0.10 m
D. 0.16 m

Passage II (Questions 148-154)

Phosphorous occurs most commonly in nature in the form of calcium phosphate [$Ca_3(PO_4)_2$] rocks, which also contain fluorapatite [$Ca_5(PO_4)_3F$]. Pure phosphorous is commercially produced by heating calcium phosphate along with silica sand and carbon.

$$2\ Ca_3(PO_4)_2(s) + 6\ SiO_2(s) + 10\ C(s) \rightarrow$$
$$6\ CaSiO_3(s) + 10\ CO(g) + P_4(s)$$

Reaction 1

There are two diverse forms of elemental phosphorous, red and white. Red phosphorous is relatively stable, while white phosphorous spontaneously ignites when exposed to oxygen.

$$P_4(s) + 5\ O_2(g) \rightarrow P_4O_{10}(s)$$

Reaction 2

When white phosphorous is heated in the presence of concentrated sodium hydroxide, phosphine, a poisonous gas, is formed. Phosphine, in turn, reacts with oxygen to form phosphoric acid.

$$P_4(s) + 3\ NaOH(aq) + 3\ H_2O(l) \rightarrow 3\ NaH_2PO_2(aq) + PH_3(g)$$

Reaction 3

$$PH_3(g) + 2\ O_2(g) \rightarrow H_3PO_4(s)$$

Reaction 4

Phosphoric acid may also be prepared by combining sulfuric acid with calcium phosphate.

$$Ca_3(PO_4)_2(s) + 3\ H_2SO_4(aq) \rightarrow 2\ H_3PO_4(aq) + 3\ CaSO_4(aq)$$

Reaction 5

When white phosphorous is heated with chlorine gas, phosphorous trichloride is formed.

$$P_4(s) + 6\ Cl_2(g) \rightarrow 4\ PCl_3(g)$$

Reaction 6

In the presence of excess chlorine gas, the phosphorous trichloride will continue to react, forming PCl_5 (phosphorous pentachloride).

GO ON TO THE NEXT PAGE.

148. Which of the following best describes the spatial arrangement of the PCl_3 molecule?

    A. trigonal planar
    B. trigonal pyramidal
    C. square planar
    D. bent

149. The reaction of sulfuric acid with calcium phosphate is best categorized as which of the following types of reactions?

    A. Combination
    B. Decomposition
    C. Single Replacement
    D. Double Replacement

150. Phosphorous and nitrogen exhibit similar chemical behavior, as they both carry 5 valence electrons. Which of the following is the most likely explanation why phosphorous forms PCl_5, but nitrogen will not form NCl_5?

    A. The greater nuclear charge of phosphorous makes it more electronegative than nitrogen.
    B. Phosphorous has d orbitals available to use in bonding, while nitrogen does not.
    C. Phosphorous has more valence electrons available for bonding than nitrogen.
    D. The greater mass of phosphorous gives it greater gravitational attraction than nitrogen.

151. If 50.0 grams of oxygen gas reacts with 50.0 grams of phosphine and the reaction proceeds to completion, which of the following statements is true?

    A. Some oxygen gas would remain because oxygen is the limiting reactant.
    B. Some oxygen gas would remain because phosphine is the limiting reactant.
    C. Some phosphine would remain because oxygen is the limiting reactant.
    D. Some phosphine would remain because phosphine is the limiting reactant.

152. In a laboratory, 10 moles of calcium phosphate are combined with 30 moles of sulfuric acid. The reaction produces 18 moles of phosphoric acid and 27 moles of calcium sulfate. What is the percent yield of the reaction?

    A. 67%
    B. 75%
    C. 80%
    D. 90%

153. A 1 mole sample of white phosphorous is exposed to air at STP and starts to combust. If air is 20% oxygen by volume, what was the volume of air necessary for the sample to be completely consumed?

    A. 22.4 L
    B. 112 L
    C. 560 L
    D. 2800 L

154. The atoms in a PH_3 molecule demonstrate:

    A. Polar covalent bonding
    B. Non-polar covalent bonding
    C. Coordinate covalent bonding
    D. Hydrogen bonding

GO ON TO THE NEXT PAGE.

Questions 155 through 157 are **NOT** based on a descriptive passage.

155. When a 0.5 kg block is hung from a spring, the spring stretches to a length of 8 cm. If a 0.4 kg block added to the system, the length of the spring increases to 10 cm. What will be the length of the spring if an additional 0.2 kg block is added?

   A.   11 cm
   B.   12 cm
   C.   14 cm
   D.   15 cm

156. Which of the following is a true statement regarding the velocity and acceleration of an object in centripetal motion?

   A.   The velocity is constant and the acceleration is constantly changing.
   B.   The acceleration is constant and the velocity is constantly changing.
   C.   Both the velocity and acceleration remain constant.
   D.   Both the velocity and acceleration are constantly changing.

157. Which of the following represents the electron configuration of a sulfur atom in the ground state?

   A. $[Ne]3s^23p^4$
   B. $[Ne]3s^23p^6$
   C. $[Ar]3s^23d^{10}3p^4$
   D. $[Ar]3s^23d^{10}3p^6$

STOP. IF YOU FINISH BEFORE TIME IS CALLED, CHECK YOUR WORK. YOU MAY GO BACK TO ANY QUESTION IN THIS TEST BOOKLET.

STOP.

58

Verbal Reasoning
Time: 20 Minutes
Questions 158–172

It is a bizarre picture. Some of its more peculiar features have been made more bizarre by time. The eyebrows are shaved, and the hairline is raised far back by plucking or shaving in accord with a fashion of the day. The costume,
5 richly theatrical to us, may also have been modish. But these are minor considerations. The serious difficulty anyone must meet in understanding the Mona Lisa is that it has been too famous for too long. Familiar legends and conjectures have accumulated around it to the point where it is im-
10 possible to see it with a fresh vision. We never see it for the first time; it has always been around.

The most irritating legend attached to the Mona Lisa is that the eyes "follow you around the room" through some secret way of painting known only to Leonardo [da Vinci]
15 and unique to the picture. Yet the eyes of any portrait where the subject looks directly at the observer appear to follow that observer, no matter how ineptly they are executed. Then there is the superstition that the lips, if stared at long enough, "begin to smile." Any object stared at to the point
20 of strain will appear to change in one way or another, especially if we expect it to. It is unfortunate, also, that the Mona Lisa is so often called the greatest picture in the world. No picture can be the greatest in the world, because there is no single standard of perfection. If such a standard
25 could exist, it is difficult to see how so ambiguous a picture as the Mona Lisa could represent it anyway.

Such difficulties explain why efforts to interpret the painting have a way of degenerating into literary maunderings like Walter Pater's notorious one, which has become
30 the standard example of what art criticism is not [or should not be]:

She is older than the rocks among which she sits; like the vampire, she has been dead many times, and learned the secrets of the
35 grave; and has been a diver in deep seas, and keeps their fallen days about her; and trafficked for strange webs with Eastern merchants, and, as Leda, was the mother of Helen of Troy, and, as Saint Anne, the mother
40 of Mary; and all this has been to her but as the sound of lyres and flutes, and lives only in the delicacy with which it has moulded the changing lineaments, and tinged the eyelids and the hands.

45 ... If Leonardo intended to make the Mona Lisa a symbol of timeless mysteries, the landscape in the background plays a major part in this expression. ... Leonardo has invented a landscape half fantastic and half logical, where both time and place are mysterious. Mona Lisa's
50 head, played against this background, partakes of its quali-

ties, just as Madame Leblanc shared the fashionable elegance of the various accessories to her portrait.

All but the youngest of us can envision the dark-haired coyly smiling woman who is the Mona Lisa. But how many
55 of us have ever seen the actual painting? Where do these visions come from? What we are seeing are recreations of film, photograph, or painted copies. It has become ubiquitous. It is no longer a picture; it is an institution: the Parthenon, the White House, the Pyramids, or the Sphinx.

158. The word *institution* (line 58) is used in the sense of:

   A.   a building.
   B.   a tradition.
   C.   a famous painting.
   D.   an anomaly.

159. What is the author's response to the story about the children playing in the neighborhood 'haunted house', who come running home to tell their parents that they had seen the figure in the painted portrait on the wall *moving*?

   A.   The children had likely been staring at the painting too long, and expected it to move.
   B.   The figure in the painting was probably the person whom the children felt was haunting the house.
   C.   If the children had been looking at the figure for a long time, it would begin to move.
   D.   The children had probably expected the painting to move because it had been 'staring' at them.

60

GO ON TO THE NEXT PAGE.

160. According to the passage, one drawback of an art object's being "too famous for too long" (line 8) is that it can:

A. lead to mischaracterization.
B. become stale.
C. preclude original ideas.
D. inhibit criticism.

161. Assume that a later, revised series of paintings by Leonardo da Vinci is discovered. Which of the following characteristics of the discovered paintings would most *compromise* the author's analysis?

A. portrayed a slowly aging Mona Lisa.
B. pictured the Mona Lisa smiling brightly.
C. showed other examples of portraits where the eyes "follow you around the room".
D. proved that the Mona Lisa background was a real landscape.

162. On the basis of the passage, it is reasonable to conclude that:

A. perfection may be in the eye of the beholder.
B. if possible, art should always be viewed firsthand.
C. interpretation of famous paintings is becoming increasingly difficult.
D. fame frequently hurts an artist more than it helps him.

163. If the author's primary criterion for judging the standard of *"perfection"* of a picture were applied to directions, which of the following directions would be *most* perfect?

A. Walk east for 720 centimeters, then turn right and go 62 centimeters.
B. Move at a brisk pace north by northeast for 7 minutes, then turn sharply left and continue for 52 seconds.
C. Run quickly 270 degrees for 1/2 mile, then turn left and walk for 129 feet.
D. Walk 352 degrees for 62 meters, then turn 20 degrees and continue for 5 meters.

164. The author's argument that the Mona Lisa "has always been around" and "is no longer a picture", depends on the acceptance of which of the following premises?

A. It can be conclusively proven that it was a da Vinci painting.
B. The picture can be dated by the fashions which the Mona Lisa is wearing.
C. The painting has been recreated innumerable times in photographs.
D. Almost anyone can recognize and envision the painting.

Passage IV (Questions 165-172)

In postwar Germany, Lynette Comber and T.G. Younger of Oxford University conducted a controlled growth study of some 160 orphans. All of these children lagged 10 to 20 months behind normal levels of growth and
5 maturity, simply because they were not getting enough to eat. Their diet provided only about 80 percent of the calories needed for the satisfactory nourishment of a growing child. For a year, Drs. Comber and Younger supplemented the children's diets with unlimited bread and other calorie-
10 rich foods, such as jam, sugar, and semolina. As might be expected, the children shot up in height and gained rapidly in weight, to become normal in both respects.

Were the children permanently damaged during the years when near-starvation hampered their growth?
15 Apparently not. Human beings have extraordinary recuperative powers. During a famine the human organism slows its growth rate and waits, as it were, for better times; it can make up the loss later if the famine does not last too long and is not too severe. Girls seem to resist malnutrition better
20 than boys. Surveys in Guam, Hiroshima, and elsewhere after World War II indicated a general retardation of growth, but all of them showed girls less retarded than boys. Similarly, the German girls studied by Drs. Comber and Younger returned to normal more quickly than the boys.
25 Either the female is tougher than the male, or she uses her biological equipment more efficiently.

Other experiments conducted by Drs. Comber and Younger have thrown light upon the relation between emotional stress and growth. Most people would assume—
30 and, as it turns out, assume rightly—that an unhappy child will not grow as fast as a happy one, all other things being equal. Normally, of course, "all other things" are very far from equal, and under normal circumstances the problem can hardly be attacked by science at all. But by using exper-
35 imental and control groups (and partly by accident) Dr. Comber made observations that establish a clear connection between emotional states and growth.

Working with children in two orphanages—we can call them orphanage A and Orphanage B—she chose a
40 group of children from Orphanage A as experimental subjects. For six months she traced their growth on the orphanage diet, to establish their "normal" growth rate. Over the next six months, she supplemented their diet in the hope of producing a growth spurt. The children in Orphanage B, serving as control subjects, received no diet supplement at all. Theoretically, the two groups should have grown at about the same rate for the first six months; then the group in Orphanage A should have shot ahead. In fact, everything seemed to go wrong from the start. During the
45 first six months, when both diets were unsupplemented, the children in Orphanage A gained more weight than the ones in Orphanage B. During the second six months, when the
50 group in Orphanage A received diet supplements, they gained less weight than the group in Orphanage B.

The explanation, when it came was simple enough. By coincidence, at the end of the first six-month period, a sternly disciplinarian headmistress had been transferred
55 from Orphanage B to Orphanage A. She ruled the children rigidly at all times. What was worse, she chose mealtimes to administer public (and often unjustified) rebukes. Under her cruel charge, the growth rates of her tense, unhappy wards went down. And, unwittingly, she confirmed the
60 researchers' conclusions in another way. She had eight favorite children, whom she took with her from Orphanage B to Orphanage A. Even in Orphanage B, these teacher's pets had gained more weight than the other children; in Orphanage A, where they received diet supplements, they
65 gained weight faster than ever. This made quite clear the link between emotional state and the rate of growth. Or, as Dr. Comber put it, in an apt quotation: "Better a dinner of herbs where love is, than a stewed ox and hatred therewith."

---

165. The claim that during the second six months of the experiment the children in Orphanage A gained less than the children in Orphanage B necessitates which of the following conclusions?

A. The children of Orphanage A weighed less than the Children in Orphanage B.

B. The proffered dietary supplements were insufficient to override the emotional stress.

C. The children of Orphanage A were not eating their supplemented meals.

D. Emotional sustenance is even more important than nutrition to growth.

166. According to the Passage, which of the following statements must be true?

A. During the first six-month period the headmistress's favorite children were at Orphanage A.

B. The headmistress probably did not favor her "pets" with much extra food.

C. At least some of the headmistress's favorite children were girls.

D. Without the food supplements, the "teacher's pets" would not have weighed more than the Orphanage A children.

167. Which of the following statements, if true, would most WEAKEN the author's contention that there is "a link between emotional state and the rate of growth" (line 66)?

- **A.** Children were not allowed to eat while being rebuked by the headmistress.
- **B.** The headmistress's favorite children were often given extra food.
- **C.** Both Comber and Younger were female and sympathized more with the children in Orphanage A.
- **D.** It was later determined that all of the headmistress's rebukes were completely justified.

168. According to the study results, during the first six months, the children with the greatest weight gain would have been:

- **A.** the females in Orphanage B.
- **B.** the females in Orphanage A.
- **C.** the female "favorites" in Orphanage B.
- **D.** the female "favorites" in Orphanage A.

169. If the passage information is correct, which of the following statements would be best supported by the fact that fifteen years later, many of the orphans were still below average in both height and weight?

- **A.** Those children had been with too little food for too long.
- **B.** These orphans must be the children in Orphanage B whom the headmistress had most severely rebuked.
- **C.** Those children had received supplementary food and a healthy diet too late.
- **D.** The new headmistress had also been a stern disciplinarian.

170. What is the most serious apparent *weakness* of the research described?

- **A.** There was no way to determine how much of the "unlimited" food the children were eating.
- **B.** There was no way to gauge the degree of the headmistress's rebukes.
- **C.** The scientists were predisposed to "find" what they had been looking for.
- **D.** There were too many variables involved in the experiments.

171. Some recent studies have concluded that in the absence of sufficient food, males of all ages are likely to give up a portion of their food to females and children. How would these studies affect the passage's assertion that girls seem to resist malnutrition better than boys?

- **A.** It would support the assertion.
- **B.** It would support the assertion if it could be shown that the girls refused the food.
- **C.** It would refute the assertion if this behavior occurred in the Guam, Hiroshima, and WWII studies, as well as the passage study.
- **D.** It would refute the assertion.

172. The author claims, "by using experimental and control groups (and partly by accident) Dr. Comber made observations that establish a clear connection between emotional states and growth" (lines 34-36). The support offered for this conclusion is:

- **A.** strong: there was a clear correlation between the amount the children ate and their growth rate.
- **B.** strong: under difficult circumstances, an important discovery was made, albeit inadvertently.
- **C.** weak: the results do not appear accidental.
- **D.** weak: the control group was not in the same situation as the experimental group.

STOP. IF YOU FINISH BEFORE TIME IS CALLED, CHECK YOUR WORK. YOU MAY GO BACK TO ANY QUESTION IN THIS TEST BOOKLET.

Biological Sciences

Time: 20 Minutes
Questions 173–188

Passage V (Questions 173-179)

Stomach ulcers were originally regarded as the result of an autoimmune disorder, which could be triggered by stress or bad diet. In the 1980's, however, two Australian scientists presented an infectious etiology for the condition. Barry Marshall and Robin Warren presented *Helicobacter Pylori* as the causative organism for gastric ulcers. Understandably, as their theory challenged the conventional understanding of ulcer genesis, it was met with great skepticism from the medical community. In order to truly support the proposed relationship between *H. Pylori* and ulcers, the scientists had to demonstrate the presence of the bacteria in all patients with ulcers, and show that ulcers could be generated from bacterial infection alone. In addition to cultivating *H. Pylori* from ulcer patients' stomachs, Marshall ingested the bacteria himself in order to personally illustrate a causal relationship. Both of these efforts were time consuming, as they depended on the cultivation of significant colonies of *H. pylori*.

Today, scientists are considering bacterial etiologies for many other autoimmune disorders, such as Rheumatoid Arthritis. *Mycoplasma* bacteria have been linked to arthritic changes in both peripheral joints and the Temporomandibular Joint (TMJ). For scientists today, however, it is easier to detect the presence of bacteria in specific regions of the body. The invention and widespread use of the Polymerase Chain Reaction (PCR) allows scientists to quickly and efficiently assess the presence of *Mycoplasma* in joint fluid. Inded, PCR has been used to detect *Mycoplasma* specific DNA sequences in the TMJ, confirming its role in diseased joints. PCR has reduced the task Marshall and Warren faced from a few days to a few hours.

PCR testing for specific bacterial species requires the careful selection of primers based on sequences of DNA that are only found in the organism of interest. Unique sequences from the genomes of three hypothetical *Mycoplasma* bacteria are listed below.

Mycoplasma roberium:

3'-TGGGAATTC...GAAACCCTT-5'
5'-ACCCTTAAG...CTTTGGGAA-3'   (520 bp)

Mycoplasma geromanium:

3'-GGTATTTTGG...CTCCTGTGA-5'
5'-CCATAAAACC...GAGGACACT-3'   (687 bp)

Mycoplasma mazerium:

3'-GAGGACACGG...AGAAGGGGCT-5'
5'-CTCCTGTGCC...TCTTCCCCGA-3'   (794 bp)

173. Which of the following pairs of primers could be used to amplify the DNA of *M. geromanium*?

    A. 5'-GTGTCCTC-3' and 5'-CATAAAACC-3'
    B. 5'-ACCCTTAA-3' and 5'-TTCCCAAAG-3'
    C. 5'-CGGCCGTA-3' and 5'-CCAAAATAC-3'
    D. 5'-AAACCTGA-3' and 5'-GGGTTACGT-3'

174. Which of the following organisms can be detected using the primers:

a) 5'-CTCCTGTG-3' and b) 5'-CAAAATACC-3' ?

    I. *M. roberium*
    II. *M. geromanium*
    III. *M. mazerium*

    A. I only
    B. II only
    C. II and III only
    D. None of the above

175. A few years following the invention of PCR, scientists switched the DNA polymerase to Taq Polymerase, which is isolated from the bacteria *Thermus aquaticus*. Which of the following statements best explains why this substitution allows for cheaper and more efficient PCR?

    A. As *T. aquaticus* is ubiquitous in nature, it is chearper for scientists to harvest the polymerase themselves than to purchase DNA polymerase from a commercial supplier.
    B. Many previously used DNA polymerases inhibit the annealing of two complementary strands, however, Taq does not.
    C. Since Taq is isolated from bacteria which inhabit hot geysers and springs, it can withstand the high temperatures involved in PCR without being denatured or deactivated.
    D. Taq is isolated from bacteria which thrive at slightly basic pH. The buffer solution which aids in primer binding is also slightly basic, and thus Taq can function better in this environment than previous polymerases.

66

176. A student tests Sinovial Fluid from an arthritic joint for the presence of *M. roberium*, *M. geromanium*, and *M. mazerium*. In order to save materials, he performs all of the PCR tests, one after another, in the same test tube. He then runs the results of his amplifications through an agarose gel, alongside known samples of the unique segments for each bacterium. Unfortunately, he forgets to label the control lane. Below is a representation of the student's gel results.

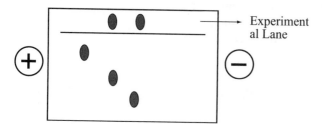

Which of the following bacteria were NOT present in the sample of synovial fluid?

A. *M. roberium and M. geromanium*
B. *M. roberium*
C. *M. geromanium and M. mazerium*
D. *M. geromanium*

177. Which of the following enzymes are absolutely necessary for PCR?

I. DNA Polymerase
II. RNA Polymerase
III. Ligase

A. I only
B. I and II only
C. I and III only
D. I, II, and III

178. A student performs PCR with a DNA template in which adenine is radioactively marked. He utililizes cytosine which is labeled with a distinct radioactive tag during the amplification process. After a 25-cycle PCR, he runs the product on agarose gel, excises the sequence, and recovers the DNA. He then tests the product for the presence of radioactive adenine or cytosine. Which of the following statements best describes his findings? (Assume the DNA sequence contains all four bases)

A. The product will test strongly positive for both radioactive adenine and cytosine.
B. The product will test weakly positive for both radioactive adenine and cytosine.
C. The product will only test positive for radioactive adenine.
D. The product will test weakly positive for radioactive adenine, and strongly positive for radioactive cytosine.

179. Another possible explanation for the presence of *Mycoplasma* in arthritic joints suggests that genes involved in inflammatory joint disorders may be linked to genes which increase susceptibility to certain bacterial infections. In this case, the presence of the bacteria, although associated, does not cause disease. Which of following scenarios would NOT support a causal relationship between *Mycoplasmsa* and joint disease?

D. A scientist elucidates the pathological cascade of inflammation resulting from *Mycoplasma* infection.
B. A doctor that treats TMJ disease solely with antibiotics reports a forty percent success rate in curing his patients.
C. *Mycoplasma* are found in the joints of an almost equal amount of disease free patients.
D. A scientist is able to raise large *Mycoplasma* colonies on joint samples he has removed from mammals.

Regulation of gene expression is complex and varied. The prokaryotic lac operon demonstrates both negative and positive control of gene expression at the transcriptional level. Operon DNA encompasses both coding and regulatory domains. The promoter (P) sequence is followed by the genes for Lac Z, Lac Y, and Lac A, three enzymes involved in the metabolism of lactose. Immediateley upstream of the promoter is an activator binding site (A). Further upstream, there is an I region, which includes the gene for Repressor (I) and its own Promotor sequence (P_i). Downstream of the lac promoter, P, is the Operator (O) region which contains the repressor binding site. The operon is depicted below.

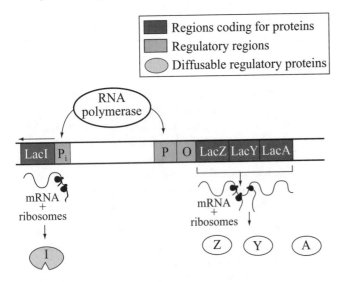

Figure 1 The lac operon

In the absence of lactose, the repressor exerts negative control by binding the operator region, and thus preventing transcription of lac enzymes. When present, lactose inactivates the repressor.

The <u>c</u>atabolite gene <u>a</u>ctivating <u>p</u>rotein, or CAP is responsible for the positive control of transcription. The CAP protein binds the A region and activates the promoter, allowing the formation of a transcription initiation complex at the P site. Activators and repressors are often themselves allosterically regulated by small molecules such as cAMP or Isopropyl-beta-D-thioglactoside (IPTG). CAP binding is, in fact, governed by cellular cAMP levels. As glucose levels fall, cAMP levels rise, activating CAP, which in turn will bind the A site and lead to lac enzyme expression. When multiple nutrients, for example both lactose and glucose, are present, slightly more transcription of lac enzymes takes place, but not as much as when only lactose is present.

In a merozygote, a diploid bacteria cell, a wildtype would look like:

$$\frac{\text{I+} \quad\quad \text{O+} \quad\quad \text{Z+}}{\text{I+} \quad\quad \text{O+} \quad\quad \text{Z+}}$$

180. mRNA transcripts of the lac enzymes would be transcribed in the presence of which of the following:

   I. lactose
  II. cAMP
 III. glucose

  A. I only
  B.. I and II only
  C. III only
  D. I, II, and III

181. Transcription factors are proteins that bind DNA in order to regulate gene expression. All of the following molecules are examples of transcription factors EXCEPT:

  A. repressor protein
  B.. CAP
  C. cortisol
  D. IPTG

182. A mutation in the O sequence would most likely result in:

  A. a change in the ratio of lac genes transcribed
  B.. a decrease in the transcription of all lac genes
  C. an increase in the transcription of all lac genes
  D. a compensatory increase in the production of repressor I

183. In a bacteria that's I- O+ Z+ / I+ O+ Z-, the mutations are:

  A. dominant, because there is no negative regulation of transcription
  B.. recessive, because the proofreading mechanism will correct
  C. dominant, because the repressor only binds to O
  D. recessive, because the repressor protein is still expressed

184. A bacteria cell that cannot metabolize lactose is colonized in a medium that contains the DNA fragments from bacteria that produce lactose digesting enzymes. Days later, the bacteria exhibits lactose metabolism as the result of which of the following processes?

  A. translocation
  B.. transduction
  C. transformation
  D. conduction

GO ON TO THE NEXT PAGE.

185. IPTG induces lac gene transcription by the same mechanism as lactose. According to the passage, IPTG must:

A. inactivate the I Region Promoter
B. inactivate repressor binding
C. enhance the formation of an initiation complex at the promoter site
D. activate CAP

186. Fluctuations in which of the following would have the greatest effect on the positive control mechanism of the lac operon?

A. DNA polymerase
B. glucose
C. lactose
D. repressor

Questions 187 and 188 are **NOT** based on a descriptive passage.

187. If PCR is performed on an isolated strand of DNA with two primers for n cycles, the result is 2^n total copies of the double-strand. If PCR is carried out on the same strand of DNA with one primer instead of two, how many total copies of the double-strand will be in the test tube after the experiment?

A. 0
B. 1
C. 1024
D. 512

188. A point mutation on one strand of the double stranded lac operon occurs in a bacteria cell just before the cell enters the S phase of the cell cycle. After 8 rounds of division, how many daughter cells will look like the original cell?

A. 0
B. 32
C. 128
D. 256

STOP. IF YOU FINISH BEFORE TIME IS CALLED, CHECK YOUR WORK. YOU MAY GO BACK TO ANY QUESTION IN THIS TEST BOOKLET.

70

16 MINI MCATS

EXAMINATION 05

Questions 189–235

Physical Sciences

Time: 20 Minutes
Questions 189–204

Passage I (Questions 189-194)

Many important scientific and industrial applications require the separation of two different gases. The process of successive effusion offers one method of performing same phase separation. In successive effusion, a mixture of gases is allowed to effuse through a series of chambers, while maintained at a constant temperature. As the gases pass through successive chambers, they separate according to Graham's law; the lighter gas concentrates in the farthest chambers as the heavier gas concentrates in the earlier chambers.

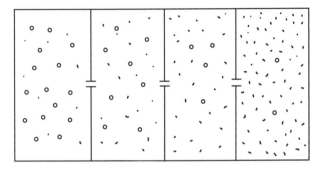

Figure 1 Chamber diagram

The separation factor, s, for any two gases is given by the formula below where M_H represents the molar mass of the heavier gas and M_L that of the lighter gas.

$$s = \sqrt{\frac{M_H}{M_L}}$$

During World War II, successive effusion was utilized to separate uranium-235, a fissionable isotope, from uranium-238, the most prevalent but less easily fissioned isotope. Both isotopes were combined with fluorine to form UF_6 gas, which then underwent successive effusion separation. Because the separation factor for the isotopes is small ($s = 1.0043$), the process had to be repeated more than a thousand times in order to achieve the required purity of uranium-235.

189. An industrial process requires the separation of fluorine and neon gases. What is the approximate separation factor for these two gases?

- **A.** 0.7
- **B.** 1.0
- **C.** 1.4
- **D.** 2.0

190. In the process of successive effusion, the lighter gas becomes more concentrated in the chambers farther along in the series because, compared to the heavier gas, it has:

- **A.** smaller average kinetic energy.
- **B.** greater average kinetic energy.
- **C.** smaller average speed.
- **D.** greater average speed.

191. Isolation of $^{235}UF_6$ was difficult and time-consuming because:

- **A.** uranium-235 is unstable.
- **B.** the molar masses of the two gases being separated are very similar
- **C.** the natural abundance of uranium-235 is so small.
- **D.** the kinetic energy of the UF_6 molecules is so large.

192. If the process of successive effusion was applied to each of the following pairs of gases, in which case would the process be most likely to be successful?

- **A.** Ar and C_3H_4
- **B.** C_2H_4 and N_2
- **C.** CO_2 and C_3H_8
- **D.** CH_4 and O_2

193. The nucleus of an atom of the most common isotope of uranium contains:

- **A.** 143 neutrons and 92 protons.
- **B.** 146 neutrons and 92 protons.
- **C.** 238 neutrons and 143 protons.
- **D.** 238 neutrons and 92 protons.

194. A closed 12 liter container holds a mixture of of helium and neon at standard temperature and pressure. If the partial pressure due to helium gas is 152 mmHg, what fraction of the gas mixture is made up by helium?

- **A.** $\frac{1}{5}$
- **B.** $\frac{1}{4}$
- **C.** $\frac{1}{3}$
- **D.** $\frac{1}{2}$

A circus strongman, with a mass of 95 kg, lifts a barbell with one hand and raises it over his head. The barbell consists of a massless bar with a length of 180 centimeters and circular solid metal plates attached to each end. He lifts the bar straight up from the ground while holding it horizontally and raises it to a height of 2.5 meters.

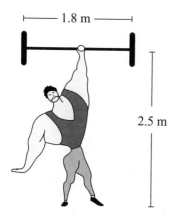

Figure 1 Strongman

It is important that the strongman grab the bar exactly at the midpoint to avoid torque that may rotate the bar and cause injury. It is also important that he bring the barbell from the ground up over his head in one quick and smooth motion. The strongman impresses the crowd by holding the barbell over his head for a long time after lifting it. When he can no longer maintain this stance, he dramatically releases the bar and steps back to stay clear of the freefalling barbell.

195. If the bar has a 60 kg metal plate attached to each end, what is the work done by the strongman in lifting it over his head?

- **A.** 1.2 kJ
- **B.** 1.5 kJ
- **C.** 2 kJ
- **D.** 3 kJ

196. After the strongman has held a barbell with a 40 kg plates for 30 seconds, he steps back and lets it fall to the ground. What is the approximate speed of the barbell at the moment before it strikes the ground?

- **A.** 4 m/s
- **B.** 6 m/s
- **C.** 7 m/s
- **D.** 10 m/s

197. The strongman attempts to lift a bar with a 50 kg plates, however, he grasps the bar 5 centimeters to the left of the midpoint. What is the magnitude of the torque on the bar when he lifts it off the ground?

- **A.** 5 Nm
- **B.** 50 Nm
- **C.** 500 Nm
- **D.** 5000 Nm

198. In one fluid motion, the strongman lifts a barbell over his head in 0.2 seconds. If the barbell has a gravitational potential energy of 2.0 kJ at the end of the motion, what is the power generated by the strongman during the lift?

- **A.** 0 kW
- **B.** 0.8 kW
- **C.** 4 kW
- **D.** 10 kW

199. The strongman holds a barbell motionless over his head for 40 seconds. If the bar has 75 kg metal plates on each end, what is the power used by the strongman to hold the bar up during this time?

- **A.** 0 kW
- **B.** 75 kW
- **C.** 150 kW
- **D.** 300 kW

200. A plate with a mass of 40 kg is placed on one end of the barbell while a 50 kg plate is placed on the other end. If the strongman is to lift the bar over his head without any rotational motion, at what distance from the 50 kg plate should he grab the bar?

- **A.** 70 cm
- **B.** 80 cm
- **C.** 90 cm
- **D.** 100 cm

GO ON TO THE NEXT PAGE.

201. Students in a chemistry lab run three trials of the reaction shown below. For each trial, they record the initial concentration of the reactants and calculate initial reaction rates. Their data is presented in Table I.

$$A + B \rightarrow C + D$$

Trial	Initial concentration of A (M)	Initial concentration of B (M)	Initial Rate
1	0.2	0.1	6.0×10^{-4}
2	0.2	0.2	1.2×10^{-3}
3	0.4	0.4	4.8×10^{-3}

Table I Reaction rates at varying reactant concentrations.

Which of the following formula correctly expresses the reaction rate?

A. rate = k[B]
B. rate = k[A][B]
C. rate = k[A]^2[B]
D. rate = k[A][B]^2

202. An archer fires an arrow straight up into the air. Which of the following best describes the change in energy from the time that the bow is fully stretched to the moment when the arrow is at its peak height?

A. kinetic to elastic potential to gravitational potential
B. gravitational potential to elastic potential to kinetic
C. gravitational potential to kinetic to elastic potential
D. elastic potential to kinetic to gravitational potential

203. What is the equilibrium expression for the reversible reaction shown below?

$$CO_3^{2-}(aq) + 2\ H_2O(l) \Leftrightarrow H_2CO_3(aq) + 2\ OH^-\ aq$$

A. $\dfrac{[H_2CO_3][OH^-]}{[CO_3^{2-}]}$

B. $\dfrac{[H_2CO_3][OH^-]^2}{[CO_3^{2-}]}$

C. $\dfrac{[H_2CO_3][OH^-]}{[CO_3^{2-}][H_2O]}$

D. $\dfrac{[H_2CO_3][OH^-]^2}{[CO_3^{2-}][H_2O]}$

204. A rocket rises through the atmosphere at a constant speed against the forces of gravity and air resistance. Which of the following is true of the net force acting on the rocket and the rocket's power?

A. Both the net force and the power are increasing.
B. Both the net force and the power are decreasing.
C. The net force is zero and the power is decreasing.
D. Both the net force and the power have constant values.

STOP. IF YOU FINISH BEFORE TIME IS CALLED, CHECK YOUR WORK. YOU MAY GO BACK TO ANY QUESTION IN THIS TEST BOOKLET.

Verbal Reasoning

Time: 20 Minutes
Questions 205–219

… Huge radar dishes ensconced deep in the jungles of South America than incessantly search the sky for radio signals are the hallmark of SETI (Search for Extraterrestrial Intelligence). But the computer side of the program is more
5 low-tech. The program now uses thousands of home PCs that are have been volunteered for consolidating the information gleaned by the giant dishes. Though almost three-quarters of the heavens have been scanned with no discernible patterns discovered, it is hoped that one day a
10 computer will unravel a radio signal from a distant civilization. As an example, early TV signals, shows like I Love Lucy and Ed Sullivan, left the earth about 40 years ago, and have traveled 40 light years, reaching several thousand nearby stars. However, these signals are relatively weak and
15 SETI is not likely to detect the equivalent of Earth type TV transmitters, even on the nearest stars. Even still, the search continues.

Behind all of man's continuing efforts to detect life elsewhere in the universe, there may lie an astounding
20 irony: perhaps humans and all other forms of life originated not here on Earth but on another world. In 1973 British biologist Francis Crick, who won a Nobel Prize as co-discoverer of the "double-helix" structure of the heredity molecule DNA, and Leslie Orgel of California's Salk insti-
25 tute, speculated that billions of years ago a sophisticated civilization on a planet circling some nearby star shipped some microorganisms to Earth. These seeds, they suggest, took hold on the then-barren planet, and proceeded to set the inexorable process of evolution in motion.

30 Two perplexing aspects of earthly life led Crick and Orgel to this idea. They note that many vital functions of organisms on Earth depend on the rare element molybde-num. Molybdenum is now considered one of our essential trace minerals. It has been found to be essential in most
35 mammals, as well as in all plants. We obtain it primarily from foods, but since it is often scarce in the earth's crust and therefore deficient in many soils, molybdenum defi-ciency can be a problem. In fact, it was recently discovered that molybdenum deficiency in the soil in an area of China
40 was responsible for the highest known incidence of esophageal carcinoma over many generations. In their view, organisms would not have placed such reliance on a rare element—unless they were descended from life forms that arose on a planet where molybdenum is more common.

45 A second puzzling feature of life, as we know it, is the fact that the same type of molecule—DNA—controls the inheritance of all organisms, as if all were descended from the same ancestors. Crick and Orgel believe that if life orig-inated on Earth, it would have arisen in many places and at
50 many different times, and this would have resulted in a diversity of genetic codes.

Most scientists would agree that the hypothesis offered by Crick and Orgel is possible. The fear that foreign living matter could proliferate in a barren world has led
55 scientists to routinely sterilize spacecrafts sent from the earth to the moon and other planets to prevent contamina-tion of alien soil—and so make sure that if modern men spread the gift of life, they do so not accidentally, but with the forethought of their progenitors.

205. Which of the following assertions is most clearly a thesis presented by the author?

A. We may be the ancestors of aliens.
B. The SETI program will eventually discover alien life.
C. Aliens intentionally spawned humankind.
D. Notable scientists believe in alien ancestors.

206. Which of the following scientific advances would most seriously *challenge* the hypothesis involving aliens?

A. Association of efforts to detect alien life with man's genetic structure.
B. Proof of ancient alien landing sites in the southwest desert.
C. The discovery of large molybdenum deposits in the earth.
D. Confirmation of TV-type transmissions emitting from another star system.

78

GO ON TO THE NEXT PAGE.

207. According to the passage information, what would happen if life had evolved spontaneously here on earth without outside intervention of any kind?

  I.   The idea of the existence of alien life forms could be dismissed.
  II. Organisms would not be dependent on a rare element.
  III. There would be different molecules controlling the inheritance of at least some organisms.

  A.   I only
  B.   II only
  C.   II and III only
  D.   I, II, and III

208. If the hypothesis of the passage is correct, one should find that relatively weak TV-type transmissions:

  A.   cannot possibly reach our planet from nearby star systems.
  B.   travel at about the same speed as light.
  C.   might be the first signal that an alien planet receives from the earth.
  D.   are what SETI has been programmed to detect.

209. Which of the following suppositions is most clearly believed by the author?

  A.   SETI will eventually detect alien transmissions.
  B.   The evolution of our species is a foregone conclusion.
  C.   Crick and Orgel were geniuses.
  D.   The "seeding" of earth was probably accidental.

210. The word *perplexing* (line 30):

  A.   detracts somewhat from the author's argument.
  B.   conveys that Crick and Orgel are the first to respond
  C.   conveys that certain aspects of earthly life have not been satisfactorily explained.
  D.   suggests that further study needs to be undertaken.

211. On the basis of the passage, it is reasonable to conclude that:

  A.   the aliens were probably "seeding" more than just one planet at a time.
  B.   the aliens did not "seed" earth intentionally.
  C.   eventually SETI may yield the reasons why aliens chose earth for seeding.
  D.   the aliens might not have known a great deal about earth.

212. Which of the following choices would the author of the passage be most likely to describe as *barren*?

  A.   a lifeless desert
  B.   a lifeless but fertile garden plot
  C.   a sterile woman without children
  D.   a massive rocky planet

Time, which is everywhere yet nowhere, which is intuitively obvious yet logically indefinable, which is as straightforward as an alarm clock yet as paradoxical as relativity, has inevitably fascinated speculative minds in almost
5 every age. For centuries, philosophers and scientists have chewed over time's puzzling properties and tried to determine what it is and where (if anywhere) it is going.

Their speculations have centered on three fundamental questions: Is time real or unreal? Does it move in one
10 direction only, or is it reversible? Does it have a beginning or an end, or is it infinite? None of these questions has yet been answered to everyone's satisfaction, and some of them may never be answered to anyone's satisfaction. Yet the mere asking of them stretches the mind, and the search for
15 answers, though it may prove unsuccessful, can still reveal much about both time and the universe we inhabit.

The first question, "Is time real?" can be quickly disposed of. For the scientist, the question is meaningless, in the sense that it cannot be answered by scientific meth-
20 ods, and also trivial, meaning that it is not worth answering. To ask whether time is real is to ask whether the changes— biological, astronomical, or atomic—by which we measure time, and which we measure by it, are real. And the scientist, whose business is precisely the understanding and
25 explanation of such changes, is compelled to assume that they—and therefore time—are real. If the changes are not real, or at least real enough to perform experiments with, he is in the wrong line of work.

Beyond this, all of us here on earth—scientists,
30 philosophers, doctors, lawyers and candlestick makers— live in a world in which time and change, real or not, must be coped with. A friend of the Russian philosopher Nikolai Berdyaev recounts how the old man would "plead passionately for the insignificance and unreality of time, and then
35 suddenly stop and look at his watch with genuine anxiety at the thought that he was two minutes late for taking his medicine!" A philosopher today who jaywalks across a superhighway, believing that the motion of the speeding cars is an illusion, will not survive very long to philosophize
40 on the matter.

To be sure, most of us, when feeling too beset by the ceaseless changes of existence, have at some point daydreamed of a place where time and change were not— of Tennyson's Lotus Land "where it was always afternoon."
45 With the Irish poet Yeats we have yearned for the Land of Heart's Desire,

Where beauty has no ebb, decay no flood,
But joy is wisdom, time an endless song.

But though in our dreams time may have a stop, it
50 starts up again in the moment of our waking.

A no less familiar chord of longing is struck by the second fundamental question, "Can time be reversed?" Who among all of us has not at some time in his life mused along the lines of the Victorian doggerel,

55 *Backward, turn backward, oh time in your flight;*
Make me a child again, just for tonight.

or wished with Shakespeare's Richard II to "call back yesterday, bid time return"? To turn back time, to be able to undo our mistakes and relive our ecstasies—that would be
60 a secret worth having! For such a magical elixir of youth, the alchemists toiled long years over their alembics, and Faust was prepared to sell his very soul.

Common sense born of experience, however, teaches
65 us that a backward-moving time is as fantastical as an unmoving time. The kettle boils only after we have set it on the stove, never before. The apple ripens only after the apple blossom has fallen. All of us grow older with time, not younger.

213. If the author's primary criterion for judging the *'realness'* of time were applied to human feelings, which of the following feelings would be the LEAST real?

A. Love
B. Hunger
C. Pain
D. Cold

GO ON TO THE NEXT PAGE.

214. On the basis of the passage, one may assume that as humans discover newer and more effective scientific methods:

   A. what was once irreversible will become reversible.
   B. what was once impossible will become possible.
   C. what was once trivial will become important.
   D. what was once meaningless will become meaningful.

215. With which of the following statements would the author most likely *disagree*:

   I. A scientist must make certain assumptions in order to do his job.
   II. We cannot rely on common sense.
   III. Philosophy is important to scientific discovery.

   A. I only
   B. II only
   C. III only
   D. II and II only

216. The author apparently believes that a philosopher may come to a conclusion that:

   A. it is possible to go back in time.
   B. defies common sense.
   C. centers on only one of the fundamental questions.
   D. cannot be taken literally.

217. According to the author, which of the following statements must not be true?

   A. Time has no beginning or end.
   B. Time must be infinite.
   C. Time can be moving and unmoving.
   D. Time is real.

218. The assertion that time is paradoxical is NOT clearly consistent with the information about:

   A. the ironies of philosophical conclusions.
   B. our yearnings for a return to a former period of our lives.
   C. time being rather easy to define.
   D. our abilities to use common sense born of experience.

219. On the basis of the passage, it is reasonable to conclude that:

   A. alchemists must have believed that time was reversible.
   B. many philosophers believe that time is an illusion.
   C. time has no beginning and no end.
   D. time is not intuitively obvious.

STOP. IF YOU FINISH BEFORE TIME IS CALLED, CHECK YOUR WORK. YOU MAY GO BACK TO ANY QUESTION IN THIS TEST BOOKLET.

 STOP.

Biological Sciences

Time: 20 Minutes

Questions 220–235

Passage V (Questions 220-225)

Medical advances in immunization have lead to a dramatic decrease in the morbidity and mortality of infectious disease. A similar trend has been noted in the incidence of many viral diseases. Viral vaccination *primes* the host immune system, so that a second exposure to the virus will initiate a rapid immune response, protecting the host from fulminant infection. Host vaccination may be accomplished with either live viruses or viral particles.

Live-attenuated viral vaccines utilize low virulence viruses, which are selected by *in vitro* cultivation under adverse conditions (i.e. low temperature). By harvesting viruses which do best in such extreme conditions, scientists decrease the chance of successful replication in the conditions of the human body. Most successful viral vaccines belong to this group.

A heterologous viral vaccine involves the use of closely related, yet less virulent, viruses. A related virus will share many antigens with the virulent organism, and thus will induce an immune response that cross-reacts with antigens of the virulent organism.

By introducing a gene coding for an immunogenic protein from a virulent organism into the genome of a non virulent virus, scientists generate live recombinant vaccines. Once introduced into the host, the recombinant organism induces a host immune response to the virulent organisms' proteins.

Killed (inactivated) viral vaccines are used when live vaccines are not feasible or unavailable. A virus is grown in bulk and inactivated, and then the protein of interest is purified and concentrated from the culture suspension. Virulent organisms are inactivated with either beta-propiolactone or formaldehyde. As these vaccines are not infectious, they are considered safer than live virus vaccines. However, they are usually of lower immunogenicity, require multiple doses to induce immunity, and are usually expensive to prepare. Subcellular viral fractions establish host immunity by directing an immune response specific to one or two viral proteins.

220. Both cowpox and vaccinia are related to the variola virus, the organism responsible for smallpox. The 18th century physician, Edward Jenner, observed that milkmaids infected with the cowpox virus were immune to smallpox. This natural vaccination is most closely related to which of the following vaccines?

   A. live attenuated vaccines
   B. live recombinant vaccines
   C. live heterologous vaccines
   D. inactivated vaccines

221. Which of the following is the LEAST important characteristic in developing a successful vaccine?

   A. eliciting a virus-specific immune responses
   B. providing life-long protection against a particular virus
   C. reproduction of a few of the salient features of wild type infection, with mild clinical disease
   D. inexpensive

222. DNA vaccines are genetically engineered plasmids with foreign DNA. Within the host cells, the plasmid transcripts are able to elicit an immune response. Which of the following enzymes is responsible for expression of the recombinant plasmid gene?

   A. DNA polymerase
   B. DNA ligase
   C. RNA polymerase
   D. RNA primase

223. During the last few months of pregnancy, mothers transfer antibodies to their unborn babies through the placenta. Maternal antibodies will protect children for up to 6 months after birth from illnesses for which the mother has been vaccinated. Based on this information, the immune system of a 3 month old baby can most accurately described as:

   A. completely unprimed
   B. completely primed
   C. unprimed to only those diseases the mother was exposed to
   D. primed to only those diseases the mother was exposed to

224. According to the passage, in order for the live recombinant vaccines to succeed, the host must have which of the following organelles?

   A. rough endoplasmic reticulum
   B. nucleus
   C. lysosome
   D. peroxisome

84

GO ON TO THE NEXT PAGE.

225. All of the following organs are involved in an "unprimed" immune response, EXCEPT:

- **A.** the bone marrow
- **B.** the spleen
- **C.** lymph nodes
- **D.** the adrenal glands

226. Both the inactived, Salk, and the live-attenuated, Sabin, forms of the polio vaccine are in widespread use worldwide. Which of the following characteristics are true of the two vaccine forms?

- **I.** Salk requires multiple doses to activate the immune system
- **II.** Sabin elicits only a minor immune response
- **III.** Sabin is less expensive to prepare

- **A.** I only
- **B.** I and III only
- **C.** II and III only
- **D.** I, II, and III

Passage VI (Questions 227-233)

Alexander Fleming discovered penicillin in 1928, and since then it has proven to be a wonder drug, saving the lives of countless people. Since then, dozens of new drugs have been discovered which have antibacterial activity similar to penicillin—a class of drugs we now call 'antibiotics'.

Unfortunately, after 85 years of antibiotic use, many bacteria have become resistant to even the most current antibiotics. Infections that were previously controllable have once again become life-threatening. The underlying factors in resistance development are numerous, including over-prescription of antibiotics and noncompliance with antibiotic regimens. Ultimately, all of these factors affect the natural selection of bacteria.

As a result, new drugs, which kill antibiotic resistant bacterial strains, are a primary focus of pharmaceutical research. One such drug currently under development, RG7, is being evaluated for its efficacy and mechanism of action. Researchers administer RG7 to cultures of *E. Coli*. Cell counts, ATP levels, and protein levels are measured before and after administration of RG7 for 3 sets of cultures. The researcher's data is presented in the table below.

Group	Condition	Cells	ATP	Protein
1	Pre RG7	40	18	7
1	Post RG7	30	16	3
2	Pre RG7	53	20	6
2	Post RG7	20	15	1
3	Pre RG7	30	16	5
3	Post RG7	29	17	4

Table 1 Relative levels of cell counts, ATP, and proteins before and after RG7 administration.

227. Using the information in the passage, what is the most likely mechanism of the action of RG7?

- **A.** Destruction of ribosomes
- **B.** Destruction of Golgi apparatus
- **C.** Disruption of Kreb's cycle
- **D.** Disruption of lysosome integrity

228. A particular antibiotic functions via the destruction of bacterial DNA. Which of the following is the most likely mechanism of action

    A.   Destruction nuclei within cells
    B.   Digestion of histone protiens
    C.   Inactivation of enzymes which cleave circular DNA
    D.   Destruction nucleoli

229. Some bacteriocidal drugs function via the formation of pores in the bacterial cell wall. Which of the following statements best explains why these drugs are not cytotoxic to human cells?

    A.   Eukaryotic cells are more efficient in repairing cell wall damage.
    B.   Human lysosomes digest the antibiotics before the drugs induce significant cytotoxicity.
    C.   Human cells produce cytoprotective molecules which are secreted on the cell surface.
    D.   Human cells lack a cell wall for the antibiotic to destroy.

230. According to the passage, many bacteria have evolved antibiotic resistance in just 85 years. Which of the following factors best explain the reason behind rapid bacterial evolution?

    A.   Rapid reproduction and low mutation rate
    B.   Slow reproduction and low mutation rate
    C.   Rapid reproduction and rapid mutation rate
    D.   Slow reproduction and slow mutation rate

231. The passage implicates noncompliance with antibiotic regimens as a key factor in the development of bacterial antibiotic resistance. Which of the following statements is NOT a factor in the relationship between patient noncompliance and bacterial resistance?

    A.   Oftentimes, patient's are relieved of the symptoms of infection before the infection is completely cleared.
    B.   Early termination of an antibiotic regimen allows a significant amount of bacteria to live.
    C.   Bacteria require exposure to antibiotics in order to develop resistance.
    D.   Older antibiotics, such as penicillin are not as effective against newer bacteria

232. Bacteria are commonly used in the synthesis of human proteins which are deficient in certain disorders, such as insulin for Type I diabetes. Unfortunately, not all proteins can be generated with the sole use of bacteria. Some portions of human proteins are added posttranslationally by an organelle not found in bacteria. Which of the following organelles is most likely for this posttranslational modification?

    A.   Nucleus
    B.   Ribosome
    C.   Peroxisome
    D.   Golgi

233. Unlike humans, bacteria are able to reproduce via a variety of mechanisms. Which of the following is NOT a mechanism of bacterial reproduction?

    A.   Mitosis
    B.   Budding
    C.   Binary fission
    D.   Sexual reproduction

234. The success of any vaccine is dependent on the integrity of the host immune system. Specifically, the host response must generate not only memory T and B cells, but also virus-neutralizing antibodies. Which of the following cells are responsible for generation of the latter?

A. T-cells
B. Plasma cells
C. Macrophages
D. Thymus cells

235. Some bacterial species are able to survive in the presence or absence of oxygen. Such bacteria are collectively known as facultative anaerobes. Which of the following bacterial processes allows survival in the absence of oxygen?

A. Oxygen extraction from water
B. Fermentation
C. Spore formation
D. Protein metabolism

STOP. IF YOU FINISH BEFORE TIME IS CALLED, CHECK YOUR WORK. YOU MAY GO BACK TO ANY QUESTION IN THIS TEST BOOKLET.

EXAMINATION 06

Questions 236–282

Physical Sciences

Time: 20 Minutes
Questions 236–251

The work done by conservative forces is path-independent. More specifically, the work on a given object accomplished by a conservative force depends only on the initial and final positions. Thus, if the work performed is known to be a function of object displacement, the force responsible can be categorized as conservative. Gravitational pull provides an oft-cited example of conservative force.

The work done by a nonconservative force, on the other hand, is path-dependent. Thus, the work done by a nonconservative force on a given object is a function of the distance the object travels. Friction is an example of a nonconservative force.

The potential energy of an object increases when work is accomplished against a conservative force, however, the same is not true when work is performed against nonconservative forces.

Example 1

A 10 kg block is moved from the ground to a height of 20 meters by the path shown below.

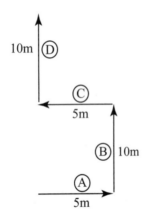

Figure 1

Example 2

A 10 kg block is pulled along a flat surface for 30 meters as depicted below. The frictional force impeding the motion of the block is 20 N.

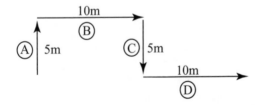

Figure 2

236. What is the gravitational potential energy of the block at the end of Example 1?

  A. 200 J
  B. 300 J
  C. 2000 J
  D. 3000 J

237. What is the distance traveled by the object in Example 2, and the magnitude of its final displacement?

  A. distance = 20 m, displacement = 20 m
  B. distance = 20 m, displacement = 30 m
  C. distance = 30 m, displacement = 30 m
  D. distance = 30 m, displacement = 20 m

238. What is the coefficient of kinetic friction between the block and the surface in Example 2?

  A. 0.1
  B. 0.2
  C. 0.4
  D. 0.5

239. If it takes the object 40 seconds to travel from the beginning to the end of the path pictured for Example 2, how much power is exerted?

  A. 15 W
  B. 40 W
  C. 300 W
  D. 2400 W

240. In Example 1, work is performed in which section (A-D)?

  A. Work is done in all four sections.
  B. No work is done in any section.
  C. Work is done only in sections A and C.
  D. Work is done only in sections B and D.

241. If the path in Example 2 required 50 seconds to complete, what was the average velocity of the object?

  A. 0.2 m/s
  B. 0.4 m/s
  C. 0.6 m/s
  D. 2 m/s

242. The work performed in Example 2 is transfered into:

  A. heat.
  B. potential energy.
  C. heat and potential energy.
  D. neither heat nor potential energy.

Nitric oxide gas reacts with bromine gas to form nitrosyl bromide gas, NOBr, according to the following reversible reaction.

$$2\ NO(g) + Br_2(g) \Leftrightarrow 2\ NOBr(g)$$

Reaction 1

At a temperature of 373 K, the equilibrium constant, K_P for the reaction is equal to 0.5.

Researchers in a chemistry lab combine nitric oxide and bromine gas in a closed container at 373 K. The reaction is allowed to equilibrate, at which point the researchers calculate the partial pressure of NOBr present. The table below presents this data, along with the initial pressures of the reactants for 5 trials.

Trial	Initial pressure of NO (atm)	Initial pressure of Br_2 (atm)	Equilibrium pressure of NOBr (atm)
1	1.0	0.25	0.21
2	1.0	0.50	0.30
3	1.0	1.0	0.39
4	1.0	2.0	0.48
5	1.0	4.0	0.58

Table 1

243. If NOBr gas is removed as it is produced, the reaction would proceed to completion. If this scenario is applied to Trial 3, which of the following gases would be the limiting reagent?

- **A.** NO
- **B.** Br_2
- **C.** NOBr
- **D.** There would be no limiting reactant.

244. What is the partial pressure due to bromine gas when the reaction in Trial 2 has reached equilibrium?

- **A.** 0.15 atm
- **B.** 0.20 atm
- **C.** 0.35 atm
- **D.** 0.50 atm

245. Which of the following is true of the total pressure in the container at equilibrium?

- **A.** It will be less than the initial total pressure in every trial.
- **B.** It will be greater than the initial total pressure in every trial.
- **C.** It will be equal to the initial total pressure in every trial.
- **D.** It will greater than the initial total pressure for some of the trials and less for others.

246. As the initial partial pressure of bromine gas is increased, the equilibrium pressure of nitrosyl bromide:

- **A.** increases and the equilibrium pressure of nitric oxide increases.
- **B.** increases and the equilibrium pressure of nitric oxide decreases.
- **C.** decreases and the equilibrium pressure of nitric oxide increases.
- **D.** decreases and the equilibrium pressure of nitric oxide decreases.

247. Which of the following expressions is equal to the equilibrium constant, K_P for Reaction 1?

- **A.** $\dfrac{\left(P_{NO}\right)\left(P_{Br}\right)}{\left(P_{NOBr}\right)}$

- **B.** $\dfrac{\left(P_{NO}\right)^2\left(P_{Br}\right)}{\left(P_{NOBr}\right)^2}$

- **C.** $\dfrac{\left(P_{NOBr}\right)}{\left(P_{NO}\right)\left(P_{Br}\right)}$

- **D.** $\dfrac{\left(P_{NOBr}\right)^2}{\left(P_{NO}\right)^2\left(P_{Br}\right)}$

248. If a sixth trial were included with initial partial pressures of 1 atm for NO and 8 atm for Br_2, what would be the value of K_P for the trial?

- **A.** 0.12
- **B.** 0.5
- **C.** 1.0
- **D.** 4.0

249. A wooden beam with a length of 14 meters and a mass of 90 kg is positioned at the edge of a ledge as shown below. How far beyond the ledge can a 60 kg man walk without tipping the beam?

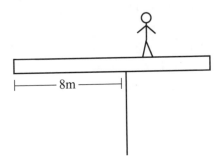

A. 0.67 m
B. 0.9 m
C. 1.2 m
D. 1.5 m

250. A reaction is first order with respect to reactant A, first order with respect to reactant B, and second order overall. The reaction rate is found to be 2.0×10^{-3} M/sec when the concentrations of both reactants is 0.2 M. What is the value of the rate constant for this reaction?

A. 8×10^{-5} M^{-1}sec^{-1}
B. 5×10^{-3} M^{-1}sec^{-1}
C. 5×10^{-2} M^{-1}sec^{-1}
D. 8×10^{-2} M^{-1}sec^{-1}

251. A sealed glass jar contains m grams of an ideal gas at a pressure P. If the temperature of the gas is increased, which of the following will occur?

A. P will increase.
B. P will decrease.
C. m will increase.
D. m will decrease.

STOP. IF YOU FINISH BEFORE TIME IS CALLED, CHECK YOUR WORK. YOU MAY GO BACK TO ANY QUESTION IN THIS TEST BOOKLET.

STOP.

Verbal Reasoning

Time: 20 Minutes
Questions 252–266

The ringing conviction of the Declaration of Independence—"We hold these truths to be self-evident: that all men are created equal..."—was challenged in 1973, not by exponents of racism, but by psychologists at two of
5 America's most prestigious universities. Both scholars published books describing their evidence that intelligence depended mainly on heredity, varied among the races, and created inherent inequalities that could not be overcome.

In *Educability and Group Differences*, psychologist
10 Arthur Jensen of the University of California at Berkeley suggested that the difference in intelligence-test results typically found between American blacks and whites could not be ascribed to social, economic or education discrimination but must be attributed to an innate intellectual inferiority in
15 blacks. He did not retreat from the controversial position he had set forth in earlier years, that compensatory education had failed and that continued efforts to improve the environment of blacks would help not at all to narrow the I.Q. gap between the races.

20 In *I.Q. in the Meritocracy*, Harvard University psychologist Richard Herrnstein accepted Jensen's idea that intelligence is largely hereditary and went on to draw disturbing conclusions. He proposed that educational equality, free social mobility and environmental enrichment for the
25 deprived of all races would lead, paradoxically, to a society of hereditary castes. His reasoning: 1) People with high I.Q.s, or high intelligence (Herrnstein believed they are the same), had already risen to the top of U.S. society, and those with the low I.Q.s and low intelligence had remained
30 at the bottom. 2) If environmental influences on I.Q. were made the same for everyone, hereditary factors would become relatively more important. 3) As high I.Q.s became increasingly determined by heredity, so would the wealth and power they so often bring, and with environmental dif-
35 ferences evened out, low I.Q. and low status would also be more and more governed by the genes. Eventually, even a tendency to be unemployed might run in a family's genes "about as certainly as bad teeth do now."

Critics of Jensen and Herrnstein—ostensible there
40 were very many and very vocal – pointed out that many psychologists believe I.Q. tests do not really measure intelligence and, in addition, are biased against blacks, reflecting not their innate mental ability but their isolation from the white middle-class culture that was the basis of the tests.
45 In addition, the critics insisted, simple factors such as nutrition can affect intelligence.

Several researchers in the early 1970's offered evidence of the effects of training on I.Q. test scores. Ones such researcher was education psychologist Phyllis
50 Levenstein of the State University of New York at Stony Brook. She reported that an experiment, with the cumber-

some name of Mother-Child Home Program of the Verbal Interaction Project, had succeeded in raising the I.Q. of deprived preschool children by an average of 17 points, and
55 that "if the children stay in the program the full two years ... they are apt to retain these gains in school." Levenstein's project used trained "toy demonstrators" to visit toddlers at home and to encourage inarticulate or illiterate parents to play and talk with their children, stimulating them to use
60 words and make observations.

One of the strongest refutations of "Jensenism," as the anti-egalitarian viewpoint was being called, came from geneticist Theodosius Dobzhansky of the University of California at Davis. In *Genetic Diversity and Human*
65 *Equality*, he explained that intelligence is not immutably fixed by heredity. What the genes really determine, he said, is how people will react to their environment: "Similar genes may have different effects in dissimilar environments," and racial differences in I.Q. are probably deter-
70 mined by differences in living conditions and educational opportunities. Additionally he did not think that class status would become hereditary. This was because high status requires not just intelligence but "energy, self-discipline ... persistence and other personal qualities."

252. On the basis of the passage, it is reasonable to conclude that:

A. the signatories of the Declaration of Independence intended that all men are of equal intelligence.
B. those who espoused Jensenism were racists.
C. even prior to 1973, attempts at compensatory education had been going on for some time.
D. intelligence is largely hereditary.

253. An important comparison is made in the passage between:

    A. environment and heredity.
    B. genetic diversity and human equality.
    C. biased testing and future performance.
    D. educability and group differences.

254. The results of the researchers, whom had succeeded in helping to raise the I.Q. of deprived preschool children (lines 47-60), are most in accord with the view that:

    A. one-on-one time with a "toy demonstrator" can raise a child's I.Q.
    B. parents play a critical role in a child's I.Q. development.
    C. intelligence and I.Q. are one in the same.
    D. the I.Q. tests were biased toward white middle-class culture.

255. Years later, in *The Bell Curve*, Herrnstein writes, "The difference in measured IQ between African Americans and Whites has remained at about 15 IQ points for decades". Passage information suggests that:

    A. the Jensenists attributed this difference to inadequate stimulation of children.
    B. without marked changes in I.Q. testing methodology, the Jensenists felt that this would not improve.
    C. Jensenism's critics argued that these results had been falsified.
    D. the opponents of Jensenism found that this difference can be overcome.

256. Which of the following statements most strongly *challenges* one of the assertions made in the passage?

    A. There is no definitive proof that an I.Q. test will accurately measure intelligence.
    B. High status within U.S. society consists of those who have wealth, power, and fame.
    C. It is genetics that can determine how a person will react to their environment.
    D. A racist is one who believes that race is the primary determinant of human traits and capacities.

257. Assume that the Jensenists *agreed* with geneticist Dobzhansky that "high status requires not just intelligence but 'energy, self-discipline ... persistence and other personal qualities'" (lines 73-75). What is the relevance of this new information to Herrnstein's theories on social stratification?

    A. Without these qualities, any attempts to raise I.Q. would probably be unsuccessful.
    B. Environmental influences would still remain relatively more important.
    C. A person with a high I.Q. will also have these personal qualities.
    D. Given a high I.Q., these qualities are unnecessary to an individual born into high society.

258. The author's attitude toward the findings and conclusions of the Jensenists is most accurately described as:

    A. favorable.
    B. neutral.
    C. mistrusting.
    D. disapproving.

Passage III (Questions 259-266)

The earliest clear examples of a society in which some people not only learned to keep records, but made it their business to do so, occurred about 5,000 years ago on the banks of the Tigris and Euphrates Rivers, among the
5 Sumerians, that singularly gifted people who evolved the first literate, urban culture. The Sumerians had the specialists for calendar making: priestly scribes who kept records on tablets of damp clay and who, doubtless, had already established themselves as professional time-reckoners.

10 In each of the small Sumerian city-states, the priests were responsible for administering the land on behalf of the gods and of the gods' earthly representative, the king. The job was not a simple one. To build a civilization out of the mixture of swamp and desert that is lower Mesopotamia re-
15 quired a network of dikes and ditches for drainage and irrigation. The construction of these works, and of the elaborate mud-brick temples over which the priests presided, required the coordinated labor of scores of men. Once built, the drainage and irrigation systems had to be kept in repair.
20 Most importantly from a time-reckoning standpoint, the irrigated fields of wheat and barley, onions and cucumbers, had to be plowed, sown, tended, and harvested at definite times of the year. Market days were held periodically in each of the small towns in the kingdom. The gods, on
25 whose goodwill the prosperity of the kingdom depended, had to be appeased with prayer and sacrifice on certain holy days – and these ceremonies had to be held on the same day in each town. For such a highly complex society a rough reckoning of the seasons would not do.

30 Our knowledge of the Sumerian calendar, unfortunately, is limited; it comes mainly from documents of the Babylonians, who succeeded the Sumerians as lords of Mesopotamia. It seems fairly certain, however, that the Sumerian priests based their original calendar on the moon,
35 dividing the year into 12 lunar months of 30 days each. This arrangement confronted them with astronomical problems that have plagued calendar makers for thousand of years.

The main problem stems from the fact that the astronomical cycles from which the day, the year, and the
40 months are derived do not fit neatly together. The year, which is based on the earth's revolution around the sun, comes to about 365 1/4 days. The month, of course, is measured by the phases of the moon, the full cycle coming to a little more than 29 1/2 days. As a result, the year is not
45 composed of 12 equal months, but of about 12 1/3. Unless the proper corrections were made, the Sumerian calendar, with its 30-day months, would have rapidly gotten out of step with the moon and the sun. The Sumerian priests must have corrected the calendar, but their exact methods have
50 been lost. We do know, however, that their Babylonian successors were able to keep the months in step with the moon by alternating 30-day months with months of 29 days, and adding an occasional extra 30-day month to make up for lost days. Similarly, they kept the year in step with the sun
55 by throwing in an extra month every three years or so.

For many centuries these calendar corrections were a matter of cut-and-try. A letter of the great Babylonian King Hammurabi, written some 1,700 years before Christ, says that the King ordered the insertion of an extra month when-
60 ever he happened to notice (or a priest called it to his attention) that "the year hath a deficiency." To the Babylonians, as well as the Sumerians and their prehistoric predecessors, the heavenly bodies were manifestations of the gods; if their motions seemed a bit capricious, who was to question the
65 gods' actions? The best that men could do was to keep track of the motions of the heavenly bodies, and pray that the gods would hold their caprices within bounds.

259. The word *astronomical* (line 36) is used in the sense of:

A. enormous.
B. planetary.
C. excessive.
D. heavenly.

260. According to the passage, the Sumerian's calendars were manufactured by:

A. priests.
B. the king.
C. each city-state administrator.
D. priestly scribes.

261. Later in the passage, the author asserts, "For many centuries these calendar corrections were a matter of cut-and-try" (lines 56-57). This assertion most likely means that:

- **A.** by the time of the Babylonians, the Sumerian's ability to make accurate calendar corrections had been lost.
- **B.** the Sumerians were no better at correcting the calendar than the Babylonians.
- **C.** during the reign of King Hammurabi, calendar corrections became even more capricious.
- **D.** there were several methods whereby a deficient calendar year might be corrected.

262. According to the passage, the Babylonians most likely continued the Sumerian practice of correcting their calendars by periodically inserting an extra:

- **A.** month.
- **B.** week.
- **C.** 29 days.
- **D.** few weeks.

263. According to the information in the passage, the problems with the lunar calendar always stemmed from:

- **I.** the calendar year being too short.
- **II.** the calendar year not being long enough.
- **III.** the whims of the king.

- **A.** I only
- **B.** II only
- **C.** III only
- **D.** II and III only

264. The author implies that the primary significance of the Sumerians was their:

- **A.** ability to create the first truly accurate calendar.
- **B.** reliance upon the lunar cycles.
- **C.** faculty for writing and recording.
- **D.** administrative and agricultural skills.

265. The author claims, "The earliest clear examples of a society in which some people not only learned to keep records, but made it their business to do so, occurred about 5,000 years ago on the banks of the Tigris and Euphrates Rivers, among the Sumerians" (lines 1-5). Thus, King Hammurabi's letter "written some 1,700 years before Christ" (line 58) would have been created:

- **A.** 3300 years afterward.
- **B.** 6700 years ago.
- **C.** 300 years after that.
- **D.** 1300 years later.

266. On the basis of the passage, it is reasonable to conclude that:

- **A.** the written documentation on the Babylonians exceeds that of the Sumerians.
- **B.** the Sumerians left behind voluminous written records of their culture.
- **C.** the Sumerians are not studied by scholars to the same extent as the Babylonians.
- **D.** the Babylonian kingdom consisted of small city-states.

STOP. IF YOU FINISH BEFORE TIME IS CALLED, CHECK YOUR WORK. YOU MAY GO BACK TO ANY QUESTION IN THIS TEST BOOKLET.

STOP.

100

Biological Sciences
Time: 20 Minutes
Questions 267–82

With the nickname "flesh-eating bacteria," the culprit of a condition known as *necrotizing fasciitis* (NF) are hard to ignore. True to its name, this bacteria voraciously consumes skin and underlying fascia, leaving internal organs exposed and extremities gangrenous. Host death may ensue in as little as 12-24 hours. Survivors of *necrotizing fasciitis* are often left with multiple limb amputations and severe disfigurement. Given the devastating potential of this bacteria, it is stunning that the very same organism is part of normal pharyngeal flora.

The bacteria responsible for *necrotizing fasciitis* is *S. pyogenes*, a Gram positive Group A streptococcus (GAS). This same bacteria also plays a role in more common illnesses, such as strep. throat, community-acquired pneumonia and scarlet fever. While it is poorly understood why *S. pyogenes* causes only minor infection in some instances and life-threatening ones in others, the mechanism of extensive tissue death has been attributed to pyogenic exotoxins. Bacterial exotoxins interfere with cell oxygenation and digest surrounding tissue. In NF, the exotoxins also elicit an autoimmune response, expediting the necrotizing process.

The treatment of NF involves immediate and aggressive antibiotic therapy. In 1952, Dr. H. Eagle conducted an experiment comparing the efficacy of penicillin and clindamycin against GAS during various phases of its growth curve. The results of this study are now referred to as the Eagle effect. They remain clinically important in the treatment of both NF and less threatening GAS infections, such as cellulitis.

Lag Phase	5 hours
Log Phase	10 hours
Stationary Phase	15 hours
Death	N/A

Table 1 Average Amount of Time Spent in Each Growth Phase for *S. pyogenes*

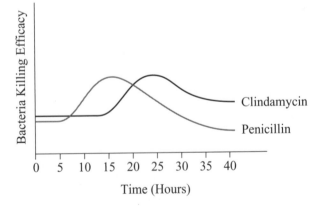

Figure 1 Efficacy of Microbial Killing: Penicillan v. Clindamycin

267. A patient is complaining of severe sore throat and fever. Culture of the throat grows *S. pyogene* in significant amounts. Microscopic examination of the culture would reveal:

    A.   Rod-shaped organisms
    B.   Round organisms organized in chains
    C.   Spiral-shaped organisms
    D.   Round organisms organized in clusters

268. According to the passage, the function of pyogenic exotoxin most resembles which of the following organelles?

    A.   the nucleus
    B.   the lysosome
    C.   the smooth endoplasmic reticulum
    D.   the golgi apparatus

269. A woman enters the hospital with severe skin cellulitis which began 24 hours prior. Her leg is swollen, red, tender to the touch, and she complains of fever. Based on the result of Eagle's study, what will you use to treat her?

    A.   Clindamycin, because this patient is likely in the log phase of her infection
    B.   Clindamycin, because this patient is likely in the stationary phase of her infection
    C.   Penicillin, because this patient is likely in the log phase of her infection
    D.   Penicillin, because this patient is likely in the stationary phase of her infection

270. Penicillin is an antibiotic that inhibits bacterial cell wall synthesis. While it is effective in killing many Gram (+) bacteria such as *S. pyogenes*, it does not affect host cell function. This is because:

    A.   Prokaryotic cells do not have cell membranes
    B.   Penicillin binds receptors found only in S. pyogenes
    C.   Eukaryotic cells do not have cell walls
    D.   Eukaryotic cells have cell membranes

271. According to the passage, *S. pyogenes* is associated with infections of the:

    A.   respiratory tract only
    B.   integumentary system only
    C.   both the respiratory and integumentary systems
    D.   neither respiratory nor integumentary systems

GO ON TO THE NEXT PAGE.

272. According to the Eagle effect, at which point on the bacterial growth curve would penicillin have the greatest efficacy?

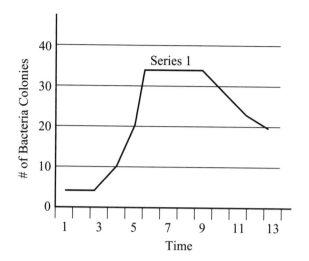

Figure 1 Bacterial Growth Curve

A. Part A
B. Part B
C. Part C
D. Part D

Although fungi are simple eukaryotes, they are more similar to complex animals than prokaryotes despite obvious chemical and structural differences. Multicellular fungi have cells that rapidly grow into filamentous structures called hyphae, which may be of different mating types. Hyphae form the structural units of the fungal body, known as a mycelium, which has a large surface-to-volume ratio adapted for nutrient absorption.

Fungal cells possess cell walls made of chitin, a linear homopolymer containing β-(1→4)-linked N-acetylglucosamine residues. Chitin fibers can be polyanionic, and interact with counterions to provide rigidity and stability to cells. Most fungal cell membranes often contain ergosterol, a sterol distinct from the cholesterol derivatives that comprise mammalian cell membranes.

Fungal infections in mammals are rare, and occur most frequently in immune-compromised states. The unique characteristics of fungi make treatment with antibacterial antibiotics ineffective. Although several antifungal therapies are now available, systemic use is accompanied by several adverse effects. The toxicity of many antifungal drugs limits their effectiveness and can include hepatotoxicity, nephrotoxicity and GI disturbance in some cases.

Fungal infection is not necessarily disadvantageous to the host, however. Fungal infection of certain plant roots forms structures known as mycorrhizae. These fungal structures increase the effective surface area of the root, thereby conferring resistance to drought and temperature extremes.

There are also many fungi that survive independent of other living organisms.

273. According to the passage, which would be a likely target for antifungal drugs?

A. Mycorrhizae
B. β-(1→4) glycosidic bonds between glucose residues in chitin
C. ergosterol in fungal cell membranes
D. 70S ribosomes.

274. Which of the following is a likely "counterion" used to provide rigidity to fungal chitin fibers?

A. Cl^-
B. PO_4^{3-}
C. N-acetylglucosamine.
D. Na^+

275. According to the passage, which of the following is not an accurate classification of fungi?

    A. autotrophic
    B. heterotrophic
    C. mutualistic
    D. parasitic

276. Which of the following is another example of a fungus involved in a mutualistic relationship?

    A. mushrooms growing from a compost pile
    B. lichen
    C. *rthrobotrys conoides* attacking a nematode
    D. bread mold

277. According to the passage, what is the likely benefit of mycorrhizae for plants?

    A. protection against parasites
    B. providing rigidity and stability to the roots.
    C. nutrient absorption.
    D. glycogen production.

278. Fungi primarily undergo asexual reproduction and occasionally undergo sexual reproduction. According to the passage, what structure is necessary for fungal reproduction, and what primary advantage does sexual reproduction confer on an organism that mainly reproduces asexually?

    A. hyphae; exchange of chromosomes by conjugation
    B. mycelium; genetic recombination
    C. hyphae; genetic recombination
    D. mycelium; excision repair.

279. The yeast *S. cerevisiae* can produce ethanol as a byproduct of anaerobic metabolism, in conditions of insufficient oxygen. Based upon this information, yeast may be best classified as:

    A. obligate anaerobes
    B. obligate aerobes
    C. facultative protista
    D. facultative anaerobes

280. Fungal cells are found in both the haploid and diploid states. However, some hyphae can adopt a different state known as the dikaryon, where the cell contains two genetically different nuclei. What is the most accurate genetic description of the dikaryotic state?

    A. *(n)*
    B. $(n + n_1)$
    C. $(2n)$
    D. (XY)

281. "The Gram stain is one of many assays used in the identification of bacteria. If *C. septicum,* a Gram (+) bacterium, is stained using the Gram stain, it would appear:

A. Red or pink, due to its thicker wall
B. Red or pink, due to its thinner wall
C. Blue, due to its thicker wall
D. Blue, due to its thinner wall

`282. Anaerobic infections are most likely to occur in all of the following locations EXCEPT:

I. Teeth and gums
II. Nail beds
III. Alveoli

A. I and II only
B. II only
C. III only
D. None of the above

STOP. IF YOU FINISH BEFORE TIME IS CALLED, CHECK YOUR WORK. YOU MAY GO BACK TO ANY QUESTION IN THIS TEST BOOKLET.

STOP.

106

EXAMINATION 07

Questions 283–329

Physical Sciences

Time: 20 Minutes
Questions 283–298

A tennis net is tightened through the use of a crank on one of the supporting poles. One end of the rope which suspends the net is wrapped around a cylindrical spindle with a radius of 2 cm. The spindle is connected to a handle with a length of 20 cm. A metal hook, which locks into a saw-toothed wheel, is used to prevent the net from slipping once it has been tightened. The locking wheel has a radius of 8 cm. The mechanism is shown in the diagram below.

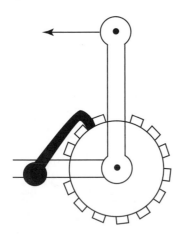

Figure 1 Tennis crank diagram

The crank mechanism operates as a machine, converting work done on the handle into work done on the net. For this machine, the ideal mechanical advantage is given by the ratio of the distance over which the force on the handle acts to the distance over which the force on the net acts. The actual mechanical advantage is given by the ratio of the force on the net (input force F_I) to the force on the handle (output force F_O). The efficiency of the machine is equal to the ratio of the actual mechanical advantage to the ideal mechanical advantage.

283. If the input force on the handle of the crank has a constant magnitude of 120 N, what is the approximate work done by the force during one complete revolution of the handle?

    A.   15 J
    B.   75 J
    C.   150 J
    D.   750 J

284. If a tennis player provides 60 N of input force,and the output force on the rope supporting the net is 480 N, what was the efficiency of the crank mechanism?

    A.   12.5%
    B.   50%
    C.   62.5%
    D.   80%

285. If the force required to maintain regulation net height is 800 N, what is the minimum force that must be exerted by the hook on the jagged wheel to hold the net's position assuming no force is exerted on the handle?

    A.   0 N
    B.   200 N
    C.   400 N
    D.   3200 N

286. Which of the following changes to the mechanism will increase the ideal mechanical advantage?

    A.   Increase the length of the handle and decrease the radius of the spindle.
    B.   Decrease the length of the handle and increase the length of the handle.
    C.   Increase the force on the handle and decrease the force on the rope.
    D.   Decrease the force on the handle and increase the force on the rope.

287. The force exerted by the rope can best be described as:

    A.   centripetal force.
    B.   centrifugal force.
    C.   friction.
    D.   tension.

288. After the court maintainence crew lubricates the crank mechanism, less force is required to tighten the net. This observation is supported by the fact that, when the mechanism is lubricated, the:

    A.   ideal mechanical advantage is decreased.
    B.   ideal mechanical advantage is increased.
    C.   efficiency is decreased.
    D.   efficiency is increased.

289. If the efficiency of the mechanism is 85%, which of the following statements is true?

    A.   The output force does more work than the input force.
    B.   The output force does less work than the input force.
    C.   The output force does the same work as the input force.
    D.   The output force does no work.

GO ON TO THE NEXT PAGE.

A chemistry student contructs a calorimeter from insulated cups and a thermometer, which she uses to determine enthalpy changes associated with various spontaneous acid-base reactions. She determines the heat capacity of the handmade calorimeter to be 15 J/°C. The specific heat of water, *c*, is equal to 4.18 J/g·°C.

The student combines various acids and bases the in calorimeter and then records the initial and final temperatures of the solutions. The details and results of her three trials are shown in Table 1 below.

Trial	Acid	Base	Initial Temp. (°C)	Final Temp. (°C)
1	50 ml of 2.0 M HCl	50 ml of 2.0 M NaOH	22	34
2	50 ml of 2.0 M HCl	50 ml of 2.0 M NH$_3$	22	32
3	50 ml of 2.0 M NH$_4$Cl	50 ml of 2.0 M NaOH	22	23

Table 1 Initial and Final Temperatures of Various Acid-Base Solutions.

290. Which of the following statements is true regarding all three of the student's trials?

A. The reactions are endothermic because energy is released into the surrounding water.
B. The reactions are endothermic because energy is absorbed from the surrounding water.
C. The reactions are exothermic because energy is released into the surrounding water.
D. The reactions are exothermic because energy is absorbed from the surrounding water.

291. Which of the following expressions represents the heat generated in trial 3?

A. $[(100)(4.18)(1) + (15)(1)]$ J
B. $[(50)(4.18)(1) + (15)(1)]$ J
C. $(100)(4.18)(1)$ J
D. $(50)(4.18)(1)$ J

292. The student measures the enthalpy change for trial 3 as −4.3 kJ/mol. If the actual enthalpy change for the reaction is known to be −5.0 kJ/mol, what is the percent error in the measured value?

A. 7%
B. 14%
C. 27%
D. 43%

293. Which of the following statements regarding the student's reaction of NH$_4$Cl with NaOH is true?

A. ΔH and ΔG are positive.
B. ΔH and ΔG are negative.
C. ΔH is positive and ΔG is negative.
D. ΔH is negative and ΔG is positive.

294. The student notices that her measured enthalpy values are consistently smaller than the textbook values. Which of the following is the most likely explanation for her observation?

A. Some of the energy released during a phase change is stored.
B. Physical agitation of the cup produces artificially high temperature readings.
C. The heat absorbed by the calorimeter was included in the measured values.
D. Some energy from the reaction was lost to the surroundings.

295. The reaction in trial 1 is depicted below. The reaction is best described as a:

$$HCl + NaOH \rightarrow NaCl + H_2O$$

A. Single displacement
B. Double displacement
C. Combustion
D. Combination

Questions 296 through 298 are **NOT** based on a descriptive passage.

296. A safety net protects trapeze artists by decreasing the force of their landing by:

   A.   decreasing the landing time.
   B.   increasing the landing time.
   C.   decreasing the impulse of the landing.
   D.   increasing the impulse of the landing.

297. Polonium-210 undergoing radioactive decay emits an alpha particle at speed v. What is the recoil speed of the remaining nuclide?

   A. $\dfrac{4v}{206}$

   B. $\dfrac{4v}{210}$

   C. $\dfrac{206v}{4}$

   D. $\dfrac{210v}{4}$

298. Which of the following is true of a chemical reaction that is spontaneous at low temperatures but becomes non-spontaneous as the temperature is increased?

   A. ΔH is negative and ΔS is positive.
   B. ΔH is positive and ΔS is negative.
   C. ΔH and ΔS are positive.
   D. ΔH and ΔS are negative.

STOP. IF YOU FINISH BEFORE TIME IS CALLED, CHECK YOUR WORK. YOU MAY GO BACK TO ANY QUESTION IN THIS TEST BOOKLET.

Verbal Reasoning

Time: 20 Minutes
Questions 299–313

Basic to the understanding of the monetary value of antiques is the fact that stated figures are purely arbitrary, and there is no such thing as a fixed price. The discussion of values is highly subjective. Social and emotional factors
5 often affect an object's worth and in some cases to a very great degree. Rarely will two experts look at a specimen and arrive at the exact same dollar value for it. Intrinsic value and monetary value are often inseparable to the collector. The highly subjective nature of the former ... pre-
10 cludes a discussion of it [here], and we shall confine ourselves purely to the latter.

According to *Webster's New World Dictionary* "value" is "...a fair or proper equivalent in money, commodities, etc., for something sold or exchanged; fair price.
15 The worth of a thing in money or goods at a certain time; market price. The equivalent (of something) in money. Estimated or appraised worth or price; valuation." The *Roget's International Thesaurus* allows interchangeable use of value with "...worth, rate, par value, valuation, estima-
20 tion, appraisement, money's worth, etc." Thus, it is obvious there are many interpretations as to what comprises value.

For the purpose of this particular work, it is important to be more specific in the use and definition of this key word. In order to do so, modification must be made to "fair
25 market value,' a more legalistic sounding term which has been strictly defined (by the Department of the U.S. Treasury in their publications concerning appraisals) as "...the price at which the property would change hands between a willing buyer and a willing seller, neither being
30 under any compulsion to buy or sell and both having reasonable knowledge of the relevant facts."

Since there are no rigid fixed rules or formulas in arriving at the price of an antique or collector's item, it may be said that the "fair market value" of such items is deter-
35 mined by considering all factors that reasonably bear on determining the price and which would be agreed upon between the willing buyer and the willing seller who were not under any pressure to act.

Having thus injected the word "price" into the discus-
40 sion, it may be logically assumed that a current value in U.S. dollars has been assigned to all antiques one might see in a store ... It may further be assumed that the dollar value shown for the respective antiques are those prices known to have been realized or accurately estimated to be realized as
45 "fair market value" when the piece changed hands between a willing buyer and a willing seller, neither of whom were under any pressure to act. In other words – based on the store owner's experience and very close acquaintance with the antique market and the highly regarded authorities in
50 the antique field, the prices reflected ... are those that each antique would bring at retail on the nationwide collectors'

market, as it now exists. However, the value is further determined by the factors: demand, rarity, and condition. With demand being of the greatest significance and condition the
55 least in order.

299. Suppose behavioral geneticists discover that many people who fall into deep credit card debt have a genetically predisposed condition, which compels them to purchase items that are on sale, or being auctioned, irrespective of their need for these items. The author of the passage would be most likely to respond to this information by:

   A. suggesting that a strictly defined 'fair market value' could still be negotiated by such persons.

   B. proposing that this situation would fall under the nature of intrinsic value.

   C. asserting that such factors are of little relevance to a discussion of value.

   D. explaining that most people probably feel some compulsion to buy to some degree or another.

300. According to the passage, when shopping for antiques, one should consider that:

   I. the price is always negotiable.
   II. the price will usually be consistent with its value.
   III. the price will usually be indicated in U.S. dollars.

   A. I only
   B. III only
   C. II and III only
   D. I, II, and III

GO ON TO THE NEXT PAGE

301. Suppose the author had inserted the following sentence at line 6: "This may be particularly true when an object has been passed down through a family for generations and is considered an heirloom by the current owner". This example would best support the author's discussion of:

A. neither the seller or the buyer being under any pressure to sell.

B. why some people might not be as willing to sell certain objects.

C. the difficulty of quantifying an object's intrinsic value.

D. the factors which will further determine the value of an object.

302. The ideas in the passage seem to derive primarily from:

A. evidence on the behavior of sellers and buyers.

B. knowledge of ongoing antique transactions.

C. speculation based on accepted theory.

D. facts observable in antique transactions.

303. At an estate sale, a relatively worthless item has been manipulated to look like a rare antique because the seller is desperate to recoup monetary losses in other areas. This situation best points out the author's emphasis that:

A. objects should be confirmed as genuine antiques.

B. situations where the seller is in desperate need of money should be avoided.

C. it is difficult to assign monetary value to an object.

D. a buyer be fully informed about the pertinent facts.

304. The author would most likely agree with which of the following statements?

A. It is unlikely that neither buyer nor seller would be compelled to actl.

B. A buyer should always begin negotiating well below the price she is willing to pay.

C. The thesaurus definition of "value" is too ambiguous to be useful.

D. One can usually count on the accuracy of an antique's the marked price.

305. What is the most serious apparent *weakness* of the Department of the U.S. Treasury's concept of "fair market value" as described?

A. The concept is based upon an unlikely set of assumptions.

B. "Legalistic sounding" does not mean that it would be legally binding.

C. As outlined, the concept is less rigorous than the Webster's definition.

D. A "fair market" does not really exist.

306. Elsewhere, the author of the passage states, "An item is only worth what someone is willing to pay for it". This statement most directly supports the passage assertion that:

A. There is no such thing as a fixed price.

B. The ultimate factor determining value is demand.

C. An item's actual price may fluctuate dramatically from day to day.

D. The price of an object should be determined before itt is put up for sale.

GO ON TO THE NEXT PAGE.

With all the gusto and curiosity that characterized raku and salt glazing more than 20 years ago, many potters and sculptors have turned to wood firing as their process of choice. Peripatetic questing, more than any other character-
5 istic or quality, seems to compel the creators and to inhabit the work itself.

Ubiquitous and eclectic, wood firing in North America has gained popularity because its enthusiasts have decided that their work demands the effects of the process. The
10 genre has had virtually no critical support. If anything, contemporary authors have ignored wood-fired ceramics; one in particular Garth Clark, in commentary on Peter Voulkos' anagama-fired work, has written: "In 1979, Voulkos began to fire the plates in a Japanese-style, wood-
15 fired anagama and produced a few masterpieces, but these pieces were generally retrogressive in their aesthetic, too dependent on the generosity of the kiln, and too imitative of Bizen, Seto and other traditional Japanese kilns." Clark's book, *American Ceramics*, contains 240 illustrations, only
20 one of which is of a wood-fired object. Elaine Levin's *History of American Ceramics* contains 352 illustrations, two of which depict pots identified as having been wood fired. No other genre of claywork is so consistently ignored.

Despite the lack of critical savvy by contemporary
25 ceramic historians, the movement has proceeded on level terrain, with neither a verbal headwind nor a boost from comprehending and appreciative writers who might have advanced the climate of acceptance for this type of work by the public at large. The result is that those ceramists who
30 fire with wood are themselves the most reliable and articulate speakers for the movement, at present. As always, the work itself is the best statement about why wood firing continues to grow in popularity among its practitioners and connoisseurs.

35 Paul Chaleff often solicits the high-risk areas of his anagama-type [wood firing] kiln for effects impossible to achieve by other means. Exposure to violent heat in or near the firebox subjects clay to great stress; objects made with this firing space in mind must be from a clay whose refrac-
40 tory qualities will be appropriate for such a tumultuous zone, yet sensitive enough to capture the fire's visual/tactile statement. Even then, a very small percentage will survive and, among those, fewer still will measure up, aesthetically. (So much for the "generosity" of the kiln.)

45 Chaleff's work often embodies values that confront established norms in our culture, that test the elasticity of our perspective. For example, must "beautiful roughness" always be an oxymoron when it comes to judging ceram-ics? Must the artist display white-knuckle control over
50 every square centimeter of an object for it to be considered a success? (Is anything else simply luck?) Will anyone dare

to admit that an artist's handling of materials can reveal the materials themselves to contain tactile and visual expres-siveness? Has status-hunger made ceramics a medium to be
55 done increasingly from the neck up rather than from the heart out?

Trust, rather than fear, characterizes the wood firer's approach to the unpredictable, for, in the words of Louis Pasteur, "chance favors only the prepared mind." The very
60 fire that can ruin our best work can also bless it beyond our best intentions. Whether we choose wood firing for purely practical or for more esoteric reasons, the wish to partici-pate in an ancient dialogue with materials characterizes much of what wood firing is about. The ghostly counter-
65 parts to these pieces lie in shard piles across the country. It is humbling to note that they could well fill a gallery from floor to ceiling as a perverse endorsement of electric kilns and their *heated* but *unfired* wares.

307. The author's comparison of wood-firing and other types of firing indicates that:

A. wood firing is the method which the author uses.
B. without wood firing, electric firing would not be possible.
C. the author has great respect for wood firing.
D. the results of wood firing are more predictable.

116

308. The author cites Garth Clark's description of the "generosity of the kiln" (line 17, and lines 42-44) to make the point that:

A. electric kilns provide a much more forgiving method of firing.

B. without different methods, most ceramics would look very similar.

C. wood kilns are relatively easy to learn to use.

D. the firing of a wood kiln can be unpredictably destructive.

309. The author is primarily concerned with demonstrating that wood firing:

A. has come a long way, in the last 20 years, towards acceptance in the ceramics community.

B. is a capricious practice requiring patience, knowledge, and strong determination.

C. is tremendously unpredictable.

D. is flourishing for good reason, despite being consistently disregarded by ceramic critics.

310. The author's characterization of wood firing and how the practitioners of this craft have been perceived suggests that the retort/comment about "electric kilns and their *heated* but *unfired* wares" (line 68) was meant to:

A. explain why a clay sculpture might break more easily in a wood kiln.

B. make clear the differences between electric and wood kiln firing.

C. convey scorn for the more controlled conditions of electric kilns.

D. communicate the pride one feels after the successful firing of a wood kiln.

311. The contention that "chance favors only the prepared mind" (line 59) can most justifiably be interpreted as support for the idea that:

A. without suitable understanding, fortune is against you.

B. if you prepare yourself well, the odds will always be in your favor.

C. without some degree of luck, you have only your intellect.

D. 'accidents' can actually assist you if you are ready for them.

312. Given the claims made in the passage, the idea that, "Despite the lack of critical savvy by contemporary ceramic historians, the movement has proceeded on level terrain, with neither a verbal headwind nor a boost from comprehending and appreciative writers who might have advanced the climate of acceptance for this type of work by the public at large" (lines 24-29), suggests:

A. The critics should realize that wood firing is fast gaining in popularity and support, rather than hinder it.

B. The popularity of wood firing has been steadily advancing despite its lack of critical acclaim.

C. Facing dismissive ignorance in the media, wood firing has nevertheless managed to gain in popularity among ceramicists.

D. Wood firing has been exploding in popularity among ceramicists with virtually no help from critics.

313. In organizing a group of ceramicists to try wood firing for the first time, the author would most likely advise them to approach wood firing with:

A. love, because fire can have such a beautiful effects on all of their wares.

B. an open-mind, because they might not initially like what little comes out of the kiln.

C. caution, because most pieces will be destroyed and many will look substandard.

D. patience, because it requires experience and an expanded perspective to obtain good results.

STOP. IF YOU FINISH BEFORE TIME IS CALLED, CHECK YOUR WORK. YOU MAY GO BACK TO ANY QUESTION IN THIS TEST BOOKLET.

STOP.

Biological Sciences
Time: 20 Minutes
Questions 314–329

Passage V (Questions 314-319)

As organisms from plants to protozoa to humans are eukaryotes, the term eukaryotic applies to an appreciably large variety of cell types. Despite the impressive range of eukaryotic cells, many cellular processes are conserved among different organisms. One such process is protein synthesis.

Generally, protein synthesis involves mRNA transcription and subsequent translation on a ribosome. The translated protein is then sent to the endoplasmic reticulum and Golgi apparatus for further modification, before reaching its final destination, be it the nucleus, lysosome, or extracellular matrix.

Our understanding of the details of these processes and their regulation is far from complete. One method of studying cellular processes is by removing or "knocking out" certain genes from a cell's genome. By analyzing cellular function before and after removal of the gene, the specific activity of the corresponding cellular protein can be explored.

Researchers in a genetic laboratory perform a "knock out" study in which gene A is known to encode a protein, and Genes B and C are somehow involved in posttranslational processing. The researchers selectively remove Genes B and C in 3 sets of mice; each set or group is comprised of 3 mice. Group 1 is missing Gene B, Group 2 is missing Gene C, and Group 3 is missing both. The researchers assess protein activity in the "knock out" mice and make comparisons to a control group. Their results are present in Table 1.

Group	Mouse 1	Mouse 2	Mouse 3
Normal	100	100	100
1	55	50	45
2	25	30	30
3	5	10	5

Table 1 Percent activity of protein after knock-out out of 100 % normal activity

314. According to Table 1, which of the following best describes the function of the protein expressed by Gene B?

   A. Glycosylates the corresponding protein of Gene A in the ER
   B. Tags Gene A's protein for its final destination in the extracellular matrix
   C. Inhibits further Gene A transcription via negative feedback as a transcription factor
   D. Cleaves and activates Gene A's protein

315. The mitochondria in eukaryotic cells is an extremely valuable organelle, in that it allows for complete oxidation of fuels. There is a growing belief that mitochondria originate from prokaryotes which survived symbiotically in eukaryotic cells. Which of the following observations regarding mitochondria is LEAST likely to support this theory?

   A. Mitochondria contain their own circular DNA
   B. Mitochondria house their own ribosomes
   C. Mitochondria may reproduce independent of cellular reproduction
   D. Mitochondria have a separate nucleus

316. According to the researchers data, which modulatory gene has a greater effect on protein function.

   A. Gene B because Group 1 shows an average decrease of 50% protein activity
   B. Gene C because Group 2 shows an average decrease of 72% protein activity
   C. Gene B because Group 2 shows an average decrease of 28% protein activity
   D. Gene C because Group 1 shows an average decrease of 50% protein activity

317. Which of the following statements best explains the magnitude of the decrease in percent protein activity observed when both genes B and C are "knocked out"?

   A. Gene C's protein adds a posttranslational component which is necessary for protein function.
   B. Gene B's protein adds a posttranslational component which is necessary for protein function.
   C. Modification by Gene B and C proteins has a synergistic effect on protein function.
   D. Modification by Gene B and C proteins has a cumulative effect on protein function.

318. A new pesticide is being developed which is effective against both eukaryotic and prokaryotic parasites. What organelle might this drug target in order to affect both?

   A. Nucleus
   B. Golgi apparatus
   C. Ribosome
   D. Endoplasmic reticulum

319. Which of the following organelles is NOT common to both plant and animal cells?

   A. Centrioles
   B. Mitochondria
   C. Vacuoles
   D. Lysosomes

GO ON TO THE NEXT PAGE.

The body's involuntary motor functions are mediated by two classes of receptors: cholinergic and adrenergic. Members of either class may be activated either pre- or post-synaptically.

Cholinergic receptors respond to acetylcholine. This neurotransmitter is degraded by the enzyme acetylcholinesterase. Cholinergic receptors can be of the nicotinic or muscarinic variety. The nicotinic receptor, which selectively binds the plant alkaloid nicotine, is also a sodium and potassium ion channel. Nicotinic receptors are found not only at the neuromuscular junction, but also within sympathetic and parasympathetic ganglia. As indicated by its name, the muscarinic receptor selectively binds the plant alkaloid muscarine. This receptor is instead coupled to G proteins and is only found at the effector cells of the parasympathetic nervous system. A few Muscarinic receptor-mediated responses are presented in Table 1.

Location	Action
iris	constriction
ciliary muscle	accommodation, opening of the canal of Schlemm
exocrine glands	increased secretion
bronchi	constriction
gastrointestinal tract	increased peristalsis and relaxation of the internal sphincter
heart	decrease heart rate and contractility

Table 1 Muscarinic Receptor Mediated Responses in effector organs

Adrenergic receptors have varying sensitivities to both norepinephrine and epinephrine. Norepinephrine is removed from the synapse by reuptake or is metabolized by monoamine oxidase and catechol-O-methyltransferase. Adrenergic receptors are even more varied than cholinergic. While α_2 receptors are generally presynaptic, α_1, β_1 and β_2 receptors are found on the effector cells of the sympathetic nervous system. Some common adrenergic receptor-mediated responses are shown in Table 2.

Location	Receptor type	Action
iris	α_1	dilation
exocrine glands	α_1	decreased secretion
bronchi	β_2	dilation
gastrointestinal tract	α_1,β_2	decreased motility and tone
heart	β_1, β_2	increased heart rate and contractility

Table 2 Adrenergic Receptor Mediated Responses in Effector Organs.

320. A woman witnesses an accident in which two cars collide into a child on a bicycle. The woman sprints over to the scene and pushes the two cars apart with her bare hands, freeing the child. The seemingly superhuman strength the woman displayed was the result of a massive release of a chemical from the adrenal glands. That same chemical may be released as a neurotransmitter from which of the following sites?

    A.   postganglionic sympathetic neurons
    B.   preganglionic sympathetic neurons
    C.   presynaptic parasympathetic neurons
    D.   postsynaptic parasympathetic neurons

321. The modern use of botulinum toxin is almost exclusively cosmetic. It is injected into muscles, paralyzing them in order decrease the appearance of wrinkles. The bacterial toxin functions by inhibiting acetylcholine release from storage vessels in the presynaptic neuron. If an individual were given a systemic overdose of botulinum toxin, which of the following side effects is most likely to occur?

    A.   shortness of breath and increased sweating
    B.   a decrease in blood pressure
    C.   pupil dilation and a deficit in close-range vision
    D.   a continuous urge to defecate

322. Which subdivision of the nervous system is delineated in the passage?

    A.   central nervous system
    B.   sensory nervous system
    C.   voluntary nervous system
    D.   autonomic nervous system

323. A cholinomimetic agent is structurally similar enough to acetylcholine that it may activate cholinergic receptors. Which of the following effects would NOT be expected following the administration of a cholinomimetic agent?

A. excitation of smooth muscle in the gastrointestinal tract

B. inhibition of conduction at the AV node

C. inhibition of skeletal muscle

D. excitation of secretions in the parotid gland

324. Many postsynaptic receptors affect changes in the intracellular environs via a secondary-messenger system. Which of the following receptors utilizes such means of affecting cellular change?

A. nicotinic receptors

B. muscarinic receptors

C. both

D. neither

325. In both the central and peripheral nervous system, neurons have a rich support network to enhance function and nutrition. Postganglionic neurons are enveloped by which of the following glial cells?

A. oligodendrocytes

B. Schwann cells

C. gray matter

D. ependymal cells

326. Monoamine Oxidases have been instrumental in the treatment of many psychiatric illnesses. They function by inhibiting the removal of which of the following neurotransmitters from the synaptic cleft?

A. adrenaline

B. noradrenaline

C. acetylcholine

D. norcholine

327. In the hydrolysis of acetylcholine, catalyzed by Cholinesterases, acetylcholine is used to acetylate a serine hydroxyl group at the enzyme active site, while choline becomes the leaving group. Activating Muscarinic receptors at the sinoatrial node will lead to the opening of potassium channels. If a cholinesterase inhibitor is present at this site, which of the following best describes the effect on heart rate?

A. increasing the rate of depolarization and increasing heart rate

B. slowing the rate of depolarization and increasing heart rate

C. slowing the rate of depolarization and slowing heart rate

D. the opening of a potassium channel will have no effect on heart rate

GO ON TO THE NEXT PAGE.

328. Microtubules perform multifarious functions within the cell. A drug which destroys microtubules is LEAST likely to affect which of the following cellular processes?

- A. Mitosis
- B. Movement of the cell
- C. Exocytosis
- D. Cellular Respiration

329. Some eukaryotes, such as plants, have a cell wall surrounding the cell membrane. What functionality might this cellular structure provide?

- A. Aid in photosynthesis
- B. Prevention of cell lysis
- C. Cellular infrastructure
- D. Telekinesis during mitosis

STOP. IF YOU FINISH BEFORE TIME IS CALLED, CHECK YOUR WORK. YOU MAY GO BACK TO ANY QUESTION IN THIS TEST BOOKLET.

STOP.

124

EXAMINATION 08

Questions 330–376

Physical Sciences
Time: 20 Minutes
Questions 330–345

The table below lists the isotopes of neon, along with the half-lives and modes of decay of the unstable isotopes. Radioactive decay occurs when an atom has an unstable ratio of protons to neutrons in its nucleus. This ratio is adjusted through the emission of a beta particle (β^-) or positron (β^+), or through electron capture. Alternatively, an alpha particle may be released to reduce the size of an nucleus whose number of nucleons makes it unstable. Many decay processes are accompanied by gamma radiation as well.

Isotope	Half-life	Mode of decay
Neon-17	0.10 sec	β^+
Neon-18	1.5 sec	β^+
Neon-19	17.5 sec	β^+
Neon-20		
Neon-21		
Neon-22		
Neon-23	37.6 sec	β^-
Neon-24	3.4 min	β^-

330. The most common isotope of neon is:

   A. Neon-19
   B. Neon-20
   C. Neon-21
   D. Neon-22

331. Neon-24 decays through the process shown below. What is the identity of isotope X?

$$^{24}_{10}\text{Ne} \rightarrow X + \beta^- + \beta^-$$

   A. Neon-26
   B. Neon-22
   C. Oxygen-24
   D. Magnesium-24

332. A sample of neon-19 is allowed to decay spontaneously. How much time does it take for at least 75% of the original sample to disappear?

   A. 17.5 sec
   B. 35 sec
   C. 52.5 sec
   D. 70 sec

333. The presence of fluorine is detected in a sample that originally contained pure neon. Which of the following decay processes could have taken place?

   I. Electron capture
   II. Beta decay
   III. Positron emission

   A. I only
   B. II only
   C. I and II only
   D. I and III only

334. The ratio of protons to neutrons in an atom of neon-20 is:

   A. 3 : 1
   B. 2 : 1
   C. 1 : 1
   D. 1 : 2

335. The most likely reason that neon-23 undergoes radioactive decay is that its:

   A. ratio of neutrons to protons is too large.
   B. ratio of neutrons to protons is too small.
   C. nucleus contains too many nucleons.
   D. nucleus contains too few nucleons.

336. Neon-20 results from the decay process shown below. What is the identity of the original isotope, X?

$$X = ^{20}_{10}\text{Ne} + \beta^+$$

   A. Sodium-20
   B. Fluorine-20
   C. Neon-21
   D. Neon-19

GO ON TO THE NEXT PAGE.

Under normal circumstances, a hydrocarbon will react with oxygen to form water and carbon dioxide. Many hydrocarbon combustion reactions are useful because they release a great deal of energy. For instance, methane (CH_4), propane (C_3H_8), and butane (C_4H_{10}) fuel stoves and lighters, while acetylene (C_2H_2) is used in industrial torches. The balanced equation for the combustion of a hydrocarbon may be derived from the formula below.

$$C_xH_y + \frac{2x+y}{2} O_2 \rightarrow xCO_2 + \frac{y}{2} H_2O$$

The follwing table lists various thermodynamic properties of some constituents of hydrocarbon combustion reactions.

Compound	ΔG°_f (kJ/mol)	ΔH°_f (kJ/mol)	S°_f (J/mol-K)
$CH_4(g)$	−74.8	−50.8	186.3
$C_2H_2(g)$	226.7	209.2	200.8
$C_2H_4(g)$	52.3	68.1	219.4
$C_2H_6(g)$	−84.7	−32.9	229.5
$C_3H_8(g)$	−103.9	−23.5	269.9
$C_6H_6(g)$	82.9	129.7	269.2
$CO_2(g)$	−393.5	−394.4	213.6
$H_2O(g)$	−241.8	−228.6	188.7

Table 1 Thermodynamic properties.

337. Which of the following is the balanced chemical equation the combustion of ethane?

A. $C_2H_6 + O_2 \rightarrow CO_2 + H_2O$
B. $C_3H_6 + 7 O_2 \rightarrow 3 CO_2 + 3 H_2O$
C. $C_2H_6 + O_2 \rightarrow 2 CO_2 + 3 H_2O$
D. $C_2H_6 + 5 O_2 \rightarrow 2 CO_2 + 3 H_2O$

338. Which of the following is most likely the value of S°_f for $H_2O(l)$?

A. 0 kJ/mol-K
B. 70.0 kJ/mol-K
C. 188.7 kJ/mol-K
D. 240 kJ/mol-K

339. In an industrial torch, Acetyline undergoes combustion according to the balanced equation shown below.

$$C_2H_2(g) + \frac{5}{2} O_2(g) \rightarrow 2 CO_2(g) + H_2O(g)$$

What is the heat of combustion for acetyline?

A. −408.6 kJ/mol
B. −854.4 kJ/mol
C. −862.0 kJ/mol
D. −1307.7 kJ/mol

340. Which of the compounds listed in Table I contains a triple bond?

A. C_2H_2
B. C_2H_6
C. C_3H_8
D. C_6H_6

341. Which of the following is true of the chemical reaction shown below, under standard conditions?

$$2 C(s) + 2 H_2(g) \rightarrow C_2H_4(g)$$

A. The reaction is exothermic and spontaneous.
B. The reaction is exothermic and non-spontaneous.
C. The reaction is endothermic and spontaneous.
D. The reaction is endothermic and non-spontaneous.

342. The balanced equation for the combustion of methane gas is shown below.

$$CH_4(g) + 2 O_2(g) \rightarrow CO_2(g) + 2 H_2O(g)$$

How many liters of oxygen gas are required for the complete combustion of 8 grams of methane gas at standard temperature and pressure?

A. 11.2 liters
B. 22.4 liters
C. 33.6 liters
D. 44.8 liters

Questions 343 through 345 are **NOT** based on a descriptive passage.

343. When a loaded pistol is fired, the person firing the gun will experience a recoil sensation in the direction opposite the bullet's motion. A pistol with a mass of 1.25 kg fires a bullet with a mass of 20 grams at a speed of 250 m/s. What is the initial speed of the pistol's recoil?

A.   1 m/s
B.   2 m/s
C.   3 m/s
D.   4 m/s

344. A carpenter attempts to loosen a bolt unsuccessfully. He decides to make a second attempt with a different wrench. To successfully loosen the bolt, the carpenter should choose a wrench with a handle that is:

A.   lighter
B.   heavier
C.   shorter
D.   longer

345. Which of the sections in the diagram below represents the enthalpy change of a reaction?

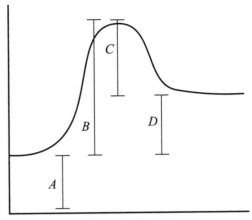

Reaction Progress

A.   *A*
B.   *B*
C.   *C*
D.   *D*

STOP. IF YOU FINISH BEFORE TIME IS CALLED, CHECK YOUR WORK. YOU MAY GO BACK TO ANY QUESTION IN THIS TEST BOOKLET.

STOP.

Verbal Reasoning

Time: 20 Minutes
Questions 346–360

Passage III (Questions 346-352)

Uri Geller could read minds, drive a car blindfolded, bend a metal fork without even touching it, and tell which of 10 canisters concealed an object from his view. Or could he? Demonstrating the psychic powers that he says he
5   possessed, the 27-year-old Israeli was so convincing that the much-respected Stanford Research Institute in Menlo Park, California, began a serious investigation of his claims. Yet magicians claimed they could duplicate or explain every one of his feats, and a Stanford spokesman at the time
10 asserted, "We've never ruled out the possibility of fraud."

Indeed, the whole history of extrasensory phenomena is tainted with deception—either deliberate trickery or the wishful thinking that makes honest experimenters see what is not there. The prevalence of such error is one reason that
15 ESP has yet to achieve general acceptance as a group of natural events like those in the traditional sciences. Underscoring the skepticism accorded psychic demonstrations that seem to contradict known physical laws, contemporary scientists like to quote 18th Century author
20 Tom Paine: "Is it more probable that nature should go out of her course, or that a man should tell a lie?"

Perhaps the classic case of fraud is provided by the Fox sisters of Hydesville, New York. In 1849 Margaret Fox, then only 10, and her sister Kate, 8, became the center of a
25 cult when their mother concluded that strange raps heard only in her youngsters' presence were spirit messages. The sisters attracted thousands of followers, among them the eminent physicist and chemist Sir William Crookes. In the 1870s Crookes wrote that he had tested the sounds made by
30 Kate and was convinced that they "were true, objective occurrences." A dozen years later, Margaret confessed that these "true occurrences" were all a "horrible deception." The sisters, she said, had made their raps by cracking their joints.

35 The Fox case is by no means the only one in which scholars were taken. In 19th Century England, the Society for Psychical Research, and its philosopher-president, Henry Sidgwick, maintained for a quarter of a century that the feats of two young men proved the reality of ESP. In
40 1882, one of the youths, Douglas Blackburn, described the "telepathic" gifts of the other, G.A. Smith: "Not only can he read numbers, words, and even whole sentences, which I alone have seen, but he rarely fails to experience the taste of any liquid or solid I choose to imagine." By 1911
45 Blackburn was writing in a different vein: "I now declare that the whole of those alleged experiments were bogus, and originated in the honest desire of two youths to show how easily men of scientific mind and training could be deceived when seeking for evidence in support of a theory
50 they were wishful to establish."

Wishful thinking misleads even the hardest-nosed experimenters in every field. Perceval Lowell, a talented astronomer, went to his grave insisting that linear markings he saw on Mars were canals dug by intelligent beings. How
55 easily such a will to believe exerts an unconscious influence on psychic research was demonstrated by Richard S. Kaufman at Yale in 1995. He set up a psychokinetic experiment in which subjects rolled dice and tried to "will" a particular result; they then took notes on how often they
60 succeeded. Using a hidden camera to film the proceedings, Kaufman found that those who believed in psychic phenomena saw far more successes than actually occurred.

The history of distortion and deceit in psychic studies once led an investigator to quip that ESP might well stand
65 for "error some place." Such jokes will proliferate until investigators succeed in doing what researchers in other fields accept as the *sine qua non* of science: experiments that lead to identical results, time after time, when repeated by different scholars in different laboratories. No one has
70 done that yet with ESP.

346. If the public reception of Einstein's theory of relativity repeated the reception that the author claims was given to the Fox sister's "occurrences", most people would:

A. accept the theory readily and quickly revise their theories about natural laws.

B. resist the theory initially but gradually modify their view of the universe.

C. claim to believe the theory but ignore its profound implications.

D. reject its version of reality as contrary to common sense.

347. On the basis of the passage, it is reasonable to conclude that:

A. Sir William Crookes was in collusion with the Fox sisters.

B. without help, the Fox sisters could not have carried out their deception.

C. the Fox sisters deception was not revealed until they were quite old.

D. Margaret and Kate deceived their mother.

348. Regarding the history of extrasensory phenomena, the passage strongly implies that:

A. there has never been a legitimate occurrence of the phenomena.

B. only a very rigorous academic institution could prove or refute claims of the phenomena.

C. several cases have proven to be highly unusual in their claims.

D. claims and occurrences of this nature will always be prevalent.

349. The passage indicates that its author would NOT agree with which of the following statements?

A. William Crookes wrote that he had actually tested the Fox sisters.

B. Stanford Research Institute is located in Menlo Park.

C. Uri Geller was an Israeli with an unusual claim to fame.

D. Henry Sidgwick apparently believed the claims of the young twins.

350. Assume that magicians were able to repeat Uri Geller's feats time after time with identical results to Geller's, and that these feats were performed in different laboratories. What is the relevance of this assumption to the author's views about the *sine qua non* of science?

A. It strengthens them by demonstrating that there are really only a few areas where ESP can be tested.

B. It is consistent with them in proving the feats are actually only illusions.

C. It weakens them by showing that ESP can still trick science and scientists.

D. It weakens them by supporting Geller's feats as provable psychic phenomena.

351. An important comparison is made in the passage between:

A. psychic studies and scientific studies of physics.

B. science of the 19th and 20th century.

C. Stanford Research Institute and the Society for Psychical Research.

D. deliberate trickery and wishful thinking.

352. Suppose the immediate relatives and family members of those who have died are much more likely to "sense" the presence of the deceased during a psychic séance than others who are present. Does this discovery support the author's argument?

A. Yes; it confirms the author's argument.

B. No; it does not affect the author's argument.

C. No; it weakens the author's argument.

D. No; it disproves the author's argument.

The painting requires long moments to take in. It is a furious chaotic flurry of activity that evokes sensations of sound, emotion, and smell: screams of agony, anger, joy and exultation: the continuous popping of rifles, war
5 whoops, hoarsely shouted orders, and thundering of war ponies: emotions of fear, resignation, excitement, and horror: the dense odor of hot prairie grass, dry winds, sweat from ponies and men, spent gunpowder, and blood. For an instant time stands still as the eye is drawn to the omnipo-
10 tent buckskin-clad figure at the center of the painting. Amidst his dying and fighting troopers, he stands defiantly with hand on hip and smoking revolver at the ready, surveying and evaluating his deteriorating situation as the storm of battle swirls around him. From the perspective of
15 historical revisionism, it would be easy to assume that he knows his end is near and is resigned to it. But that assumption would be false.

George Armstrong Custer has now become a name associated with notoriety; questionable cowardice, certain ig-
20 norant pride, poor decision-making, and finally ignominious defeat. But the true nature of the man is more complex.

Custer graduated from West Point near the bottom of his class, and his fame, and the respect that he held with his fellow army officers began only later during the Civil War.
25 As a cavalry officer, he repeatedly distinguished himself by his commanding presence, courage in battle, and tactical abilities. He once fought the legendary Confederate cavalryman, Jeb Stuart, to a standstill. And, lest it be believed that Custer's Civil War accomplishments were aberrations,
30 it must be remembered that courage ran in the Custer's blood; Tom Custer, George Armstrong's brother, won the Congressional Medal of Honor during the Civil War before following him into the Little BigHorn.

On that day, it was Custer's impetuous side that came
35 to the fore and caused him to ignore his Crow scout's warnings regarding the size of the Indian force he was facing. Custer was concerned that, as so many times before, the Indians might escape and he would be unable to bring his forces to bear upon them .... And certainly, there had never
40 been before, and never would be again, such a tremendous gathering of Indians. Thousands of them had come from all across the plains in response to Sitting Bull's entreaties and prophecies, and the encampment was so large that there were few if any sentries since the Sioux believed a camp of
45 this size impervious to attack.

Unknowingly, it was against this indomitable force that Custer split his forces, and then split them again, in order to ensure that no Indians would escape. The small force of cavalrymen led by Custer was the last to strike the
50 huge Indian camp, but they were quickly repulsed as the enraged Sioux turned to meet them. The skirmishers dis-

mounted at the base of a long sloping hill as they attempted to maintain a semblance of discipline against the ever-increasing number of warriors coming at them. But they were
55 quickly pushed back up towards the brow of the hill and broken into smaller and smaller groups as the war ponies swirled and surged around them, until at the last, they stood no more.

For those who cling to the thought that Custer was a
60 coward, they would do well to hearken to what the Indians themselves knew of the man. As the historian Stephen Ambrose noted, the great chief Sitting Bull received a report from some of his Sioux warriors immediately following the engagement and related the story to a New York
65 *Herald* reporter one year later:

Sitting Bull: Up there where the last fight took place, where the last stand was made, the Long Hair stood like a sheaf of corn with all the ears fallen around him.
Reporter: Not wounded?
70 Sitting Bull: No.
Reporter: How many stood by him?
Sitting Bull: A few.
Reporter: When did he fall?
Sitting Bull: He killed a man when he fell. He
75 laughed.
Reporter: You mean he cried out.
Sitting Bull: No, he laughed. He had fired his last shot.

353. Suppose the author had inserted the following sentence at line 21: "Though the terrible and notorious massacre of the Cheyenne chief Black Kettle and his peaceful contingent on the banks of the Washita rightfully supports some of these accusations, it is anecdotal and not necessarily indicative of the man." This example would best illuminate the author's discussion of:

A. Custer's tactical Indian-fighting capabilities.
B. false assumptions about Custer.
C. Custer's poor decision-making.
D. why Custer was misunderstood.

354. The assertion that Custer ignored his Crow scout's warnings about the size of the Indian force is NOT clearly consistent with the information about:

A. Custer's lacking awareness of the situation as he split his forces.
B. the size of Indian encampments in future years.
C. Custer's courage in battle.
D. why Custer was so intent on destroying the Indians.

355. The author most likely believes that modern historians:

A. have an agenda.
B. know little about what actually happened at the Little Bighorn.
C. treat the subject of Custer unfairly.
D. focus solely on Custer's accomplishments.

356. Which of the following findings would most *compromise* the author's conclusions about George Armstrong Custer?

A. Custer believed that the Indians could never defeat him.
B. Jeb Stuart's forces had been surprised by Custer.
C. The moment 'captured' in the painting occurs just before Custer is killed.
D. Custer was shot in the back attempting to run away from the battle.

357. Which of the following conclusions is best supported by the passage?

A. George Custer was a supreme military tactician.
B. George Custer's achievements were legendary.
C. George Custer simply did not have enough information about the size of the Sioux gathering.
D. George Custer was not a coward.

358. The author probably mentions that there had never been before or ever would be again, such a large gathering of Indians (lines 41-43) in order to:

A. demonstrate the weakness of the information that Custer was getting from his scouts.
B. provide an example of the types of gatherings the Indians arranged in later years.
C. illustrate the persistence of the myths about Custer.
D. support the idea that Custer was not a foolhardy commander.

359. According to the Passage, which of the following statements must be true?

A. Custer's forces could not have defeated the Sioux on that day.
B. Tom Custer also graduated from West Point.
C. George Custer's Civil War victories were not aberrations.
D. Sitting Bull saw Custer being killed.

360. According to the author, why did Custer repeatedly split his soldiers into smaller groups before attacking the Indian encampment?

A. To ensure that the Indians were completely surrounded
B. To enable them to capture Sitting Bull
C. To reduce the chances that the Indians could escape from his soldiers
D. To follow the advice of his scouts

STOP. IF YOU FINISH BEFORE TIME IS CALLED, CHECK YOUR WORK. YOU MAY GO BACK TO ANY QUESTION IN THIS TEST BOOKLET.

136

Biological Sciences
Time: 20 Minutes
Questions 361–376

Passage V (Questions 361-367)

Alcoholic fermentation, the conversion of sugar to alcohol by yeast, has been utilized for thousands of years in the making of alcoholic beverages and leavened bread. Ancient Egyptian tombs indicate evidence of beer and leavened bread as early as 3000 B.C. True to its extensive history in many cultures, the fermentation process has been thoroughly investigated by scientists all over the world. The word '*gas*' was first used to describe the bubbles released by yeast in the fermentation process by van Helmont in 1610. Approximately 300 years later, Scientist Eduard Buchner received the Nobel prize for his work on yeast and the isolation of the 'cell-free mixture' that catalyzes the conversion of sugar to ethanol.

The conversion of glucose to ethanol by Baker's yeast (the Emden-Meyerhoff-Parnas scheme) is shown below.

Enzyme catalyzing the conversion of compound 1 to compound 11 can operate under aerobic or anaerobic conditions; the conversion of compound 11 to compound 13 operates only under anaerobic conditions. Dihydroxyacetone phosphate (5) is converted to glyceraldehyde- 3-phosphate (6) by triosphophate isomerase providing a second mole of glyceraldehydes-3-phosphate for conversion to 1,3-diphophoglyceric acid (7). The entire fermentation process produces 31kcal of heat per mole of glucose consumed.

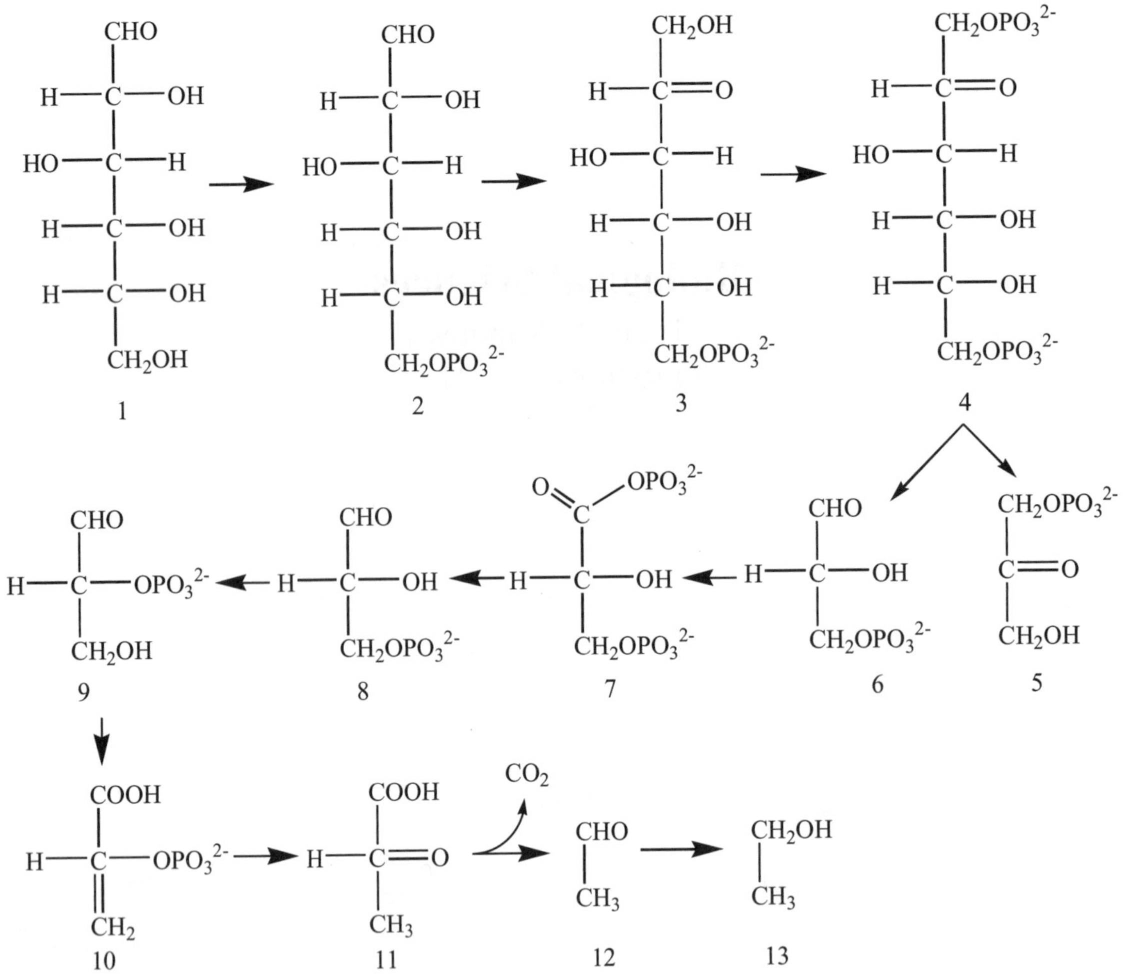

361. What is the maximum number of optically active isomers for fructose-6-phophate (3)?

A. 0
B. 3
C. 8
D. 9

362. The absolute configuration of the Carbons in Molecule 3, from top to bottom is:

A. R, R, S
B. S, R, R
C. R, S, S
D. S, S, S

GO ON TO THE NEXT PAGE.

363. When leavened bread is made with Bakers yeast, the kneaded dough "rises" as the fermentation process progresses. The gas that is most likely responsible for this phenomena is:

A. hydrogen
B. water vapor
C. carbon monoxide
D. carbon dioxide

364. As presented in the Emden-Meyerhoff-Parnas scheme, Molecule 12 is converted to 13 by yeast alcohol dehydrogenase (YAD). This reaction can be best describes as:

A. the conversion of an alcohol to a ketone.
B. the conversion of a ketone to an alcohol.
C. the conversion of an alcohol to an aldehyde.
D. the conversion of an aldehyde to an alcohol.

365. When oxygen supply does not meet the oxygen demand, human muscle cells function under anaerobic conditions. In these circumstances, muscle cells convert glucose to pyruvic acid (11), which is then converted to lactic acid via fermentation. The structure of L-lactic acid is shown below. The spatial representation of the L-lactic acid is best described as:

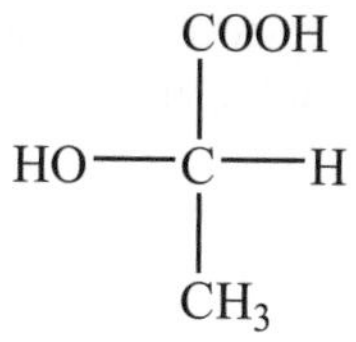

$$\begin{array}{c} COOH \\ | \\ HO{-}C{-}H \\ | \\ CH_3 \end{array}$$

A. Bent
B. Square pyramidal
C. Square planar
D. Tetrahedral

366. The build up of lactic acid in muscle cells is responsible for the feeling of soreness in overworked muscles. The functional group of lactic acid, as compared to pyruvic acid, confers:

A. a greater oxygen:hydrogen ratio.
B. double the oxygen: hydrogen ratio.
C. a lower oxygen: hydrogen ratio.
D. half the oxygen: hydrogen ratio.

367. The fermentation of glucose by Baker's yeast produces 62 kcals of heat. Assuming no other heat energy source for the reaction, how many moles of ethanol will be produced by this reaction?

A. 1 mole
B. 2 moles
C. 3 moles
D. 4 moles

GO ON TO THE NEXT PAGE.

Thalidomide (shown below) was first prescribed in Germany during the late 1950's for its sedative properties. The drug subsequently received FDA approval in the United States and became widely used in the treatment of nausea as well. Thalidomide's high efficacy combined with its low side effect profile led to widespread use worldwide. Unfortunately, many years passed before the drug was found to be responsible for limb dysgenesis in children with *in utero* exposure. Thalidomide's teratogenicity led to discontinuation of its use for many years. Recently, however, the drug has once again been approved for use in treating inflammatory conditions, including leprosy. Currently, the drug is under consideration for the treatment of cancers which are sensitive to anti-inflammatory medications.

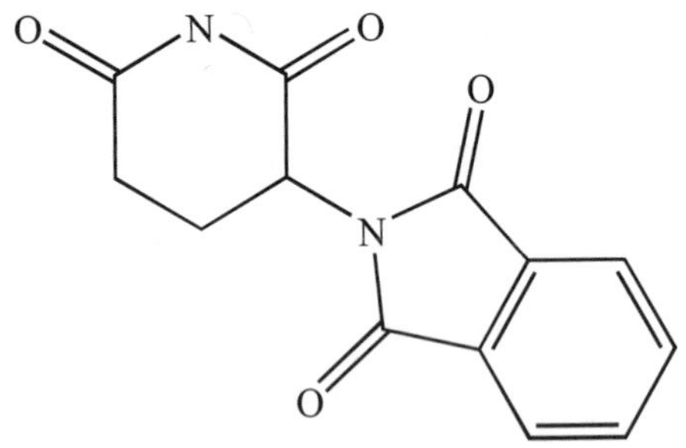

Interestingly, research has shown the "R" enantiomer to be responsible for the teratogenic effects of the drug, while the "S" enantiomer confers thalidomide's healing properties. Although production of the therapeutic isomer alone is possible, thalidomide undergoes racemization at the pH of the human body. Research continues in an attempt to find a comparable molecule without the pejorative effects on fetal development.

368. Thalidomide contains thirteen carbon molecules. How many of these are optically active?

A. 0
B. 1
C. 4
D. 13

369. If the R isomer of thalidomide is synthesized in an optically pure form, what would be true of a solution of this isomer at neutral pH?

A. The solution will rotate polarized light clockwise.
B. The solution will rotate polarized light counterclockwise.
C. The solution will not rotate polarized light.
D. The solution will produce polarized light.

370. Which of the following statements regarding the isomer of thalidomide shown below are true.

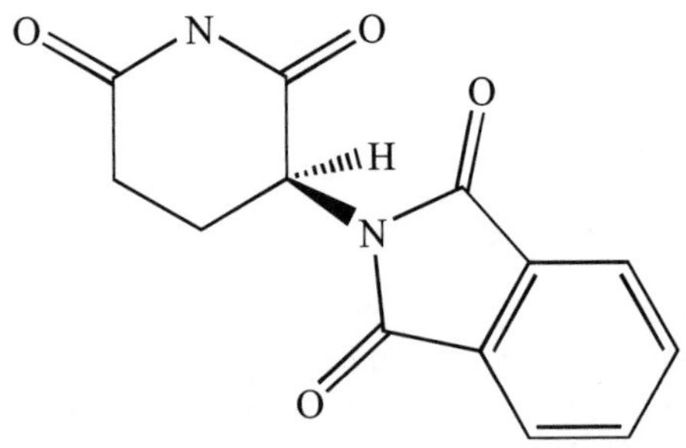

I. has sedative properties
II. when taken by humans, may result in birth defects
III. has anti-inflammatory applications

A. I
B. I and II
C. I and III
D. I, II, and III

371. Scientists often change functional groups in an attempt to modulate the physical properties of a drug. In this manner, they isolate drugs with the greatest efficacy and least adverse effects. If the topmost nitrogen atom in the figure above were replaced with an oxygen atom, what functional group would result?

A. hemiketal
B. acetal
C. carbonyl
D. anhydride

372. What is the hybridization of the atoms adjacent to the Nitrogen atoms of thalidomide?

A. sp
B. sp^2
C. sp^3
D. s

373. Which of the following is <u>not</u> a resonance structure of thalidomide?

A.

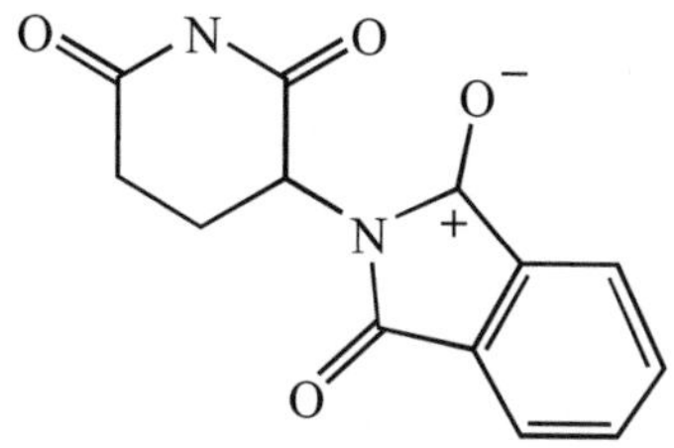

B.

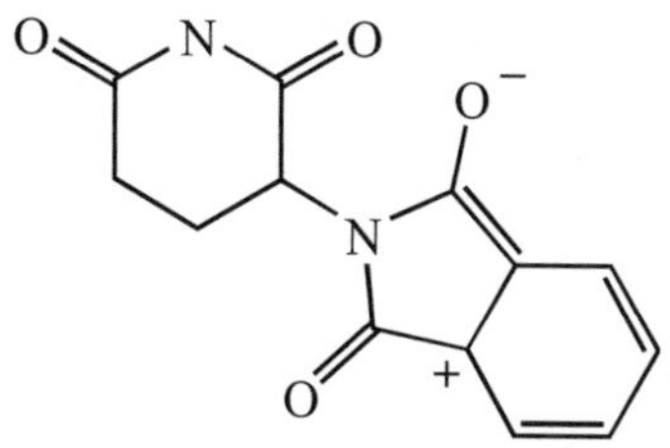

C.

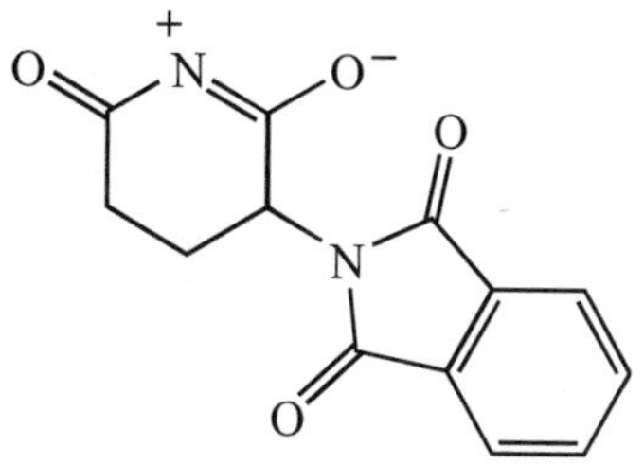

D.

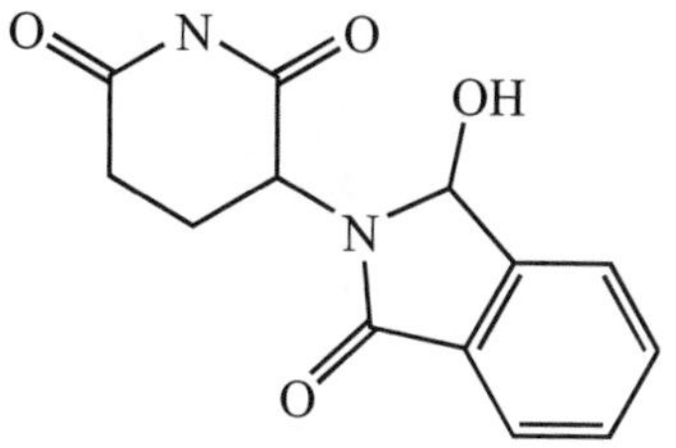

374. Which of the following best describes the relationship between the two thalidomide enantiomers?

A. geometric isomers
B. epimers
C. stereoisomers
D. structural isomers

Questions 375 and 376 are **NOT** based on a descriptive passage.

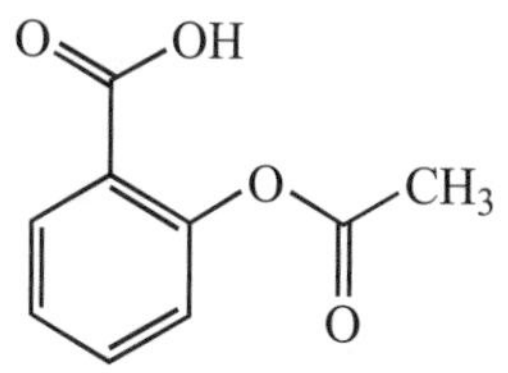

Figure 1 Aspirin

375. Aspirin is a commonly used anti-inflammatory medication. The drug (Figure 1) also inhibits platelet aggregation, an important property in the management of cardiovascular disease. At neutral pH, a solution of aspirin will:

A. The solution will rotate polarized light clockwise.
B. The solution will rotate polarized light counter-clockwise.
C. The solution will not rotate polarized light.
D. The solution will produce polarized light.

376. Which functional groups are present in aspirin?

A. ether, alcohol, ketone
B. ester, carboxylic acid
C. ketone, aldehyde
D. ether, ester, aldehyde

STOP. IF YOU FINISH BEFORE TIME IS CALLED, CHECK YOUR WORK. YOU MAY GO BACK TO ANY QUESTION IN THIS TEST BOOKLET.

EXAMINATION 09

Questions 377–423

Physical Sciences

Time: 20 Minutes
Questions 377–392

A small object can be placed on the surface of a fluid and remain there without sinking, even though the object is significantly more dense than the fluid. The object creates a depression in the fluid that is countered by the fluid's surface tension. More specifically, the surface tension responds by exerting an upward force on all sides of the object at an angle to the surface. A force diagram is shown below for the end view of a needle resting on the surface of a fluid.

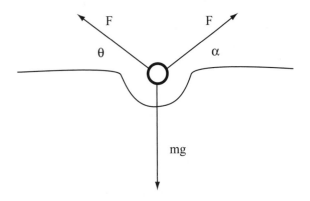

Figure 1 needle force diagram

The surface tension, γ, of a fluid is defined as $\gamma = \dfrac{F}{L}$, where F is the force exerted by the liquid and L is the length over which the force acts. For the needle shown in the diagram, the value of L is twice as large as the length of the needle because the surface tension acts on both sides of the needle.

In capillary tubes, the adhesive forces between a fluid and the tube walls cause the fluid to climb the tube against the force of gravity. The height to which a fluid will climb in a cylindrical tube is given by the formula below.

$$h = \frac{2\gamma\cos\phi}{\rho g r}$$

where γ is the surface tension, ρ is the density, g is the acceleration due to gravity, $9.8\ \text{m/s}^2$, r is the radius of the tube, and ϕ is the angle the surface of the fluid makes with the walls of the tube.

In fluids such as mercury, where the cohesive forces within the fluid are stronger than the adhesive forces between the fluid and the walls of the tube, the fluid will move down the tube, below its normal height. The formula above may also be used to calculate the downward displacement for other similar fluids.

The table below gives the density and surface tension for various fluids.

Fluid	Density (kg/m³)	Surface tension (N/m)
Ethyl alcohol	0.8×10^3	0.022
Mercury	13.6×10^3	0.465
Water (20° C)	1.0×10^3	0.073
Water (100° C)	1.0×10^3	0.059
Soapy water (20° C)	1.0×10^3	0.025

Table 1

377. Surface tension may be measured by recording the force required to remove a circular wire from a fluid. Which of the following expressions represents the surface tension of a fluid which exerts a force F on a wire ring with a radius r?

    A. $\dfrac{F}{2\pi r}$

    B. $\dfrac{F}{4\pi r}$

    C. $\dfrac{F}{\pi r^2}$

    D. $\dfrac{F}{2\pi r^2}$

378. The surface tension of which of the following fluids will be able to support the heaviest object?

    A. Pure cold water
    B. Pure hot water
    C. Soapy cold water
    D. Soapy hot water

379. Distilled water and ethyl alcohol are placed in identical capillary tubes under the same conditions. Which fluid will climb higher?

    A. Ethyl alcohol, because it has lower surface tension.
    B. Ethyl alcohol, because it has lower density.
    C. Water, because it has greater density.
    D. Water, because it has greater surface tension.

380. Which of the following diagrams most accurately reflects the appearance of mercury in a capillary tube?

A.

C.

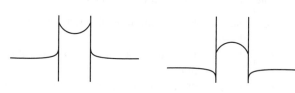

B.

D.

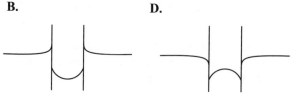

381. A sample of water climbed to a height of 2 cm. in a cylindrical capillary tube. If the tube is then replaced with a cylindrical tube of twice the original radius, what is the height of the water in the second tube?

A. 1 cm.
B. 2 cm
C. 4 cm
D. 8 cm

382. Ethyl alcohol has lower surface tension than water. The most likely explanation for this observation is that ethyl alcohol:

A. is less dense than water.
B. is more dense than water.
C. has weaker intermolecular forces than water.
D. has stronger intermolecular forces than water.

Passage II (Questions 383-389)

Lead iodide is only slightly soluble, dissolving according to the following endothermic reaction.

$$PbI_2(s) \rightarrow Pb^{2+}(aq) + 2\ I^-(aq)$$

Reaction 1

In an experiment designed to measure the solubility product for lead iodide, a student mixes 6.0 ml of 0.030 M potassium iodide with 10.0 ml of 0.015 M lead nitrate in the presence of 4.0 ml of 0.200 M potassium nitrate. The test tube containing the solution is shaken vigorously for ten minutes, then the lead iodide precipitate is allowed to settle to the bottom. The potassium nitrate does not take part in the reaction, but its presence promotes better crystal formation in the precipitate. The experiment is performed at a temperature of 25° C.

After the precipitate is filtered out, the supernatant is combined with acidic potassium nitrite solution to produce the reaction below.

$$2\ I^-(aq) + 2\ H^+(aq) + NO_2^- \rightarrow I_2(aq) + NO(g) + H_2O(l)$$

Reaction 2

Iodide ions are colorless in solution. However, as diatomic iodine is brown in aqueous solution, its concentration may be measured with a spectrophotometer. Once the concentration of I_2 is measured, the concentrations of the lead and iodide ions can be calculated and the solubility product can be found.

383. Which of the following equations represents the solubility product for lead iodide?

A. $K_{sp} = [Pb^+][I^-]$
B. $K_{sp} = [Pb^{2+}][I^-]$
C. $K_{sp} = [Pb^+][I^-]^2$
D. $K_{sp} = [Pb^{2+}][I^-]^2$

384. How many moles of Pb^{2+} ions are initially present in the test tube?

A. 1.5×10^{-4}
B. 1.5×10^{-1}
C. 6.6×10^{-1}
D. 1.5×10^0

385. Reaction 2 is necessary in order to find solubility product because:

A. the precipitate must be removed before the ion concentrations are measured.
B. the concentration of iodide ions cannot be measured with a spectrophotometer.
C. excess nitrate ions must be removed before the ion concentrations can be measured.
D. hydrogen ions act as a catalyst in the dissociation of lead iodide.

386. In order for the solubility product to be calculated most accurately, which of the following reactants must be the limiting reagent in Reaction 2?

A. I^-
B. I_2
C. H^+
D. NO_2^-

387. Which of the following would be the most likely effect of raising the solution temperature to 35°C?

A. The solubility of lead iodide would increase, but the solubility product would remain the same.
B. The solubility of lead iodide would decrease, but the solubility product would remain the same.
C. The solubility of lead iodide and the solubility product would increase.
D. The solubility of lead iodide and the solubility product would decrease.

388. Suppose that after the test tube was shaken and the precipitate was allowed to settle, solid potassium iodide was added to the test tube, which was then shaken once more. The addition of KI would most likely:

A. increase the concentration of I^- ions and Pb^{2+} ions in the solution.
B. decrease the concentration of I^- ions and Pb^{2+} ions in the solution.
C. increase the concentration of I^- ions and decrease the concentration of Pb^{2+} ions in the solution.
D. decrease the concentration of I^- ions and increase the concentration of Pb^{2+} ions in the solution.

389. A sample of lead iodide is placed in distilled water and the concentration of iodide ions is found to be 2.8×10^{-3} M. What is the concentration of lead ions in this solution?

A. 1.4×10^{-3} M
B. 2.8×10^{-3} M
C. 4.2×10^{-3} M
D. 5.6×10^{-3} M

GO ON TO THE NEXT PAGE.

390. All of the following statements are true for an ideal flow system EXCEPT:

    A. Volume flow is the same at all points.
    B. The flow is without turbulence at all points.
    C. Fluid velocity is the same at all points.
    D. The density of the fluid is the same at all points.

391. Which of the graphs below best demonstrates the relationship between fluid pressure, P, and depth below the surface, y?

A.

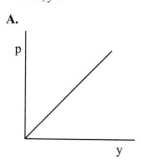

B.

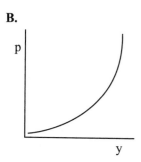

C.

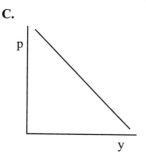

D.

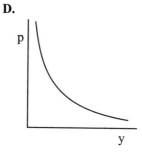

392. Which of the following solutions will best conduct electricity?

    A. 0.1 M NaCl
    B. 0.1 M NaNO$_3$
    C. 0.1 M MgS
    D. 0.1 M MgCl$_2$

STOP. IF YOU FINISH BEFORE TIME IS CALLED, CHECK YOUR WORK. YOU MAY GO BACK TO ANY QUESTION IN THIS TEST BOOKLET.

Verbal Reasoning
Time: 20 Minutes
Questions 393–407

Richmond Enquirer, Saturday Morning, March 23, 1861: "The issue to be decided by the people of Virginia is clearly stated in the following resolution, adopted by public meeting in the county of Dinwiddie: ... "Resolved, ... The
5 old Union being irreparably dissolved, there is no option left us, (the people of Virginia,) save to unite our destinies with our sister Southern States—or, to remain a useless appendage to the Northern Confederacy—the latter alternative being utterly repugnant to ALL TRUE SOUTHERN
10 MEN."""

While northern industrial opportunity attracted scores of immigrants from Europe in search of freedom, the South's population stagnated. Even as slave states were added to the Union to balance the number of free ones, the
15 South found that its representatives in the House had been overwhelmed by the North's explosive growth. More and more emphasis was now placed on maintaining parity in the Senate. Failing this, the popular paranoia suggested the South would find itself at the mercy of a government in
20 which it no longer had an effective voice. Jefferson Davis, at the time a Senator from Mississippi, summed up the sectionalist argument himself. Speaking, in effect, to the people of the North concerning slavery, "It is not humanity that influences you... it is that you may have a majority in the
25 Congress of the United States and convert the Government into an engine of Northern aggrandizement... you want by an unjust system of legislation to promote the industry of the United States at the expense of the people of the South." From such a position it was a short step to the proposition
30 that if a state or section of the country no longer felt itself represented by, or fairly treated by, the Federal Government, then it had the right to dissolve its association with that government. It could secede from the Union. No provision had been made for such an eventuality in the
35 Constitution. The use of force to stop a state from seceding was, the argument went, unconstitutional, since the Union itself was a creature of the states. They had wholly created it.

Ironically, Davis came, over time, to regard the estab-
40 lishment of a strong central authority as essential to the survival of the Confederacy, in spite of his virulent States' Rights rhetoric before the war. This gradual change of position brought him increasingly into conflict with States' Rights advocates throughout the Confederacy. Yet in his at-
45 tempts to weld the Confederacy into a cohesive union that could defend itself against the North's attempts at reunion, and at the same time offer itself as a legitimate trading partner to its European allies, Davis realized that a binding set of guidelines and rules—a strong central government—was
50 a necessity, not an option. From this perspective the States' Rights advocates seemed to be promoting a virtual states' anarchy; a system whereby each State was the law unto itself and could pick and choose whether it wished to any

longer be a part of the loosely knit organization called the
55 Confederacy. Though Abraham Lincoln had, by this time, long passed from the earth, one can imagine him smiling gently, if not reproachfully, at his Southern counterpart who came too late to see the wisdom of a strong central government.

393. Which of the following conclusions can justifiably be drawn from the Richmond Enquirer excerpt (lines 1-10)?

   A. Only the men of Virginia believed that their state should secede.
   B. By this time Virginia had seceded from the Union.
   C. Virginia was probably not the first state to secede from the Union.
   D. One of the last states to secede from the Union was Virginia.

394. Each state is allotted Representatives according to state population, along with two Senators per state. Given the information in the passage, if increasing "emphasis was now placed on maintaining parity in the Senate" (lines 17-18) the South could probably only have accomplished this by:

   A. increasing each state's population.
   B. adding even more states to the Union.
   C. electing Jefferson Davis as their President.
   D. seceding from the Union.

395. The author would argue that an understanding of the factors which led the South to form the Confederacy is important to the study of Civil War because it:

A. provides a basis for understanding the importance of a strong central government.

B. explains the reasoning behind Jefferson Davis's decision to form the Confederacy.

C. indicates the strength of the feelings Southerners had about being forced into the Union.

D. illustrates how little can be gained through violent resistance when other options are available.

396. The author's discussion regarding the position of the southern states in the Union could most reasonably be extended to:

  I. citizens of a country.

 II. auto workers in a factory.

III. sailors at sea on a warship.

A. I only

B. III only

C. I and II only

D. I and III only

397. Which of the following objections, if valid, would most *weaken* the argument made for the use of force in maintaining the Union being unconstitutional?

A. No means other than force could be found that would hold the Union together.

B. An amendment to the Constitution authorizing the use of force in cases of secession had not been passed.

C. The citizens of the states, not the states, had created the Union.

D. Jefferson Davis gradually changed his views on slavery in the South.

398. The author's characterization of Jefferson Davis suggests that his reference to Davis as Lincoln's "Southern counterpart" (line 57) meant that:

A. Davis was, for a short time, the President of the Confederacy.

B. slavery repulsed Davis in the same manner it had repulsed Lincoln.

C. Davis had tried desperately to overcome Lincoln's attempts at outlawing slavery.

D. Davis in some ways mirrored Lincoln's role in the North.

399. Which of the following conclusions about the Constitution can be inferred from the passage?

A. The Constitution explicitly authorizes the use of force to prevent state's secession.

B. The use of force to prevent secession was arguably unconstitutional.

C. The authors of the Constitution did not foresee a state's wish to secede.

D. A state had a Constitutional right to secede from the Union.

GO ON TO THE NEXT PAGE.

One of the oldest methods of preserving foods is dehydration. Dehydrated foods resist spoilage because both enzymes and microorganisms require moisture. But while preserving food, dehydration also affects its taste – usually
5 adversely, though prunes and raisins, which are dehydrated plums and grapes, have agreeable flavors – and it almost always causes some loss of nutritional quality. A few vitamins, particularly, tend to be destroyed or depleted by the light of sun-drying.

10 These disadvantages are far outweighed by dehydration's usefulness and simplicity. Sun-drying was invented at about the same time as agriculture. In Mesolithic Denmark and China, people sun-dried fish, meat, and fruit to save them for another day. As long ago as the 13th Century, men
15 were using dried food that could be reconstituted in somewhat the same way modern milk powder is. The nomadic warriors of Genghis Khan, who spent long hours on horseback, sun-dried mare's milk to a lightweight powder, and put some of the powder in a water-filled saddle bottle at the
20 beginning of each day's journey. Stirred throughout the day by the jogging of the horse, the mixture became a thin porridge by nightfall.

Today, sun-drying for preservation is especially important in under-developed nations. In modern Turkey, for
25 example, many villagers eat a complex sun-dried mixture called *tarhana*, based on powdered yogurt made of cow or buffalo milk. To the yogurt are added wheat flour and bits of carrots, beans, or peppers. The resultant chalky powder can be stored almost indefinitely. It is reconstituted by boil-
30 ing it in water to produce a stew containing most of the original nutrients – except for vitamin C, which is destroyed by the light of the sun.

In industrialized nations, some of this loss of nutritional quality and flavor is prevented by newer drying tech-
35 niques. Foods are frozen, then placed for varying periods of time in a chamber from which the air has been exhausted. With air pressure reduced to the vanishing point, the water in the food evaporates quickly, preserving much of the flavor and nutrients of even such delicate fruits as strawberries.

40 Only in comparatively recent times have new preservative methods been devised to rival cooking and dehydration. The canning of food was developed little more than 200 years ago, by a man who set out to solve a specific problem in the spirit of modern science and technology. In
45 the 1790s, during the wars that followed the French Revolution, the armies of France fought on battlefronts all over Europe. Thousands of soldiers in those armies were disabled, not in combat, but by slow starvation and by deficiency diseases induced by a diet of smoked fish, salt meat,
50 and hardtack. In desperation, the French government offered 12,000 francs (nearly a half a million dollars today)

for a practical way to preserve enough food to supply a large, constantly moving army.

An inventor named Nicolas Appert took up the chal-
55 lenge. A man of many food trades, Appert had been variously a chef, confectioner, wine maker, brewer, and distiller and had dabbled in food preservation. Now, spurred by the prize offer, he embarked upon a series of tests that occupied him for more than a decade. Appert knew nothing of en-
60 zymes or bacteria, nor did anyone else in his day. He did know one fact – that heat neutralizes whatever it is that causes food to spoil – and he set out to make this neutralization permanent. After 14 years of trial and error, he arrived at a process that did the job. The food – vegetables,
65 fruits, fish, or meat – was sealed in stoppered bottles and the filled bottles were immersed in boiling water; the heat sterilized bottles and contents alike. The food then remained edible until the bottles were opened. The technique was effective enough to win Appert his prize in 1809; he started a
70 canning factory and went on to found a family canning dynasty that continued the business into the 20th Century.

---

400. According to information in the passage, a loss of nutritional value would be likely to occur when food is:

   A. slowly cooked to remove moisture.
   B. dried in the sun.
   C. dehydrated by almost any means.
   D. bottled or canned.

401. The author of the passage apparently associates the degree of development in nations, such as Turkey (lines 33-39), with:

   A. industrialization.
   B. their method of drying food.
   C. the nutritional value of their food.
   D. agriculture.

402. The assertion that the "canning of food was developed little more than 200 years ago, by a man who set out to solve a specific problem in the spirit of modern science and technology" (lines 42-44) is NOT clearly consistent with the information about:

- **A.** the methods of sun-drying in use at that time.
- **B.** what difficulties would need to be overcome in order to be successful.
- **C.** Appert's family legacy.
- **D.** what actually led Appert to begin his tests.

403. According to the passage, one drawback of dehydrating food that has been ameliorated by more modern techniques of dehydration is:

- **A.** simplicity.
- **B.** the need for sunlight.
- **C.** rehydration.
- **D.** loss of flavor.

404. Which of the following conclusions regarding the method of canning, for which Nicolas Appert was awarded a prize by the French government in 1809, can be inferred from the passage?

- **A.** The 'stoppers' were probably made from natural cork.
- **B.** Cans were not actually used in the process.
- **C.** The technique would have worked at any altitude.
- **D.** Appert invented the method too late to help his countrymen.

405. Based on passage information, the most effective situation for sun-drying food would be found during:

- **A.** a hot sunny day in a desert.
- **B.** a hot sunny day high on a mountain.
- **C.** a cold sunny day high on a mountain.
- **D.** a cold sunny day in a desert.

406. Apparently, an attractive benefit of dehydration which has been lost through modern processes is:

- **A.** usefulness.
- **B.** flavor.
- **C.** simplicity.
- **D.** nutritional value.

407. Though both processes preserved foods, the sun-drying and canning methods of food preservation described in the passage differed in that one of them did not:

- **A.** adversely affect flavor.
- **B.** resist spoilage as well.
- **C.** eliminate moisture.
- **D.** require a vacuum.

STOP. IF YOU FINISH BEFORE TIME IS CALLED, CHECK YOUR WORK. YOU MAY GO BACK TO ANY QUESTION IN THIS TEST BOOKLET.

STOP.

Biological Sciences

Time: 20 Minutes
Questions 408–423

Passage V (Questions 408-414)

The parathyroid glands sense low blood calcium levels and respond with PTH secretion. Parathyroid hormone (PTH) elicits effects in the kidneys, bone, and intestine to regulate serum calcium levels. The action of PTH on the kidney is twofold. First, it stimulates calcium reabsorption in the thick ascending loop of Henle and distal tubule of the nephron. This salvages the calcium that is filtered by the kidney and reduces the amount of calcium that is excreted in the urine. Second, PTH upregulates the conversion of 25-(OH)D to 1,25-(OH)$_2$D by renal cells. 1,25-(OH)2D is the active form of vitamin D which promotes the active transport of calcium through the microvilli of intestinal epithelium. Thus, PTH works indirectly, through 1,25-(OH)$_2$D, to maximize calcium absorption.

Both PTH and 1,25-(OH)$_2$D act on the bone to release stored calcium into the bloodstream. Osteoclasts dissolve bone matrix by secreting acid and collagenase onto the bone surface, thereby releasing calcium. In the presence of PTH and 1,25-(OH)$_2$D, the maturation of osteoclasts is accelerated, resulting in increased resorption of bone and a release of calcium from the bone mineral compartment.

408. In DiGeorge syndrome, there is defective embryonic development of the parathyroid glands. Children with this syndrome would be expected to have:

- **A.** high serum calcium
- **B.** low serum calcium
- **C.** high serum PTH
- **D.** low serum thyroid hormone

409. Hormone secretion is often regulated by negative feedback inhibition. A negative feedback signal for PTH is:

- **A.** low bone density
- **B.** high serum PTH
- **C.** high serum phosphate
- **D.** high serum calcium

410. PTH most likely acts on target cells by:

- **A.** upregulating the production of the secondary messenger cAMP
- **B.** upregulating the transcription of 1,25-(OH)$_2$D
- **C.** upregulating Na$^+$ entry into the cell
- **D.** downregulating Na$^+$ entry into the cell

411. Although converted in renal cells, 1,25-(OH)$_2$D acts on sites as distant as the intestine and peripheral bone. 1,25-(OH)$_2$D may be best classified as:

- **A.** an enzyme
- **B.** a neurotransmitter
- **C.** a hormone
- **D.** a coenzyme

412. Albright's osteodystrophy is a hereditary disease in which serum calcium levels are low, despite elevated serum PTH levels. Which of the following is the most likely basis of the disorder?

- **A.** a deficiency of the nuclear receptor which couples PTH to the parathyroid transcription factor.
- **B.** autostimulation of osteoblastic cells.
- **C.** a deficiency of the G$_s$-protein which couples the PTH receptor to adenyl cyclase.
- **D.** a defect in osteoclastic secretion of digestive enzymes.

413. The precursor to 1,25-(OH)$_2$D is 7-Dehydrocholesterol. Cholesterol derivatives are also precursors of:

- **A.** cortisol and aldosterone
- **B.** epinephrine and norepinephrine
- **C.** prolactin and oxytocin
- **D.** adenine and guanine

414. Tight regulation of serum calcium is crucial for proper nervous system function. Low blood calcium levels may result in numbness and tingling in the hands and feet, referred to as the "stocking-glove" effect. Insufficient serum calcium would have the greatest affect which of the following neuronal structures?

- **A.** dendrites
- **B.** axon hillock
- **C.** axon
- **D.** axon terminal

GO ON TO THE NEXT PAGE.

Passage VI (Questions 415-421)

Although ovulation does not occur until puberty, the human ovary contains all the eggs needed for reproduction at the time of birth. During each menstrual cycle many eggs begin to mature, though usually only one is ovulated. The egg which first completes maturation is released from the ovary, and passes into the fallopian tube for fertilization.

The female reproductive cycle is delicately orchestrated by leutinizing hormone (LH) and follicle stimulating hormone (FSH), both secreted by the anterior lobe of the pituitary gland. Fertility disorders in women often result from imbalances in these hormones.

New drugs which mimic the actions of LH and FSH are first line treatments in many female reproductive disorders. Researchers in a pharmaceutical laboratory investigate two such newly developed drugs. Drug A binds to LH receptors, while Drug B binds to FSH receptors. The researchers randomize 15 rats with fertility disorders into three study groups. Rats in group A receive Drug A, while rats in group B receive Drug B, and rats in group C receive a placebo. After 1 month, the researchers perform oophorectomies and count number of developing follicles in the rat ovaries. An average female rat will have a maximum of 10-12 developing follicles at any given point in the cycle.

Subject	Group A	Group B	Group C
1	5	6	5
2	15	7	7
3	5	12	4
4	6	9	10
5	10	10	5

Table 1 Number of developing follicles per rat 1 month after treatment

415. According to the passage, which of the following conditions is LEAST likely to result in infertility:

A. Mutation in the FSH gene
B. Multiple follicular release
C. Downregulation of LH receptors
D. Inflammation of the fallopian tube

416. For subject 4 in Group C, which of the following treatment conditions is most likely responsible for the number of maturing follicles harvested?

A. Stimulation of the LH receptor
B. Inhibition of the FSH receptor
C. Unassociated with the treatment
D. Stimulation of the pituitary gland

417. When a follicle bursts and an egg is released, the remnant of the follicle forms the corpus luteum and induces thickening of the uterine wall. This endometrial hyperplasia is triggered by release of which of the following hormones from luteal cells?

A. Progesterone
B. Human chorionic gonadotropin
C. Luteinizing hormone
D. Gonadotropin releasing hormone

418. The rats identified as Subject 2 in all three groups have the same reproductive disorder. According to the study data, which of the following conditions is the most likely reason behind Subject 2s' infertility?

A. Overproduction of LH
B. Insensitivity of FSH receptors to FSH
C. Mutation in the LH gene
D. Functional pituitary adenoma

GO ON TO THE NEXT PAGE.

419. Reproductive therapies often result in multiple pregnancies. Overstimulation of follicular development increases the probability of multiple ovulation. Which of the subjects in the study best demonstrates this phenomenon?

A. Group A, Subject 5
B. Group C, Subject 4
C. Group B, Subject 3
D. Group A, Subject 2

420. Eggs within a human ovary are frozen in the middle of meiosis I until activation during follicular maturation. Once the oocyte does complete this division, which of the following daughter cells result?

A. Two haploid cells of equal size
B. Two diploid cells of equal size
C. One haploid cell and one polar body
D. One diploid cell and one polar body

Questions 421 and 423 are **NOT** based on a descriptive passage.

421. Which of the following represents the correct progression of spermatogenesis?

A. spermatogonia → spermatids → spermatocytes → spermatozoa
B. spermatogonia → spermatozoa → spermatids → spermatocytes
C. spermatogonia → spermatocytes → spermatids → spermatozoa
D. spermatids → spermatogonia → spermatozoa → spermatocytes

422. Which of the following conditions would LEAST likely result in male infertility?

A. Inability to produce microtubules
B. Defect in the acrosomal enzymes
C. Lack of testosterone
D. Defect in mitochondria

423. Osteoclasts are responsible for bone resorption. The precursors of these cells are:

A. monocytes
B. erythrocytes
C. osteoprogenitor cells
D. chondrocytes

STOP. IF YOU FINISH BEFORE TIME IS CALLED, CHECK YOUR WORK. YOU MAY GO BACK TO ANY QUESTION IN THIS TEST BOOKLET.

STOP.

EXAMINATION 10

Questions 424–470

Physical Sciences
Time: 20 Minutes
Questions 424-439

Passage I (Questions 424-439)

A rooftop water storage tank provides water to a series of cylindrical pipes which lead to three different spigots as shown below. The cross-sectional radius of each spigot is 0.5 cm and the radius of the cylindrical tank is 4 m. The radius of the pipe at point D is 5.0 cm and the radius at point E is 2.5 cm. The tank is large enough that any motion of the water in the tank as it drains may be ignored.

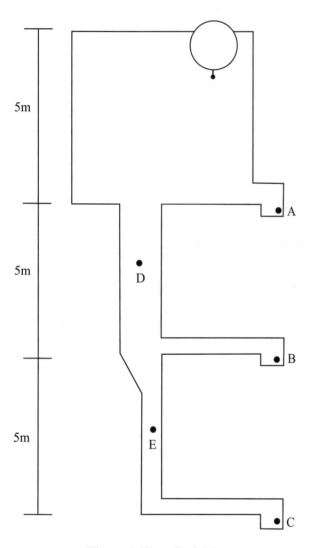

Figure 1 Water Tank Diagram

A spherical sensor floats at the top of the water in the tank. When the water level lowers to a certain point, the sensor touches the bottom of the tank and triggers a signal which indicates that the tank needs to be refilled. The sensor has a specific gravity of 0.8 and a volume of 300 cm³. The density of water is 1000 kg/m³. Flow in the system is ideal.

424. What is the mass of the water displaced by the sensor at any given moment?

- **A.** 240 g
- **B.** 300 g
- **C.** 375 g
- **D.** 700 g

425. Spigot A and spigot C are opened at different times under the same conditions. Which of the following statements best describes the relationship of the volume flow rates and flow speeds for spigot A and spigot C?

- **A.** The flow rates will be the same but the flow speeds will be different.
- **B.** The flow rates will be different but the flow speeds will be the same.
- **C.** The flow rates and the flow speeds will be the same.
- **D.** The flow rates and the flow speeds will be different.

426. When spigot C is opened and spigot B is closed, water flows past point D at a speed of v. What is the speed of the water as it flows past point E?

- **A.** $\dfrac{v}{4}$
- **B.** $\dfrac{v}{2}$
- **C.** $2v$
- **D.** $4v$

427. If the tank is full, what is the approximate speed of the water as it escapes spigot B?

- **A.** 7 m/s
- **B.** 10 m/s
- **C.** 14 m/s
- **D.** 20 m/s

428. When all of the spigots are closed, what is the pressure difference between point C and the surface of the tank?

- **A.** 1.0×10^4 Pa
- **B.** 1.5×10^4 Pa
- **C.** 1.0×10^5 Pa
- **D.** 1.5×10^5 Pa

429. What is the approximate mass of the water in the storage tank when it is full?

- **A.** 8.0×10^4 kg
- **B.** 2.5×10^5 kg
- **C.** 4.8×10^5 kg
- **D.** 7.5×10^5 kg

430. When spigots B and C are opened simultaneously, the volume flow at point E will be:

- **A.**   greater than the flow at point D.
- **B.**   less than the flow at point D.
- **C.**   equal to the flow at point D.
- **D.**   equal to zero.

Passage II (Questions 431-437)

Halide anions typically form soluble salts with metal cations. Among the exceptions to this are the salts formed between halogen and silver or lead ions. The table below shows the solubility products for silver and lead salts at 25° C.

Salt	Solubility product, K_{sp}
PbF_2	2.7×10^{-8}
$PbCl_2$	1.6×10^{-5}
$PbBr_2$	4.0×10^{-5}
PbI_2	7.1×10^{-9}
AgF	soluble
AgCl	1.8×10^{-10}
AgBr	5.3×10^{-13}
AgI	8.3×10^{-17}

Table 1. Solubility products

431. A sample of solid silver chloride is placed in distilled water at 25° C. The solid equilibrates with the dissociated ions in solution. Which of the following expressions gives the concentration of Ag^+ ions in the solution?

- **A.** $\sqrt{1.8 \times 10^{-10}}\ M$
- **B.** 1.8×10^{-10} M
- **C.** $(1.8 \times 10^{-10})^2$ M
- **D.** $(3.6 \times 10^{-10})^2$ M

432. Which of the following statements is best supported by the data presented in Table 1?

- **A.**   The solubility of silver halogen salts increases with increasing atomic radius of the halogen.
- **B.**   The solubility of silver halogen salts decreases with increasing atomic radius of the halogen.
- **C.**   The solubility of lead halogen salts increases with increasing atomic radius of the halogen.
- **D.**   The solubility of lead halogen salts decreases with increasing atomic radius of the halogen.

433. A sample of solid lead bromide is placed in a 0.2-molar NaBr solution and allowed to reach equilibrium. What is the concentration of Pb^{2+} ions at equilibrium?

- **A.** 1.0×10^{-7} M
- **B.** 2.0×10^{-6} M
- **C.** 5.0×10^{-4} M
- **D.** 1.0×10^{-3} M

434. A chemist mixes 50 ml of a 0.1 M $AgNO_3$ solution with 50 ml of 0.1 M $Pb(NO_3)_2$ solution. Then the chemist slowly adds dilute NaCl solution to the mixture. Which of the following statements is true?

- **A.** NaCl will precipitate out of solution first.
- **B.** $PbCl_2$ will precipitate out of solution first.
- **C.** AgCl will precipitate out of solution first.
- **D.** No precipitate will appear.

435. The solubility product for silver chloride is 1.3×10^{-9} at 50° C. Which of the following statements is true regarding the solvation of AgCl?

- **A.** ΔH and ΔS are positive.
- **B.** ΔH and ΔS are negative.
- **C.** ΔH is positive and ΔS is negative.
- **D.** ΔH is negative and ΔS is positive.

436. A student dissolves 12.7 grams of silver fluoride in 2.0 liters of water. What is the concentration of fluorine ions in the solution?

- **A.** 0.01 M
- **B.** 0.05 M
- **C.** 0.1 M
- **D.** 0.2 M

> Questions 437 through 439 are **NOT** based on a descriptive passage.

437. A drain cover, with an area of 0.20 m^2, sits at the bottom of a swimming pool. If the drain cover is 3 meters below the surface of the water, what is the force exerted on the cover by the water in the pool? (The density of water is 1000 kg/m^3.)

- **A.** 600 N
- **B.** 3000 N
- **C.** 6000 N
- **D.** 150,000 N

438. A cylindrical wire lengthens by 2% when subjected to a stretching force. If the radius of the wire were doubled, the same stretching force would result in an increase of:

- **A.** 0.5%
- **B.** 1%
- **C.** 4%
- **D.** 8%

439. When a volatile solute and a non-volatile solvent are combined in ideal solution, the vapor pressure of the solution will be:

- **A.** greater than the vapor pressure of the solute.
- **B.** greater than the vapor pressure of the solvent.
- **C.** equal to the vapor pressure of the solute.
- **D.** equal to the vapor pressure of the solvent.

STOP. IF YOU FINISH BEFORE TIME IS CALLED, CHECK YOUR WORK. YOU MAY GO BACK TO ANY QUESTION IN THIS TEST BOOKLET.

GO ON TO THE NEXT PAGE.

Verbal Reasoning

Time: 20 Minutes
Questions 440-454

GO ON TO THE NEXT PAGE.

As an agent of erosion, the wind is secondary, but as a medium for transporting sand and other light material across the desert, it builds and tears down land forms all on its own. Impeded not at all by vegetation and very little by
5 topography, winds dehydrate the soil—and all living things as well—and accentuate every effect of drought. On a hot, gusty day a desert traveler can be almost sick with the oppressive heat yet never feel a drop of perspiration, so rapid is the evaporation; actually he may be perspiring at
10 the rate of nearly a quart of water an hour.

Both duststorms and sandstorms, which are not the same thing, are whipped up by robust winds. A good blow can lift clouds of dust particles, so thick they blot out the sun, thousands of feet in the air. But sand, being heavier and
15 coarser, rarely gets more than a few feet off the ground. A sandstorm often starts with a mist of suspended dust and sand. When the mist clears, the heavier particles remain as a low, thick cloud, gliding over the desert like a great moving carpet. The air above it is clear, and the heads of
20 people can project out of the cloud as if they were walking chin-deep in water. The abrasive, sandblast effect is great-est at ground level and insignificant above a height of 18 inches. Projecting rocks are carved into strange, top-heavy shapes, and telegraph poles are neatly amputated at their
25 bases unless specially sheathed in metal, and even then they last only a few years.

In the wake of the winds, large areas of many deserts are left sand-free. The surface is composed of small rocks fitted together like a smooth, hard mosaic. This "desert
30 pavement," laid down by flowing water and exposed by winds, is often highly polished by abrasion, by oxidation of metal in the stones or both. The pavement or armor is spread over what is called "gibber plain" in Australia, serir in Libya and reg in the Sahara, in contrast to erg, the vast
35 area where sand accumulates.

The deserts are not the only place where the wind builds sand piles. There are dune fields on many ocean and lake shorelines, on the leeward sides of rivers crossing semiarid lands, like the Arkansas and the Platte, and in
40 places where loose sandstone deposits are weathering and disintegrating, like Nebraska's Sand Hills. There is such an incalculable amount of sand—wet and dry—in the world that geologists have had a hard time accounting for it. Sandstone is a minor source; most sand starts as tiny crys-
45 tals of quartz which break off granite and other hard igneous rocks. Gypsum is still another source; some of the dunes at White Sands National Monument in New Mexico are almost pure gypsum from a dried-up lakebed.

Wind-borne sand particles scud along the ground,
50 colliding with each other, bouncing off obstructions and wearing off their rough irregularities. Eventually, smoothed

and rounded, they approach a perfectly spherical shape – and may keep it, without further wearing, for millions of years. It was once believed that sand grains were rounded
55 while washing down riverbeds, but laboratory experiments showed they are too lightweight to abrade each other in water. A cube of quartz a fiftieth of an inch in diameter, it was estimated, would have to be transported by water a distance equivalent to 50 times around the world before it
60 became fully rounded, but wind abrasion would round it off 100 to 1,000 times more rapidly.

440. Assume that only the 'felsic' compositional group of igneous rock is composed mostly of quartz. Based upon this new information:

   A.   the author has made an error.
   B.   White Sands is an abundant source of felsic rock and rock particles.
   C.   most sand would have to come from some other type of igneous rock.
   D.   most sand would probably come from felsic rock.

441. Which of the following conclusions is best supported by the author's description of how sand particles change shape?

   A.   Heavier rocks in water would abrade more quickly than smaller windblown particles.
   B.   Most of the rounded sand grains in the world have been exposed to wind abrasion at one time or an-other.
   C.   Weight seems to be more significant than size in de-termining particle shape.
   D.   Most sand particles are spherical in shape.

442. Which of the following assertions is most clearly an idea presented by the author?

- **A.** Windblown sand is capable of eroding metal.
- **B.** Large areas of the desert are relatively uninhabited.
- **C.** Most areas of a desert are actually polished and free of sand.
- **D.** Gypsum is only found in dried-up lakebeds.

443. The passage suggests that the heavier particles of wind-blown sand:

- **A.** cannot usually be lifted above the ground.
- **B.** produce the most significant erosion effects.
- **C.** are sometimes compacted into a "gibber plain".
- **D.** are not eroded by water.

444. During an interview on desert life, a zoologist remarks that the desert-dwelling Stenocara beetles' ability to collect water from wind-borne fogs is being emulated in certain devices which will be used to collect water for drinking and irrigation in the desert, to collect vapors in industrial condensers, and even to dispell fog at airports. This information would most weaken the passage assertion that:

- **A.** wind essentially renders the desert devoid of any water.
- **B.** the desert offers nothing in the way of usable water.
- **C.** desert winds dehydrate all living things.
- **D.** deserts are devoid of any sizeable vegetation.

445. The contention that, "As an agent of erosion the wind is secondary …" (line 1), can most justifiably be interpreted as support for the idea that:

- **A.** the crucial cause of erosion is movement.
- **B.** the principal agent of erosion is water.
- **C.** the chief means of erosion is wind.
- **D.** the key player in erosion is sand.

446. According to the passage, one may conclude that in the desert, above a height of 18 inches:

- **A.** wind-blown sand is essentially non-existent.
- **B.** there is significantly less erosion.
- **C.** it may be easier to breathe in a duststorm.
- **D.** the air is much cooler.

GO ON TO THE NEXT PAGE.

Passage IV (Questions 447-454)

A ship has six different motions that must be dealt with. These are: roll (tipping from side to side); pitch (seesawing up and down); yaw (fishtailing to produce a zigzag course); heave (lifting up and down); surge (speed-
5 ing up and slowing down as the ship rides a wave); and sway (moving of the whole ship to one side or the other). Of these, rolling and pitching present the greatest problems.

Every ship has its own rolling period – the time it takes to roll freely from starboard to port and back again, a
10 measure of its own internal rhythm. It can roll just a little, or it can roll wildly, until its rail goes under; but the time the roll takes will be the same. In this respect it is like a pendulum; the farther the pendulum swings, the faster it goes.

A ship's rolling period is determined by the shape of
15 its hull, its beam, and the distribution of weight. Rolling becomes a matter of concern when wave periods coincide with a ship's natural rolling period. When the waves are fairly regular, a minor change of course or speed usually ends synchronous rolling. However, as the sea grows
20 rougher and more irregular an interesting phenomenon frequently takes place: the ship begins to respond to compo-nent waves with frequencies that match its own internal rhythm. In such circumstances these particular wave trains hit the side of the ship just as it is starting its roll, and under
25 this constant nudging [rolling] soon builds to a dangerous degree. The principle is the same as that used by a man giving his child a ride in a swing, when he builds up the arc of the swing by giving it a small push each time that its downward motion starts. When the sea does this to a ship a
30 much more drastic change of course or rate of speed must be made to break the motion.

To counteract this motion most modern vessels are equipped with antirolling devices of one kind of another. The most effective of those now in use are gyro-controlled
35 stabilizing fins, standard equipment on all but a few of the large liners now in service. The mechanism functions on the same principle as the ailerons of an airplane.

Pitching, an uphill-downhill movement when a ship is riding the waves, is a far more serious problem than rolling
40 and is the crux of the problem of achieving completely reli-able, all-weather scheduling for shipping. The problem is not one of driving the ship forward harder and harder as the waves try to beat it back, but of designing hull forms that will pitch less when speeding into a rough head sea.
45 Interestingly, waves shorter than the ship will not make it pitch, even though they are in synchronism with its natural pitching period.

Therefore, a designer can forget about all waves in the spectrum that are shorter than the hull he is designing, and
50 worry only about the ones that are as long or longer.

Furthermore, he knows that the longer he can make his ship the faster she can go before pitching becomes violent. Theoretically, then, all ships should be very long. However, length is expensive, and there is a practical limit to the size
55 of most vessels.

447. According to information in the passage, rolling would be less likely to occur when a seagoing liner:

  I. is driving into the oncoming waves.
  II. is beset by rough and irregular waves.
 III. has a longer hull.

  A. I only
  B. II only
  C. III only
  D. I and III only

448. According to the passage, the ship's rolling period is con-sidered a result of all of the following factors EXCEPT:

  A. the shape of the ship's hull.
  B. the length of the ship.
  C. the distribution of the ship's weight.
  D. the beam of the ship.

GO ON TO THE NEXT PAGE.

449. The ideas in the passage seem to derive primarily from:

    A. facts observable in a ship's log.
    B. evidence on the behavior of ships and waves.
    C. speculation based on an accepted theory.
    D. knowledge of ongoing hydrology studies.

450. The ideas discussed in this passage would likely be of most use to:

    A. a ship designer.
    B. a captain of a large liner.
    C. a sailing hobbyist.
    D. a competitive yachtsman.

451. In 1928, the clipper Ellis Spethman broke apart in heavy seas with a loss of all hands. Subsequent investigation revealed that her back had broken due to excessive pitching. Given the information in the passage, this result was probably due to:

    A. not immediately changing her speed and course.
    B. the ship heading straight into the oncoming waves.
    C. poor design.
    D. the clipper encountering waves that were longer than her hull.

452. Assume that all vessels are now required to have antirolling devices when they are built. This assumption necessitates which of the following conclusions?

    A. It was most likely determined that roll was more serious than pitch.
    B. The requirement apparently does not apply to all vessels.
    C. Vessels without the devices were probably determined to have long enough hulls.
    D. Those vessels without the devices had been built before the requirement.

453. The passage presents an important relationship between:

    A. airplanes and ships.
    B. pendulums and swings.
    C. wave regularity and minor speed changes.
    D. hull length and rolling period.

454. According to the passage, pitching is, in part, a function of a ship's:

    A. weight distribution.
    B. speed.
    C. date of manufacture.
    D. beam.

STOP. IF YOU FINISH BEFORE TIME IS CALLED, CHECK YOUR WORK. YOU MAY GO BACK TO ANY QUESTION IN THIS TEST BOOKLET.

172

Biological Sciences
Time: 20 Minutes
Questions 455-470

The reaction of allyl chloride with a chloride anion may proceed via any one of four possible reaction mechanisms. The four possible pathways are presented in Figure 1 below. The preferred pathway is a function of the polarity of the reaction solvent. Although all four mechanisms involve substitution, each results in a distinct product.

Researchers in a University laboratory calculated the free energies of activation ($\Delta G^{\ddagger}$) in kcal mol^{-1} for the different pathways in two different solvents. Their data is shown in Table 1. In addition, the researchers found the $\Delta G^{\ddagger}$ for the reaction of three allyl chloride congeners with the chloride anion (via all four pathways). This data is also presented in Table 1. The structures of the congeners are shown in Figure 2.

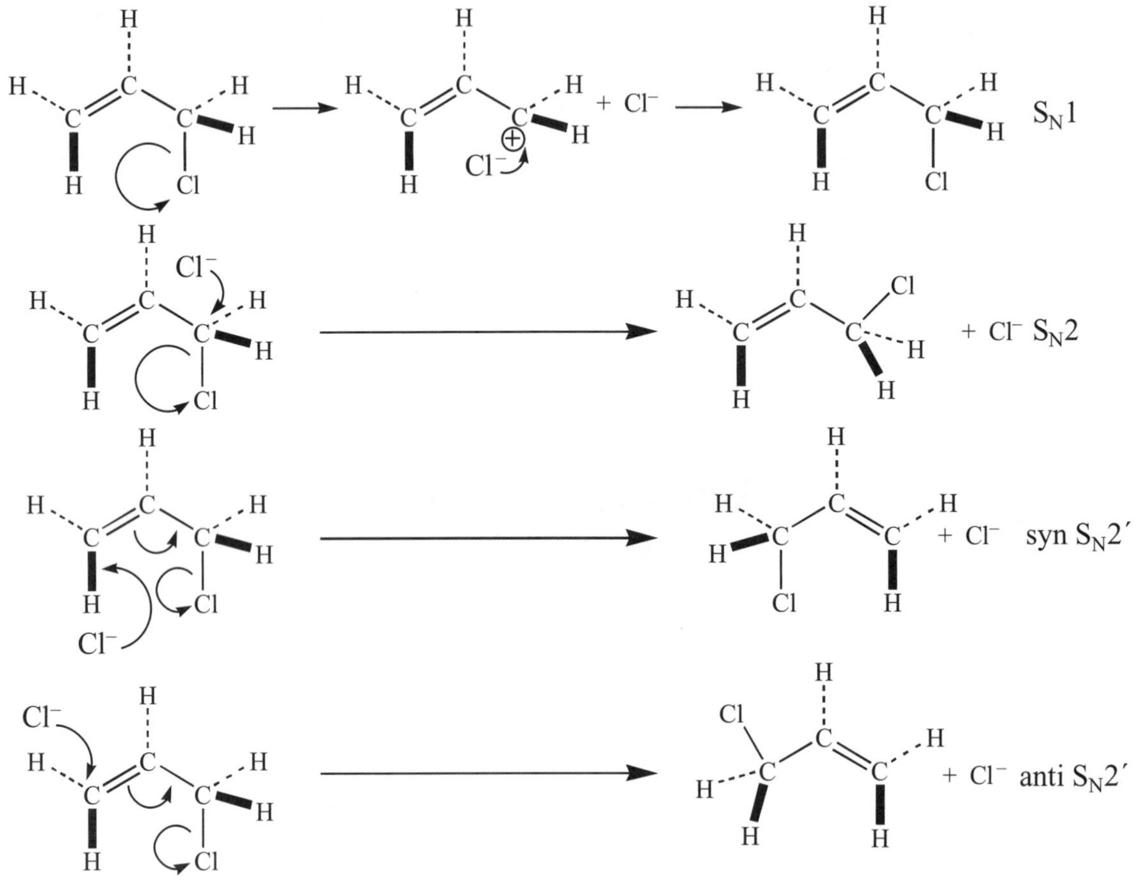

Figure 1

Pathway	Allyl	Z-crotyl	E-crotyl	Isoprenyl
CCl_4				
S_N1	88.7	78.7	77.0	70.2
S_N2	23.0	21.5	22.6	21.0
Syn S_N2'	30.3	31.1	33.2	33.0
Anti S_N2'	28.3	27.5	28.1	27.8
H_2O				
S_N1	25.8	18.7	16.7	12.2
S_N2	31.7	30.2	29.3	25.4
Syn S_N2'	37.0	32.5	NA	NA
Anti S_N2'	36.0	30.6	NA	NA

NA = Information is not available.

Table 1

GO ON TO THE NEXT PAGE.

The researchers discovered that the preferred pathway in organic solvents for all the reactions listed in table 1 is S_N2. However, the difference in energy between the pathways narrows as the polarity of the solvent increases. The data in table 1 indicates that in water the preferred pathway, based on a lower energy of activation, is S_N1. The calculated values show the anti S_N2' as the preferred alternative pathway in all cases.

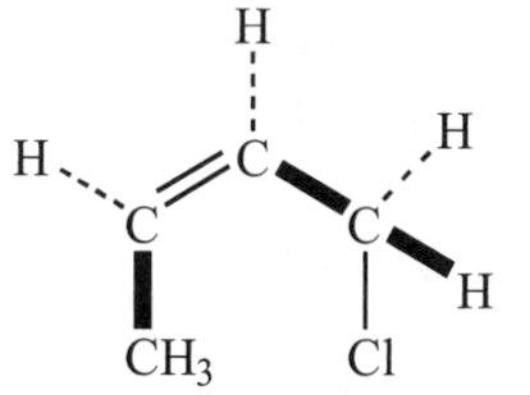

Z-crotyl chloride

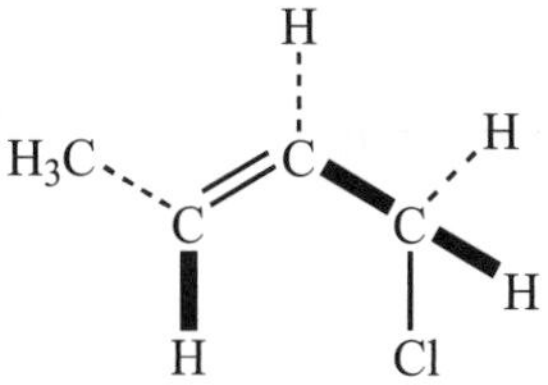

E-crotyl chloride

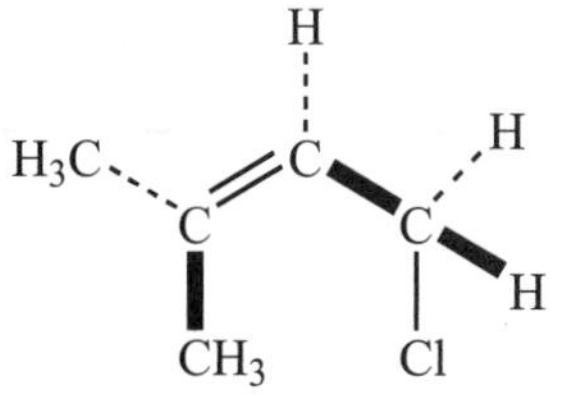

Isoprenyl chloride

Figure 2

455. Which of the following reagents, when reacted with allyl chloride, will produce an alcohol with the hydroxyl group on C3?

A. Concentrated H_2SO_4
B. HB_3
C. HBr
D. Ethanol

456. What hypothesis can the researchers present to explain the change in preferred pathway (in Figure 1) when the solvent is changed from carbon tetrachloride to water?

A. The hydrogen bonding of the aqueous solvent stabilizes the transition state of the SN_2 pathway.
B. The hydrogen bonding of the aqueous solvent stabilizes the transition state of the anti SN_2' pathway.
C. The hydrogen bonding of the aqueous solvent stabilizes the transition state of the syn SN_2' pathway.
D. The hydrogen bonding of the aqueous solvent stabilizes the transition state and intermediate of the SN_1 pathway.

457. If the researchers instead react a bromide anion with the molecule shown below in carbon tetrachloride, what the major product will be formed?

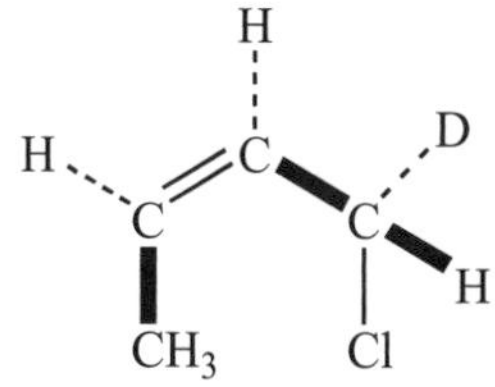

A.

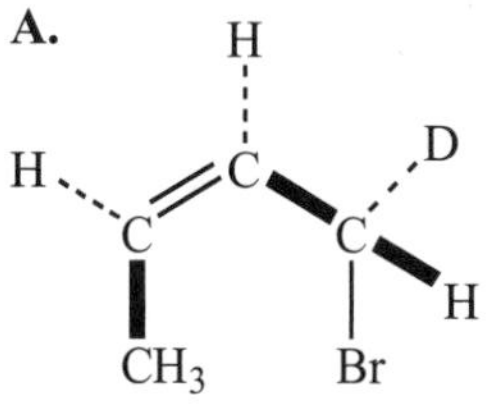

B.

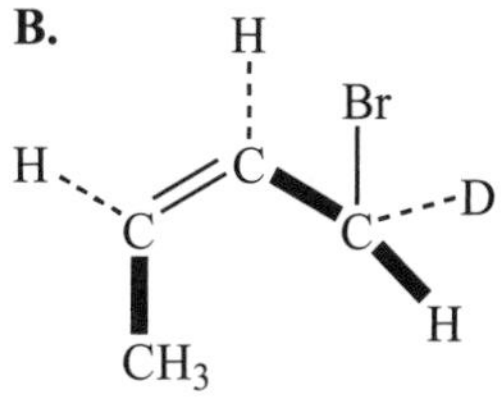

C.

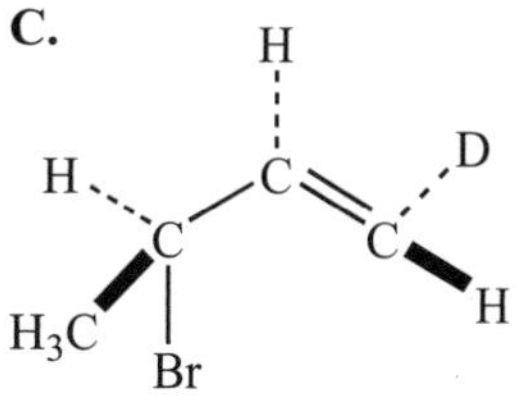

D.

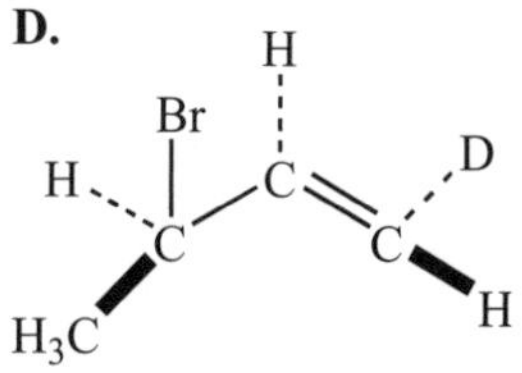

458. Which of the following congeners forms the most stable carbocation following the loss of the chloride ion?

A. allyl chloride
B. Z-crotyl chloride
C. E-crotyl chloride
D. isoprenyl chloride

459. Which of the following statements is NOT true regarding the reaction of Z-crotyl chloride with the chloride anion in carbon tetrachloride?

A. the reaction is bimolecular
B. the reaction goes with inversion
C. the rate can be increased by increasing the concentration of the chloride anion
D. the reaction occurs in two steps

460. Which of the following statements regarding the reaction of isoprenyl with the chloride anion in water is supported by the passage?

A. A carbocation is formed.
B. The reaction goes with inversion.
C. A strong nucleophile is required.
D. The reaction occurs in one step.

461. The researches can form a saturated haloalkane when they react which of the following reagents with E-crotyl chloride?

A. Concentrated H2SO4
B. H_2, Pd
C. 1) O_3, 2)Zn, H_2O
D. BH_3

Passage VI (Questions 462-468)

Citronellol is an alcohol that is found in many plant oils, including geranium and rose oils. It has been shown to be effective as a moth repellant when sprayed on fabrics. A related molecule, pulegone, is also found in plant oils and has an odor reminiscent of peppermint and camphor. As with citronellol, pulegone is believed to aid in repelling insects. The conversion of Citronellol to Pulegone is shown in the figure below.

Citronellol is first converted to isopulegone using pyridinium chlorochromate (PCC) in dichloromethane. PCC is formed by the reaction of pyridine with chromium trioxide. The formation of reaction intermediates, citronellal and isopulegols, may be followed via layer chromatography. The final conversion to pulegone is achieved by reacting the isopulegones with sodium hydroxide in ethanol. If the PCC is deposited on alumina before reacting with citronellol, the reaction will only proceed to the formation of Citronellal.

Citronellol → Citronellal → Isopulegols → Isopulegone → Pulegone

462. What is the relationship between isopulegone and pulegone?

- **A.** enantiomers
- **B.** diasteromers
- **C.** geometric isomers
- **D.** structural isomers

463. In the absence of a buffer, PCC functions as an acid to promote the cyclization of the citronellal. Why must an acidic proton be present for this to occur?

- **A.** The protonation of the double bond makes it a stronger nucleophile.
- **B.** The protonation of the carbonyl makes it a better electrophile.
- **C.** The acid cleaves the double bond.
- **D.** The acid oxidizes the carbonyl.

464. What is the absolute configuration of C3 in citronellal?

- **A.** R
- **B.** S
- **C.** cis
- **D.** trans

465. In converting Isopulegone to Pulegone, sodium hydroxide functions to:

- **A.** convert a less thermodynamically stable double bond to a more stable one.
- **B.** convert a more thermodynamically stable double bond to a less stable one.
- **C.** cataylze ring closure.
- **D.** oxidize an alcohol.

466. Why is PCC a better choice of oxidant for the conversion of citronellol to citronellal than cold dilute $KMnO_4$?

   A. PCC is a stronger oxidant so it can achieve the conversion with higher efficiency.

   B. PCC is stronger oxidant so it will oxidize the alcohol to the carboxylic acid.

   C. PCC is a weaker oxidant so it does not oxidize the alkene to an alkyne.

   D. PCC is a weaker oxidant so it will not oxidize the alcohol to the carboxylic acid.

467. Which of the following structures is the most likely product when Citronellol is heated with sulfuric acid?

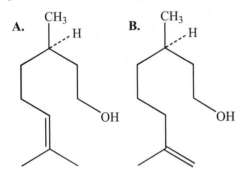

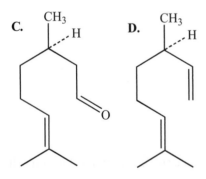

468. If distillation were used to separate citronellol from ethanol, which product would distill first?

   A. cintronellol

   B. ethanol

   C. They would come across at the same time.

   D. The order cannot be determined.

Questions 469 and 470 are **NOT** based on a descriptive passage.

469. What is the IUPAC name for isoprenyl chloride?

   A. 1-chloro-3-methyl-2-butene

   B. 4-chloro-2-methyl-3-butene

   C. 1-chloro-3,3-dimethyl-2-propene

   D. 4-chloro-1,1-dimethyl-2-propene

470. Hydrogenation of an alkene is a type of addition reaction. In order for hydrogenation to occur at an appreciable rate, a heterogeneous catalyst may be employed. Which of the following statements is FALSE regarding this type of reaction?

   A. Both Hydrogen atoms and the reactant alkene interact with the surface of the catalyst.

   B. The catalyst may exist in a different phase from the reactants

   C. The reaction is endothermic

   D. Hydrogenation proceeds via syn addition

STOP. IF YOU FINISH BEFORE TIME IS CALLED, CHECK YOUR WORK. YOU MAY GO BACK TO ANY QUESTION IN THIS TEST BOOKLET.

 STOP.

EXAMINATION 11

Questions 471–517

Physical Sciences
Time: 20 Minutes
Questions 471–486

A device which demonstrates the occurrence of interference between sound waves is depicted in the diagram below. Sound waves travel from the speaker through tube A and tube B and then superimpose at the receiver. The length of tube B may be increased or decreased with the use of a sliding section. A change in the length of tube B will, in turn, affect the phase relationship of the waves superimposed at the receiver. The length of tube A is fixed at 7.0 m.

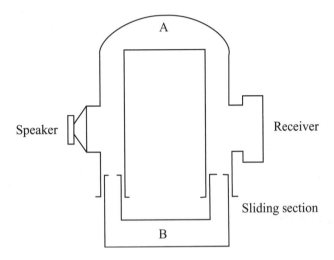

Figure 1 Wave Speaker-Receiver

The speed of sound varies according to the medium through which the sound wave passes. Wave speed increases as the resistance to compression of the medium increases, and decreases as the density of the medium increases.

The speed of sound in a gas, v, is given by the relationship below.

$$v = \sqrt{\frac{\gamma RT}{M}}$$

where γ is the adiabatic constant for the gas ($\gamma = 1.4$ for air), R is the gas constant, 8.314 J/mol-K, T is the absolute temperature, and M is the molar mass of the gas in kg/mol (M for air is 0.029 kg/mol)

The speed of sound in various media are provided in the table below.

Medium	Wave speed (m/s)
Air (273 K)	331
Air (298 K)	346
Air (373 K)	366
Helium (273 K)	972
Water (298 K)	1493
Iron	5130

Table 1 Sound wave speed in various media.

The loudness of a sound wave is described by the decibel scale, which relates the intensity of a sound, I, to the intensity at the threshold of hearing, I_o. ($I_o = 10^{-12}$ W/m^2)

$$dB = 10\log\left(\frac{I}{I_o}\right)$$

The decibel levels of some common sounds are given in the table below.

Sound	dB
Threshold of hearing	0
Whisper	30
Normal conversation	50
Busy traffic	80
Lawn mower	100

Table 2 Decibel levels of common sounds.

471. A sound wave with a wavelength of 1.0 meter is generated by the speaker in the interference device. At what length-setting for tube B will there be no signal at the receiver?

    A.   8.0 m
    B.   8.5 m
    C.   8.75 m
    D.   9.0 m

472. A signal generated by the speaker takes 0.0200 seconds to reach the receiver through tube A. If the medium in the tubes is air, what is the approximate temperature of the air?

    A.   265 K
    B.   295 K
    C.   305 K
    D.   395 K

473. Identical sound waves are generated in air and helium. How does the sound wave traveling through air compare with the sound wave traveling through helium?

- **A.** The waves will have the same frequencies and wavelengths.
- **B.** The waves will have different frequencies and wavelengths.
- **C.** The waves will have the same frequencies and different wavelengths.
- **D.** The waves will have the same wavelengths and different frequencies.

474. What is the intensity of a whisper?

- **A.** 10^{-15} W/m²
- **B.** 10^{-12} W/m²
- **C.** 10^{-9} W/m²
- **D.** 10^{-4} W/m²

475. Which of the following is the most likely explanation for the observation that sound waves travel faster in water than in air?

- **A.** water is more resistant to compression than air.
- **B.** water is less resistant to compression than air.
- **C.** water is more dense than air.
- **D.** water is less dense than air.

476. On a piano, the wave frequency produced by the F key, just below middle C, is 174 Hz. What is the approximate wavelength of this wave in air at room temperature?

- **A.** 0.5 m
- **B.** 1.0 m
- **C.** 1.5 m
- **D.** 2.0 m

477. The speed of sound in seawater at 298 K is about 1530 m/s and the specific gravity of seawater is about 1.025. Given this information, which of the following statements is true?

- **A.** The same wave will have a higher frequency in seawater than in fresh water.
- **B.** The same wave will have a lower frequency in seawater than in fresh water.
- **C.** Seawater is more resistant to compression than fresh water.
- **D.** Seawater is less resistant to compression than fresh water.

478. Helium and argon gases have the same adiabatic constant, $\lambda = 1.67$. What is the approximate speed of sound in argon at 273 K?

- **A.** 97 m/s
- **B.** 307 m/s
- **C.** 972 m/s
- **D.** 3073 m/s

Passage II (Questions 479-483)

Freezing point depression and boiling point elevation are colligative phenomena. Both are typically calculated using a constant and the molality of dissolved particles in solution. The boiling point elevation constant for water is 1.86° C/mol and the freezing point depression constant is 0.52° C/mol.

Predicted values for boiling and freezing points of aqueous solutions containing ions from dissociated salts are sometimes inaccurate. Predictive inaccuracy is particularly common for concentrated solutions, as charged particles will pair together and behave as a single particle. The effect of ion pairing is taken into account by the Van't Hoff factor, which adjusts the multiplier used to calculate colligative properties for ionic solutions.

$$i = \frac{\text{actual number of particles after dissociation}}{\text{number of particles expected from formula unit}}$$

The Van't Hoff factors for various 0.05 M salt solutions at 25° C are provided in the table below.

Salt	i (Van't Hoff)
NaCl	1.9
HCl	1.9
$MgSO_4$	1.3
$MgCl_2$	2.7
$FeCl_3$	3.4

Table 1 Van't Hoff factors.

479. The Van't Hoff factor for $MgSO_4$ is smaller than that of NaCl. The most likely explanation for this observation is that $MgSO_4$ dissociates into:

   A. particles with greater mass.
   B. particles with greater ionic radius.
   C. particles with greater charges.
   D. more particles.

480. What is the boiling point of a solution containing 9.5 grams of magnesium chloride in 1 kg of water?

   A. 100.1° C
   B. 100.5° C
   C. 101.1° C
   D. 101.5° C

481. A 1 *m* solution of which of the following salts will have the highest freezing point?

   A. NaCl
   B. $MgSO_4$
   C. $MgCl_2$
   D. $FeCl_3$

482. As the concentration of an ionic solution increases, what is the resultant effect on the Van't Hoff factor?

   A. It would decrease due to increased interaction between oppositely charged ions.
   B. It would increase due to increased interaction between oppositely charged ions.
   C. It would decrease due to decreased interaction between oppositely charged ions.
   D. It would increase due to decreased interaction between oppositely charged ions.

483. A student is conducting experiments in boiling point elevation and freezing point depression using magnesium sulfate. The student is unaware of the Van't Hoff effect and expects his results to correspond to complete dissociation of the salt based on the formula unit. The boiling point recorded by the student will be:

   A. lower than the expected value and the freezing point will be lower than the expected value.
   B. higher than the expected value and the freezing point will be lower than the expected value.
   C. lower than the expected value and the freezing point will be higher than the expected value.
   D. higher than the expected value and the freezing point will be higher than the expected value.

GO ON TO THE NEXT PAGE.

484. The specific heat of copper is 0.39 J/g-°C and the specific heat of gold is 0.13 J/g-°C. If a sample of copper and a sample of gold are each subjected to the same amount of heat and experience the same change in temperature, which of the following statements is most likely true?

    A.   The gold sample was one-ninth as massive as the copper sample.

    B.   The gold sample was one-third as massive as the copper sample.

    C.   The gold sample was the same mass as the copper sample.

    D.   The gold sample was three times as massive as the copper sample.

485. Which of the following is NOT a colligative property?

    A.   osmotic pressure

    B.   freezing point depression

    C.   pH

    D.   vapor pressure depression

486. The reason sailors cannot drink ocean water is that salt water consumption creates an osmotic pull for:

    A.   water to move into the body.

    B.   salt to move into the body.

    C.   water to move out of the body.

    D.   salt to move out of the body.

STOP. IF YOU FINISH BEFORE TIME IS CALLED, CHECK YOUR WORK. YOU MAY GO BACK TO ANY QUESTION IN THIS TEST BOOKLET.

STOP.

186

Verbal Reasoning

Time: 20 Minutes
Questions 487–501

With the exception of a handful of progressive lines, the railroads remained grossly neglectful until the middle of the 1880s, when they came under the combined fire of George Westinghouse, Eli Janney, and a bearded fanatic
5 named Lorenzo Coffin, Commissioner of Railroads for the State of Iowa. By this time Westinghouse had improved his air brake, which automatically and simultaneously closed the brakeshoes on all the cars of a train. Prior to this train brakes were still simple, hand-powered affairs. In an emer-
10 gency, when the engineer gave the signal—his brakemen darted from one car to another, twisting on the horizontal handwheels of each car, which slowly brought iron shoes into contact with the wheels. It was an uncertain process, and in a real pinch, it could not be done fast enough. Janney,
15 in turn, had strengthened and improved his automatic coupler. Whiling away the time, he had found the answer in his hands. By cupping them and hooking together the fingers of the opposite hands, he had the basis of an auto-matic, knuckle-jointed coupler which could be pushed
20 together but not pulled apart. By closing his thumbs over the outsides of the curved knuckles, he locked the hands so that the fingers would not slide off to one side or the other. As for Coffin, he was enraged at the powerful railroad magnates' shoulder-shrugging, act-of-God attitude toward
25 accidents which sent casualties up to 30,000 per year. By pleas, threats and a deafening peal of oratory, Coffin persuaded the Master Car Builders Association to hold a series of trials on long freight trains. One of those freights was equipped with Westinghouse brakes and Janney
30 couplers. The climax came on a summer day in 1887 outside Burlington, Iowa. "An immense train was hurled down the steep grade into Burlington at 40 miles an hour," wrote one observer. When the brakes were set, "the train came to a standstill *within 500 feet* and with hardly a jar."
35 At the glorious sight, old Lorenzo Coffin burst into tears and shouted, "I am the happiest man in all Creation."

Hardly less happy were George Westinghouse, whose brakes had done the job, and Eli Janney, whose tight-fitting coupler was judged by many observers to be not only
40 marvelous in itself but also the prerequisite for the air brake, which demanded a tight, reliable connection between the cars. Together the brake and coupler were difficult for calloused railroad conservatives to ignore, for it gave them the means of silencing the everlasting hue and cry about
45 safety and slaughter on the rails. Far more important to the profit-minded group, however, it would mean that longer trains could be operated reliably and economically on much tighter schedules. In other words, more freight, more passengers and, after an initial investment for the brakes
50 and couplers, much more revenue. Nevertheless, there was a formidable bloc of holdouts—But they were flogged into line in 1893, when President Benjamin Harrison signed the Safety Appliance Act which required automatic couplers and air brakes on all trains. Whereupon Eli Janney settled
55 down to live off his royalties on the sort of Virginia farm which would soothe the soul of any retired Confederate major who had served 20 years as a dry-goods clerk and poor inventor. This was not the case for George Westinghouse. He was the archetype of the 19th Century
60 captain of industry, who could put together big corporations like Westinghouse Air Brake Company and, later, the mammoth Westinghouse Electric Corporation and run the business with the same sure instinct he used in perfecting his original invention. "Like a lion in the forest," reported
65 an awed contemporary, "he breathed deep and with delight the smoky air of his factories…He was transformed into a giant when confronted with difficulties which seemed insurmountable."

487. Evidence shows that until 1889 about 20,000 rail employ-ees were killed or injured each year, a third of them while stepping between cars to connect the primitive link and pin couplers. This fact tends to support the hypothesis concerning railway safety because:

A. Westinghouse had not yet come up with a solution to this problem.

B. automatic brakes were invented before automatic couplers.

C. it is clear that the powerful people who ran the rail-roads cared only about money.

D. up until this time automatic couplers were not in use.

GO ON TO THE NEXT PAGE.

488. It is possible to determine if the railroads actually were able to increase their scheduling after instituting the improvements of Westinghouse and Janney by closely examining their yearly accident reports and taxes. Such information would support the author's mention of increased revenue by:

A. demonstrating that due to the improvements the railroads made more money.

B. vvdemonstrating that more money could be made by marketing safety to passengers.

C. proving that the automatic braking and coupling systems actually worked.

D. proving that tighter scheduling made more money.

489. According to the passage information, what would have been most likely to happen if the automatic air brakes had been used *without* the automatic couplers?

A. Without the slack between the automatic couplers, the cars would have been too stiffly joined.

B. Without a tight coupling, the cars brakes would only have worked on a few of the cars.

C. Without a reliable connection, the trains might have stopped in a jerky manner.

D. With only the air brakes, each car would be stopping on its own.

490. The author would most likely agree that the owners of the railroads had a vested interest in:

I. making the most money possible.
II. silencing complaints.
III. avoiding litigation.

A. I only
B. II only
C. I and II only
D. I and III only

491. Which of the following statements most strongly challenges one of the assertions made in the passage?

A. Westinghouse's device might have been much less effective without Janney's invention.

B. Lorenzo Coffin did not actually invent anything.

C. The use of the automatic brakes and couplers did not result in the saving of many lives.

D. After the successful trial of 1887, almost all of the owners opted to institute the brakes and couplers.

492. According to the passage, which of the following is most likely to be true about the relationship between the 1887 trial of the automatic safety devices, and the state of Iowa?

A. It was in this state that all of the trials for railroad safety equipment were performed.

B. Burlington, Iowa, was where Janney planned to retire.

C. Lorenzo Coffin was Commissioner of Railroads there.

D. This was the most visible place to perform the test with the long freight trains.

493. At the age of 22, George Westinghouse saw a wreck in which two trains had crashed together on a smooth, straight, level stretch of track in broad daylight. "What was the matter? Wouldn't the brakes work?" demanded Westinghouse of an employee. "Sure," said the man, "but there wasn't time." The author would most likely use this anecdote to:

A. expand on the dangers of train travel prior to the safety devices.

B. explain why Westinghouse invented air brakes.

C. justify the costs of forcing railroad owners to institute the automatic brakes.

D. clarify why Westinghouse went from a railroad owner to an inventor.

189

The story of digitalis is one of the most fascinating in the history of pharmacology. This drug was long an old wives' remedy; it was first prescribed by a physician for heart trouble nearly 200 years ago. Nevertheless a century
5 and a half passed before its effects and proper use were understood. The halting progress of digitalis from potion to modern prescription illustrates how inadequate knowledge of pharmacology can nullify the value of even an effective drug.

10 In 1775, an English physician named William Withering was asked his opinion of a folk remedy esteemed, not for its effect on the heart, but for its ability to relieve the swelling of dropsy. The recipe, he was told, "had long been kept a secret by an old woman in Shropshire, who
15 had sometimes made cures after the more regular practitioners had failed." The medicine, like many of the period, was a complicated concoction, with more than 20 different ingredients. Withering, however, was sophisticated enough to recognize that many of the components were merely
20 window dressing. From his knowledge of botany, he suspected that the active principle of the mixture was to be found in only one of the ingredients – the leaves of the foxglove, whose pretty purple flowers dot English gardens in early summer. Accordingly, he began to treat dropsical
25 patients with a tea made with foxglove leaves. In many cases it did indeed relieve them of excess fluid by markedly increasing urine output.

Withering studied the drug for 10 years. He learned to obtain leaves of uniform potency by gathering them at a
30 particular stage of the plant's growth, and he determined the most effective dosage. In 1785, he published his observations. His book, *An Account of the Foxglove and Some of its Medical Uses,* is a classic of painstaking scientific investigation.

35 Unfortunately, the book was ahead of its time. Its basic trouble was one that has beset many studies besides Withering's: lack of information on precisely what the drug did in the body. Withering had carefully catalogued most of the foxglove's externally observable effects: increased urine
40 flow, nausea, purging, disorders of vision and a slowed pulse. ("It has," he noted, "a power over the motions of the heart to a degree yet unobserved in any other medicine.") But neither he nor his successors for generations afterward had either the knowledge or the techniques to determine the
45 effects of the drug inside the body—and therefore the diseases for which it could best be used. Later promiscuously used as a "remedy" for all forms of edema, and sometimes for totally unrelated conditions, the foxglove's effects were so uncertain that many physicians stopped
50 using it entirely.

By 1855, at least one basic fact had become clear: digitalis, as the drug came to be known, did not act directly on the kidneys; its virtues, whatever they might be, lay in what Withering had called its "power over the heart." A
55 French physiologist, Edme Vulpian, thought he knew the nature of the power: digitalis, he said, benefited the patient with an enlarged heart by improving the "tone" of the heart muscle—that is, by increasing its ability to contract— thereby reducing the size of the organ. He concluded,
60 therefore, that the time to use the drug was after the heart had become enlarged—but that course of action was rather like trying to lock the door when the horse was halfway out of the stable. Vulpian was confusing cause and effect. In congestive failure, the heart is not inadequate because it is
65 enlarged; it becomes enlarged because it is inadequate.

494. According to passage information, the "old woman in Shropshire" (lines 14-15) was most likely attempting to:

A. alleviate her patients heart problems.
B. ease swelling in her patients.
C. relieve her patients of excess fluid.
D. teach the more legitimate practitioners.

495. Which of the following statements is the most reasonable conclusion that can be drawn from the author's description of the foxglove?

A. This plant could be harvested at almost any time of the year in England.
B. This plant had been relatively unknown for its medicinal properties.
C. In England the plant was only available in early summer.
D. Digitalis was derived from the leaves of the plant.

496. If the author of the passage was asked, "When is the most effective time to treat a patient with digitalis?" The author's most likely response would be:

A. prior to the heart becoming enlarged.
B. when urine output drops below normal.
C. after verifying initial indications that the heart is becoming enlarged.
D. before swelling has advanced beyond the limbs.

497. Dropsy occurs when "fluid is drawn from the blood into the tissues when there is a higher osmotic pressure in the tissues than in the blood." From this information we can assert that digitalis most likely:

A. equalizes the osmotic pressure in the blood and tissues.
B. decreases the osmotic pressure in the blood.
C. increases the osmotic pressure in the tissues.
D. decreases the osmotic pressure in the tissues.

498. It is little known fact that the English physician was honored for his work in botany when his name was given to a common plant malady. His name is most likely used to describe:

A. the results of a plant going without water for too long.
B. the petals of the foxglove.
C. when a plant has some medicinal value.
D. a plant that has grown too large.

499. Assuming all of Dr. Withering's discoveries were novel, then prior to Withering which of the following properties of digitalis was unknown:

A. that the drug worked primarily on the kidneys.
B. how to obtain an unvaryingly potent form of the drug.
C. in what form the drug should be given.
D. why the drug also caused increased urine output.

500. According to the passage, "Vulpian was confusing cause and effect" (lines 63-64). What distinction is implied in the passage between "cause and effect", respectively?

I. enlarged and inadequate
II. inadequate and enlarged
III. congestive failure and enlarged

A. I only
B. II only
C. III only
D. I and III only

501. Derived from the information contained in the passage, an appropriate theory of pharmacological research for new medicines would state that discovering new medicines involves:

I. understanding the full spectrum of effects associated with that medicine.
II. experiencing the effectiveness of a medicine through native research.
III. communicating the needs of the medical community to local herbalists and natural healers.

A. I only
B. II only
C. I and III only
D. II and III only

STOP. IF YOU FINISH BEFORE TIME IS CALLED, CHECK YOUR WORK. YOU MAY GO BACK TO ANY QUESTION IN THIS TEST BOOKLET.

GO ON TO THE NEXT PAGE.

Biological Sciences

Time: 20 Minutes
Questions 502-517

With the dramatic increase in the percentage of obese Americans over the past several decades, research in satiety and dietary factors has also greatly increased. Satiety is a complex phenomenon governed by several factors, such as the rate of gastric emptying, choleocystokinin (CCK) release, fat content of food ingested (which slows the rate of gastric emptying), and volume of food ingested. Blockade of any one of these factors, however, will not necessarily have any impact on satiety because of the redundancy of mechanisms involved.

Caseins are dietary peptides found in dairy products which are speculated to cause premature meal termination. Once ingested, these peptides are absorbed intact by the small intestine and thought to bind with opioid receptors there. Once bound, the opioid receptors slow gastrointestinal motility, thereby decreasing the rate of gastric emptying, and stimulating a sense of premature satiety. Therefore, administration of a pre-load of casein prior to a meal may reduce overall meal size.

In the following experiment, 80 male white rats were divided into two groups of 40. One group received a pre-load administration of casein prior to feeding, while the other received a pre-load of composite amino acids in solution. In the casein group, half of the rats were also given an intramuscular injection of an opioid antagonist. Half of the rats in the composite amino acid group are also given an IM injection of opioid antagonist. The opioid antagonist used was naltrexone (1mg/kg BW). Overall food intake by each of the four groups is presented in the figure below:

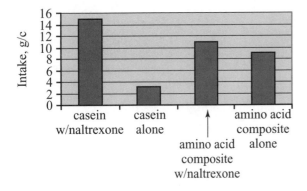

Figure 1 Bar graph of food intake.

502. Heroin is an opioid that is, unfortunately, both highly addictive and commonly abused. Based on the results of the experiment above, it can be inferred that administration of an opioid such as heroin would have what effects on satiety?

 A. Increase satiety, decrease overall food intake
 B. Increase satiety, increase overall food intake
 C. Decrease satiety, decrease overall food intake
 D. Decrease satiety, increase overall food intake

503. Administration of an opioid antagonist alone would most likely have what effect on food intake?

 A. Increase overall food intake
 B. Decrease overall food intake
 C. Decrease gastric motility
 D. No effect

504. According to the passage, satiety is dependent on the stimulation of which of the following systems?

 A. Endocrine
 B. Nervous system
 C. Digestive
 D. Musculoskeletal

505. Morphine is another type of opioid used clinically for its painkilling properties. Which of the following side effects would be seen in an individual who is chronically using morphine-based painkillers?

 A. Depression
 B. Stomach pain
 C. Headache
 D. Constipation

GO ON TO THE NEXT PAGE.

506. Which of the following cell types initiates casein digestion?

- **A.** Epithelial cells of the esophagus
- **B.** Goblet cells of the stomach
- **C.** Chief cells of the stomach
- **D.** Duodenal cells of the small intestine

507. Cholecystokinin (CCK) is released from cells of the duodenum in response to food entering the small intestine. CCK then stimulates the release of digestive enzymes from both the pancreas and bile from the gallbladder. Which of the following foods would most likely elicit the greatest release of CCK?

- **A.** cheeseburger
- **B.** tossed salad with oil-based dressing
- **C.** 2% milk
- **D.** apple

508. Which of the following measures would most strengthen the validity of the study results?

- **I.** An increase in the number of subjects (N)
- **II.** Increased casein dosage
- **III.** Inclusion of another group of rats which receives a saline pre-load
- **IV.** The use of an alternative opioid antagonist

- **A.** I only
- **B.** I and III
- **C.** II only
- **D.** I, III and IV

509. According to the passage, consumption of which of the following may aid in curbing one's appetite?

- **A.** fruit
- **B.** high-fat foods
- **C.** cheese
- **D.** high fiber vegetables

GO ON TO THE NEXT PAGE.

Diuretics are an important class of antihypertensives as they have a relatively benign side effect profile. Simply stated, diuretics increase the amount of urine excreted, thereby reducing the intravascular volume. Although different diuretics act on different segments of the nephron, all diuretics block salt reabsorption in the kidney. As even conventional wisdom would predict, water movement mirrors salt movement and thus water reabsorption is also inhibited.

The mechanisms of action of three major diuretics are depicted in Figure 1. The first diuretic, furosemide, acts by blocking the $Na^+/K^+/2Cl^-$ cotransporter found on the luminal side of the thick ascending loop of Henle. The second diuretic,

hydrochlorothiazide, functions via inhibition of the Na^+/Cl^- cotransporter in the distal convoluted tubule. In normal physiologic conditions, both the ascending loop of Henle and the early distal convoluted tubule are highly permeable to salt and significantly impermeable to water. By blocking salt reuptake in these segments, both furosemide and hydrochlorothiazide compromise the ability of the nephron to dilute the luminal filtrate, resulting in hyperosmotic filtrate being in the collecting tubule.

The third diuretic, spironolactone, antagonizes aldosterone receptors in the kidney.

Aldosterone promotes sodium reuptake in the nephron by stimulating the Na^+/K^+ exchanger in the late distal tubule and collecting tubule.

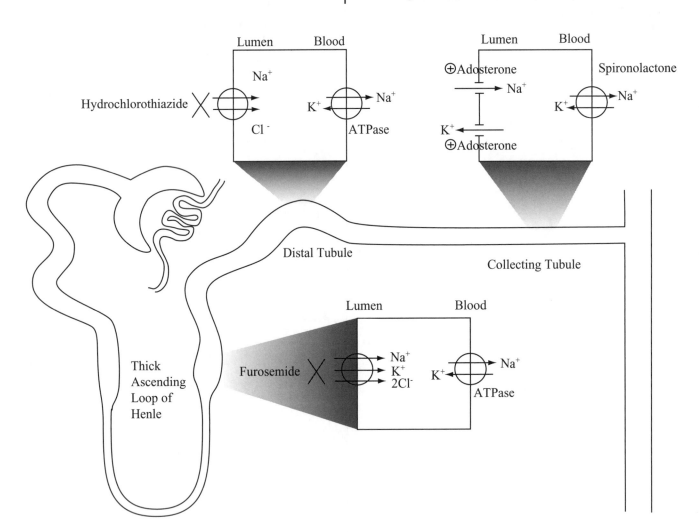

Figure 1 Mechanisms of Action of Three Major Diuretics

GO ON TO THE NEXT PAGE.

510. Serum potassium levels must be monitored when using diuretics. Which of the following diuretics would be expected to raise serum potassium levels?

- **A.** hydrochlorothiazide
- **B.** furosemide
- **C.** spironolactone
- **D.** acetazolamide

511. Sodium and chloride ions enter the cells of the distal convoluted tubule via:

- **A.** primary active transport
- **B.** secondary active transport
- **C.** passive diffusion
- **D.** pinocytosis

512. Angiotensin II stimulates the release of aldosterone and the subsequent increase in sodium retention. Angiotensin II is most likely upregulated in which of the following circumstances?

- **A.** hemorrhage
- **B.** high blood pressure
- **C.** high salt diet
- **D.** high cholesterol diet

513. In the thick ascending loop of Henle, the movement of Na^+, K^+, and Cl^- across the plasma membrane has which of the following effects on membrane potential?

- **A.** increase by 80 mV
- **B.** increase by 40 mV
- **C.** increase by 20 mV
- **D.** increase by 0 mV

514. The diuretics discussed above affect intravascular volume change by modulating salt reuptake in the kidney. Which of the following hormones modulates water reuptake in the kidney?

- **A.** ADH
- **B.** ACTH
- **C.** oxytocin
- **D.** angiotensin I

515. The primary function of the medullary loop of Henle is:

- **A.** amino acid reuptake
- **B.** glucose reuptake
- **C.** volume contraction
- **D.** toxin secretion

516. As discussed above, furosemide blocks the salt reabsorption in the thick ascending loop of Henle. The decrease in salt reabsorption causes an increase in the volume of filtrate that reaches the distal tubule. This volume change is monitored by the:

- **A.** vasa recta
- **B.** juxtaglomerular apparatus
- **C.** Bowman's capsule
- **D.** renal pelvis

197

Question 517 is **NOT** based on a descriptive passage.

517. Aldosterone is produced in the:

    A.   adrenal medulla
    B.   adrenal cortex
    C.   anterior pituitary
    D.   posterior pituitary

STOP. IF YOU FINISH BEFORE TIME IS CALLED, CHECK YOUR WORK. YOU MAY GO BACK TO ANY QUESTION IN THIS TEST BOOKLET.

STOP.

EXAMINATION 12

Questions 518–564

Physical Sciences

Time: 20 Minutes

Questions 518–533

A block attached to a spring, in the absence of friction, will vibrate back and forth across the point of origin in simple harmonic motion. An expression for the speed of the block at any given moment can be derived from the law of conservation of mechanical energy.

$$v = \sqrt{\frac{k}{m}\left(A^2 - x^2\right)}$$

where v is the speed of the block, k is the spring constant for the spring, m is the mass of the block, A is the magnitude of maximum displacement, and x is the displacement from rest at the moment in question.

The period of motion of the block, T, may be calculated using the mass of the block, m, and the value of the spring constant, k.

$$T = 2\pi\sqrt{\frac{m}{k}}$$

The displacement of the block at any given time may be derived from the basic equation for simple harmonic motion.

$$x = A\cos\left(\sqrt{\frac{k}{m}}\right)t$$

where x is the displacement of the block, A is the magnitude of maximum displacement, k is the spring constant, m is the mass, and t is time measured in seconds.

518. The minimum speed of a block in simple harmonic motion is attained when:

    A. $x = 0$
    B. $0 < x < A$
    C. $x = A$
    D. $x > A$

519. Which of the following expressions represents the frequency of motion of a mass vibrating on a spring?

    A. $f = 2\pi\sqrt{\dfrac{m}{k}}$

    B. $f = 2\pi\sqrt{\dfrac{k}{m}}$

    C. $f = \dfrac{1}{2\pi}\sqrt{\dfrac{m}{k}}$

    D. $f = \dfrac{1}{2\pi}\sqrt{\dfrac{k}{m}}$

520. A mass on a spring is pulled to the point of maximum displacement and released. If the mass subsequently vibrates in simple harmonic motion, which of the following diagrams represents the displacement of the block over time?

A.
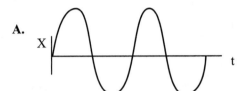

B.
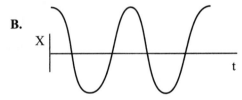

C.
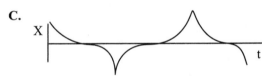

D.
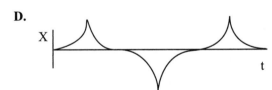

GO ON TO THE NEXT PAGE.

521. In an experiment, four different blocks are attached to four different springs as described in the table below. Once set in harmonic motion, the number of vibrations in one minute are recorded for each trial. Which trial produced the greatest number vibrations?

Trial	Spring constant k (N/m)	Mass m (kg)
1	0.3	0.5
2	0.4	0.4
3	0.5	0.3
4	0.6	0.2

A. Trial 1
B. Trial 2
C. Trial 3
D. Trial 4

522. Which of the following modifications to a block and spring system will result in increased vibration frequency?

A. Increasing the initial displacement of the block.
B. Decreasing the initial displacement of the block.
C. Increasing the mass of the block.
D. Decreasing the mass of the block.

523. At the point of zero displacement, the energy of the block and spring system can best be described as:

A. kinetic.
B. elastic potential.
C. kinetic and elastic potential.
D. kinetic, elastic potential, and heat.

Passage II (Questions 524-530)

Water covers approximately 72 percent of the surface of the Earth. Of the Earth's water, more than 97 percent is salt water found in the oceans, 2 percent is found in polar ice, and less than 1 percent is fresh water. Because of water's high specific heat, 4.184 J/g-°C, the Earth's oceans tend to exert a moderating influence on climate. The specific gravity of seawater varies between 1.02 and 1.03.

Although sodium and chloride make up the majority of the saline ions found in seawater, there are many other ions present in small quantities. The table below delineates the most abundant constituents of the Earth's natural waters.

Ion	g/kg seawater	Molality, m	Molarity, M
Cl^-	19.4	0.57	0.55
Na^+	10.8	0.49	0.47
SO_4^{2-}	2.7	0.029	0.028
Mg^{2+}	1.3	0.055	0.054
Ca^{2+}	0.4	0.011	0.010
K^+	0.4	0.011	0.010

The boiling point elevation constant for water is 1.86° C/mol and the freezing point depression constant is 0.52° C/mol. The heat of fusion of water is 6.01 kJ/mol and the heat of vaporization for water is 40.79 kJ/mol.

524. The climate of a city in the center of a large landmass would be expected to differ from the climate of a coastal city. The city in the center of the landmass:

A. will be warmer in the summer and cooler in the winter.
B. will be cooler in the summer and warmer in the winter.
C. will be warmer in the summer and winter.
D. will be cooler in the summer and winter.

525. What is the approximate freezing point of seawater?

A. –4.32° C
B. –2.16° C
C. –1.21° C
D. –0.60° C

526. Which of the following processes could be used to recover fresh water from seawater?

A. filtration
B. neutralization
C. distillation
D. decomposition

203

GO ON TO THE NEXT PAGE.

527. The quantity of ions present in seawater is often conveyed in parts-per-million (ppm). If 1 ppm is equal to 1 mg/kg, what is the quantity of magnesium ions in seawater?

A. 0.0013 ppm
B. 1.3 ppm
C. 130 ppm
D. 1300 ppm

528. Which of the following statements best describes the vapor pressure of a fresh water lake in comparison to the vapor pressure of the ocean at the same temperature?

A. Vapor pressure is greater for the lake because the ocean has a greater concentration of dissolved particles.
B. Vapor pressure is smaller for the lake because the ocean has a greater concentration of dissolved particles.
C. Vapor pressure is greater for the lake because the ocean has greater exposed surface area.
D. Vapor pressure is smaller for the lake because the ocean has greater exposed surface area.

529. Molarity is a measure of moles per volume of solution, whereas molality is a measure of:

A. grams per mass of solvent.
B. grams per mass of solution.
C. moles per mass of solvent.
D. moles per mass of solution.

530. Which of the following best describes the energy change when 180 g of water freezes?

A. 60 kJ of energy is absorbed by the water.
B. 60 kJ of energy is released by the water.
C. 400 kJ of energy is absorbed by the water.
D. 400 kJ of energy is released by the water.

Questions 531 through 533 are **NOT** based on a descriptive passage.

531. A guitar player tunes her A-string by comparing its frequency to a pure tone with a frequency of 440 Hz. When the two waves are superimposed, a beat frequency of 4 Hz is heard. The frequency of the guitar string is most likely:

A. 110 Hz
B. 436 Hz
C. 438 Hz
D. 440 Hz

532. Which of the following phase changes is most likely to occur when the pressure on a sample of H_2O is increased at constant temperature?

A. sublimation
B. melting
C. freezing
D. vaporization

533. A 3.0 meter long organ pipe is closed at one end. What are the wavelengths of the first three harmonics?

A. 12 m, 4 m, 2.4 m
B. 12 m, 6 m, 3 m
C. 6 m, 3 m, 2 m
D. 6 m, 2 m, 0.5 m

STOP. IF YOU FINISH BEFORE TIME IS CALLED, CHECK YOUR WORK. YOU MAY GO BACK TO ANY QUESTION IN THIS TEST BOOKLET.

STOP.

Verbal Reasoning

Time: 20 Minutes
Questions 534–548

With such masterful dexterity the hand moves when attended by weathered experience and cooled deliberation. The tyro most often sports neither advantage. In a doyens grip, the scalpel seems little more than a painter's brush
5 dancing in choreographed movements sharp, abrupt, and swift. The neophyte, on the other hand, must resign himself to cavort in leaden shoes.

When an empty canvas lies before an artisan in training, it is generally agreed that the hardest stroke evoked is
10 the first. The cold, dead stare of the cadaver, the distinct, permeating stench of formaldehyde in the lab, the loud, steady buzzing of tube lights overhead- all of these are of little consequence. However, one must not be tempted to assume that once in progress, the quandaries of dissection
15 resolve themselves. Rather, they only continue.

The first difficulty is in determining the degree of pressure that is to be applied, or more precisely, how deep to make any given cut. In the anterior neck region, deep incisions would obviate any opportunity to appreciate the
20 extremely superficial platysma muscle that lies almost immediately subjacent to the skin, and extends inferiorly in a fan like shape to drape over the superior quadrants of the anterior thoracic wall. In the lower extremities, on the other hand, superficial dissection will be of little benefit to the
25 dissector other than keeping him in the lab until much after everyone else has left.

Then there is always the issue of navigating between the veins, arteries, and nerves that lattice the bony-muscular regions of the body in what feels like almost a vine like
30 fashion. What lies immediately underlies the area under question is hardly known. It is veritably like treading landmined terrain. Netter lying on the gurney, soaked in formalinesque solution is of little aid to the bewildered student. The spatial complexities that associate themselves
35 with dissection yield exceeding reluctantly to resolution via reference to two-dimensional images.

What else can be said of dissection? One should be well prepared to find himself, or herself, in almost the same state of affairs, no structures located, no vasculature identi
40 fied, and yet an entire hour having passed with only random, hesitant pokings to show for the tedious moments thus passed. Doing one's best being the raison d'etre for staying; dissection is a slow process. What is more, the lab manual is of questionable assistance. "Make an incision 5
45 cm from the point demarcating a position 1 cm medial to the coracoacromial joint toward the sternal notch making sure to stay parallel to the clavicular contour and keeping the scalpel superficial to the facial plane of the pectoralis major..." A student is not left entirely to his own devices
50 though. There are his colleagues and hovering lab instructors that many times will eventually dissect the body for

those less experienced and demonstrate relevant lab structures. Somehow, in the end, some learning does occur.

At the heart of the difficulties that rhizomatically gird
55 the dissection process, lies the challenge of taking capacious amount of knowledge and applying it outside the context of rote recall. The fledgling dissector, as I must invariably be categorized, is driven to use his yet fragile knowledge of anatomy to provide markers in guiding him
60 through the thousands of three-dimensional spatial decisions that present at every turn of the scalpel. However, as the days steady his hand and labor his markers, the student's scalpel too begins to swing, just a bit.

534. The author of this passage is most likely a(n)

    A.   Anatomy lab instructor
    B.   Editor for a dissection manual
    C.   A medical student
    D.   A board-certified physician

535. The author would be most likely to agree that dissection is

    A.   a tedious process
    B.   an acquired art*
    C.   a fun pastime
    D.   loathsome experience

GO ON TO THE NEXT PAGE.

536. According to the passage above, to become an apt and dexterous dissector requires

    A.   A strong knowledge base, experience, and patience*

    B.   Patience and a passion for anatomy

    C.   A strong knowledge base and steady, skillful hand

    D.   Ability to discern how deep to cut the cadaver and navigate around vasculature

537. "Netter" (line 32) is most likely

    A.   a lab instructor

    B.   an anatomy student

    C.   an author of an anatomy atlas*

    D.   the name of the cadaver

538. If the anatomy lab in discussion were to be remodeled to provide a warmer, more relaxing ambiance, this would

    A.   make the dissection process less stressful and distasteful

    B.   increase the efficiency with which dissection is done in the lab

    C.   facilitate the application of anatomic knowledge in spatial decision making

    D.   make little or no difference*

539. According to the author, most first time dissectors feel

    A.   bewildered because they do not have a strong foundational knowledge of anatomy

    B.   frustrated by an inability to make appropriate and/or definitive decisions during the dissection process *

    C.   excited by the challenge and promise of dissecting a cadaver

    D.   angst because of the long hours required of anatomy lab

540. In the author's perspective, which of the following changes would result in the greatest benefit to new dissectors?

    A.   More lab instructors to dissect out and demonstrate important lab structures*

    B.   More colleagues per cadaver

    C.   Shorter laboratory sessions

    D.   Better ancillary reading materials

541. From the author's tone, it can be most directly inferred that the lab dissection manual is

    A.   Helpful but verbose

    B.   Circumlocutory

    C.   Difficult to read and apply *

    D.   Well written but too advanced for starting dissectors

GO ON TO THE NEXT PAGE.

To all monomaniacs seeking acceptance in the world, I reiterate the advice of a certain sea-captain: "Hark ye yet again,—the little lower layer." It is of singular import for all those who traverse the capricious road of life, to understand
5 the nature of that which they traverse. What is greater, such an understanding does not simply elucidate what is, but more importantly guides one to what should be. This is the intent.

In our reality, there is no concept of a static existence,
10 for we are continually moving. Our motion is both physical and metaphysical. Newton concerned himself with laws that govern the former. Enumeration of his three laws of motion would be mundane, so simple allusion will be deemed sufficient in the ensuing analysis of metaphysical
15 motion. First, in observing the behavior of those who are content and those who are not, we find that he who is content remains in that state until he sees something that he wants. Once his wants are set in motion, he will continue to want. An outside force will either give impetus to this desire
20 or mitigate it. Secondly, the change in desire is directly proportionate to the magnitude of the outside force. Knowledge that man cannot fly palliates his desire to, say, jump from a tenth story window. Lastly, for our every action there is an equal and opposite, not necessarily negative,
25 reaction. If there were not, what would motivate us to do? We expect with our every action to receive something that is at least equal to what we expend.

In Newton's ideal laws, we do find but one imperfection. His physical laws fold at extreme velocities. Similarly,
30 our "Newtonian" metaphysical laws fail in cases of extreme human behavior. Einstein asserted that there was an interchange between the mass and energy. On the metaphysical level, this corresponds to the interchange, the conversion rather, of that which is material into that which is spiritual.
35 He who commits suicide is willing to accept the material opportunity cost of losing his life for the spiritual liberation from turmoil. Now we have a something of unified theory of human behavior that accounts for both the commonalities and the peculiarities of man's nature.

40 This nature is residence to man's denizen want to acquire the regard of others. Man strives to remove himself from isolation, to gain not just acceptance, but favor, in the eyes of others. The current "outside forces" of various media and popular culture act in the same direction as this
45 want—giving it impetus, accelerating it. This desire now underlies all society's actions. Of what worth is a mansion if there be no one to admire you for it? Why do not we dress up at home on Saturday mornings?

In this age of reason over emotion, in this modern
50 reliving of neo-classicism, all our levels of our logic are concentric about the above desire. It is the rationalizing

exponent of all that we do. We, like the Frankenstein monster, absolve ourselves from accountability by reasoning that our unacceptance by society at large is substantial
55 reason to do as we will to gain that acceptance. We justify; we use Frankenstein logic.

If Newton is an idealist, Victor Frankenstein a genius, and Einstein an interchange proponent who favors the spiritual over material, then I cannot much argue with David
60 Russell when he states that we "live in a Newtonian world of Eisteinian physics ruled by Frankenstein logic." However, I, for one, would much rather live in an Einsteinian world of Frankenstein physics ruled by Newtonian logic.

542. From the first paragraph we can infer that the author

    I. is an enthusiast of literature from the Romantic genre
    II. feels that society must actively participate in their existence
    III. believes that life is unpredictable

    A. I and II
    B. II and III*
    C. I, II, and III
    D. only II

543. According to the framework set up by the passage, an ascetic monk who has no worldly desire or wants would most like be characterized by

    A. "Newtonian" metaphysics
    B. "Einsteinian" metaphyics*
    C. Frankenstein logic
    D. Such an individual does not fit into the framework of this passage

544. What is the role of the "outside forces" of media and culture (line 43-44)?

- **A.** They accelerate human wants according to Newtonian metaphysics
- **B.** The "outside forces" are a metaphysical manifestations of the Frankenstein monster
- **C.** The "outside forces" reinforce man's desire to be wanted and in doing so form a basis on which he can rationalize otherwise unethical behaviors
- **D.** A and C are both correct

545. "If an individual likes chocolate, seeing a chocolate ice cream cone will be more motivating than a vanilla ice cream cone." This statement illustrates which of the author's Newtonian metaphysical principles?

- **A.** The first Newtonian metaphysical principle
- **B.** The second Newtonian metaphysical principle
- **C.** The third Newtonian metaphysical principle
- **D.** It doe not illustrate any of the Newtonian metaphysical principles presented by the author

546. Which of the following most directly challenges the author's views?

- **A.** Victor Frankenstein was not a genius
- **B.** The Frankenstein monster is a symbol of society's readiness to overlook the morality of means in their eagerness to acquire a certain end.
- **C.** The underlying motivator of people's action is not to gain the favor of others, but rather to ultimately avoid incurring physical harm
- **D.** Newtonian physical and metaphysical laws are not absolute

547. What world does the author refer to when he states that he would rather "live in an Einsteinian world of Frankenstein physics ruled by Newtonian logic?"

- **I.** The present world as defined by postmodernist theory
- **II.** A world in which spiritual goals are primary and metaphysics are subordinate to this goal
- **III.** A world in people action are guided by logical and constrained by the parameters of normative human behavior

- **A.** I and III
- **B.** II and III*
- **C.** I, II, and III
- **D.** None of the above

548. The author's purpose in writing this passage is best delineated by which of the following statements?

- **A.** to offer a conceptual framework to help the reader understand human nature
- **B.** to equate physical laws to their corresponding metaphysical realities
- **C.** to define the rules of logic
- **D.** to convince the reader of the author's worldview

STOP. IF YOU FINISH BEFORE TIME IS CALLED, CHECK YOUR WORK. YOU MAY GO BACK TO ANY QUESTION IN THIS TEST BOOKLET.

Biological Sciences
Time: 20 Minutes
Questions 549–564

The Hinsberg Test may be utilized to distinguish a primary amine from a secondary amine. In this assay, an unknown amine is reacted with benzenesulfonyl chloride to form a benzenesulfonamide (Reaction 1).

Reaction 1

If the unknown is a primary amine, the benzesulfonamide formed will have an acidic proton. The reaction solvent, sodium hydroxide, will subsequently remove this acidic proton forming a charged, soluble product. As a result, the assay will produce a product from the primary amine that is soluble in the sodium hydroxide solvent. The benzenesulfonamide formed from a secondary amine, however, does not contain an acidic proton and will thus precipitate out of solution. A primary amine will also result in an insoluble solid once the reaction mixture is acidified.

In a similar reaction to the Hinsberg Test, both primary and secondary amines react with benzoyl chloride (Reaction 2) to produce an insoluble benzamide derivative.

Reaction 2

Scientists in a research lab perform both assays on five unknown amine compounds. After they form the benzenesulfonamide and benzamide derivatives, the scientists reference the melting points of these compounds to elucidate the identity of the original amine. Their conclusions and data are presented in Table I below.

Compound	Structure	Boiling Point	Melting Point Benzenesulfonamide	Melting Point Benzamide
1		200	124	144
2		196	79	63
3		185	88	105
4		185	101	120
5		129	118	75

549. A benzamide is formed by reaction of an amine with benzyol chloride. What type of compound is benzoyl chloride?

A. ketone
B. aldehyde
C. acid chloride
D. alkyl halide

550. If compound 3 is dissolved in water, what would be true of the pH of the solution?

A. 0 pH
B. $pH > 7$
C. $pH < 7$
D. $pH = 7$

551. The Hinsberg assay's ability to differentiate primary and secondary amines depends on the removal of an acidic Hydrogen from primary amine benzenesulfonamide derivatives. In Reaction 2, however, the benzamide derivative of a primary amine is not deprotonated in similar reaction conditions. The sulfonamide proton must be more acidic than the amide proton because:

A. Sulfonamides have higher molecular weight.

B. The sulfonamide has an extra oxygen, which is electron donating.

C. The benzamide anion has more resonance structures delocalizing negative charge

D. The benzenesulfonamide anion has more resonance structures delocalizing the negative charge

552. If the scientists reacted compound 4 with benzoyl chloride in sodium hydroxide, the product would be:

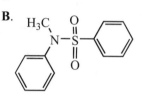

553. Which of the following compounds would form a white solid when reacted with benzenesulfonyl chloride in sodium hydroxide?

A. 1
B. 2
C. 3
D. 4

554. An unknown amine is reacted with benzenesulfonyl chloride in sodium hydroxide. After the reaction, the solution remains clear until the scientists add HCl. The solution then becomes cloudy and a white solid is isolated and dried. The melting point of the crude solid is found to be 82. From Table I, the unknown amine is most likely:

A. Compound 2
B. Compound 3
C. Compound 4
D. Compound 5

555. When forming the benzamide derivatives, the benzoyl chloride is added to the amine and then the sodium hydroxide is added. If the sodium hydroxide reacts with benzoyl chloride instead of the amine, which product would result?

A. benzamide
B. benzenesulfonamide
C. benzoic acid
D. methyl benzoate

Methyl benzoate undergoes hydrolysis in the presence of sodium hydroxide and acetone to yield benzoic acid (shown below). Students in an organic chemistry lab follow the reaction by removing aliquots of the reaction solution, ceasing the reaction with the addition of acid, and measuring the respective amounts of reactants and products. They repeat this procedure at several time intervals. The students obtain the concentration of benzoic acid present in each aliquot using titration. Through stoichometry, the students calculate the concentration of methyl benzoate, and then extrapolate the reaction rate from their data.

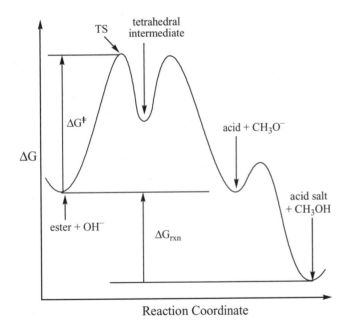

Reaction 1

The rate-determining step for the reaction is the formation of the tetrahedral intermediate when the hydroxide ion attacks the carbonyl. The reaction coordinate diagram shows that the largest activation energy is for formation of this transition state.

tetrahedral
TS intermediate

$\Delta G^{\ddagger}$

acid + CH_3O^-

ΔG

acid salt
+ CH_3OH

ester + OH^-

ΔG_{rxn}

Reaction Coordinate

Figure 1

The students discover that the rate of the reaction may be modulated via the addition of substituents to the benzyl ring. The rate-determining transition state generates a negative charge. Thus substituents that destablize the charge slow down the reaction while electron-withdrawing-substituents increase the reaction rate. Such manipulation of reaction rates allows therapeutic applications, such as the time release of medications.

556. What is the structure of the tetrahedral intermediate for the reaction of benzoic acid?

A.

B.

OH

C.

D.

OH

557. Which of the following substituents would speed up the hydrolysis when added to the benzyl ring?

A. para nitro
B. para methoxy
C. para hydroxy
D. para methyl

558. The students most likely used which of the following reagents to stop the hydrolysis reaction?

A. NaOH
B. NH_3
C. NaCl
D. HCl

559. According to the reaction coordinate diagram, which of the following steps in the hydrolysis reaction proceeds fastest?

A. formation of the tetrahedral intermediate
B. formation of the methoxyl group
C. formation of acid salt
D. nucleophilic attack of the carbonyl

560. The students correctly assert that the final reaction step is thermodynamically favored as a result of the benzoate anion's stability. Why is the benzoate anion more stable than that of the methoxide?

- **A.** The benzoate anion has a higher molecular weight.
- **B.** The methyl group of methoxide is electron withdrawing.
- **C.** The methoxide anion has a lone pair of electrons.
- **D.** The negative charge is resonance stabilized in the benzoate anion.

561. Benzoic acid may also be synthesized from toluene. Which of the following reagents should the students utilize to achieve this conversion?

- **A.** any oxidizing agent
- **B.** H_2/Pd
- **C.** HCl
- **D.** NaOH

562. Methyl benzoate may be formed by reacting methanol with benzoic acid. Which of the following reaction conditions would NOT increase the formation of methyl benzoate?

- **A.** the addition of sodium hydroxide to the reaction mixture
- **B.** The use of methanol as a solvent
- **C.** the removal of water from the reaction mixture
- **D.** the substitution of benzyl chloride for benzoic acid

Questions 563 and 564 are **NOT** based on a descriptive passage.

563. Which of the following nucleophiles is most likely to react with propyl benzoate to form a new product?

- **A.** CH_2OH
- **B.** NH_3
- **C.** CH_3COOH
- **D.** Cl^-

564. If optically pure L-lactic acid has a rotation of $-12.5°$, which of the following values represents the rotation of plane polarized light by its enantiomer?

- **A.** $-12.5°$
- **B.** $+12.5°$
- **C.** 0
- **D.** $+25°$

STOP. IF YOU FINISH BEFORE TIME IS CALLED, CHECK YOUR WORK. YOU MAY GO BACK TO ANY QUESTION IN THIS TEST BOOKLET.

EXAMINATION 13

Questions 565–611

Physical Sciences

Time: 20 Minutes
Questions 565–580

Passage I (Questions 565-571)

Designers of electric circuits rely on the fact that the resistance of electrical conductors is not constant, but varies with length, cross-sectional area, and temperature. The dependence of resistance on length and area is demonstrated by the equation:

$$R = \rho \frac{L}{A}$$

where R is the resistance of a wire, ρ is the resistivity of the conductor, L is the length of the wire in meters, and A is the cross-sectional area of the wire in m^2.

The equation below shows resistance as a function of temperature:

$$R = R_o[1 + \alpha(T - T_o)]$$

where R_o is the resistance at some reference temperature T_o, α is the temperature coefficient of resistivity, and R is the resistance at temperature T.

The table below provides some data for various conductors.

Conductor	ρ^a (Ω–m)	α (1/K)	R^b (Ω)
Copper	1.7×10^{-8}	3.9×10^{-3}	0.05
Aluminum	2.8×10^{-8}	3.9×10^{-3}	0.09
Platinum	1.1×10^{-7}	3.9×10^{-3}	0.34
Lead	2.2×10^{-7}	3.9×10^{-3}	0.68
Iron	1.1×10^{-7}	5.0×10^{-3}	0.31
Tungsten	5.6×10^{-8}	4.5×10^{-3}	0.17

[a] Resistivity values are given for a temperature of 293 K.
[b] Resistances are given for a cylindrical wire with a radius of 0.32 mm and a length of 1 m at a temperature of 293 K.

Table 1

Some conductors show a dramatic zeroing of resistance below a critical temperature, and are accordingly termed, "superconductors". Lead, for example, becomes a superconductor at temperatures below 7.18 K. Because the resistance in a superconductor is effectively equal to zero, once a current is established, it will continue to flow without any need for applied voltage. Currents have been observed to flow in superconducting circuits for months to years without energy loss.

Note: Assume all wires have a radius of 0.32 mm unless otherwise specified.

565. An increase in which of the following variables will result in increased wire resistance?

   I.   Temperature
   II. Length
   III. Area

   A.   II only
   B.   I and II only
   C.   I and III only
   D.   II and III only

566. Which of the following conductors, when used for an electrical application, would requires the LEAST amount of power?

   A.   Copper
   B.   Aluminum
   C.   Platinum
   D.   Iron

567. What is the resistance of a 1 meter-long iron wire at a temperature of 273 K?

   A.   0.21 Ω
   B.   0.28 Ω
   C.   0.34 Ω
   D.   0.39 Ω

568. Resistance thermometers are sometimes used to measure boiling and freezing points. The greater the change in resistance over the given temperature range, the more accurate the resistance thermometer will be. Which of the following metals will make the most accurate resistance thermometer?

   A.   Copper
   B.   Aluminum
   C.   Iron
   D.   Tungsten

569. A current of 10 A is transmitted over a kilometer-long copper wire with a radius of 0.32 mm. How much power is lost in transmitting the current through the wire?

   A.   5 W
   B.   50 W
   C.   500 W
   D.   5000 W

GO ON TO THE NEXT PAGE.

570. A one meter long tungsten wire with a radius of 0.32 mm is placed in a circuit so that it conducts a current of 4 A. If the wire is replaced by a one meter long tungsten wire with a radius of 0.64 mm, what is the current conducted by the new wire?

A. 1 A
B. 2 A
C. 8 A
D. 16 A

571. What is the resistance per meter of a cylindrical aluminum wire with a cross-sectional area of 0.96 mm?

A. 0.01 Ω/m
B. 0.03 Ω/m
C. 0.27 Ω/m
D. 0.81 Ω/m

Passage II (Questtons 572-579)

Aqueous salt solutions may be acidic or basic depending on the properties of the anions and cations present. Salts such as $NaC_2H_3O_2$ will produce basic aqueous solutions while others, such as NH_4Cl, will produce acidic solutions. Salts which are made from the conjugates of a strong acid and a strong base, such as NaCl, will produce neutral solutions.

The base dissociation constants for various anions are given in the table below.

Anion	Base constant K_b
$C_2H_3O_2^-$	5.6×10^{-10}
ClO^-	3.3×10^{-7}
F^-	1.5×10^{-11}
HS^-	1.8×10^{-7}
S^{2-}	7.7×10^{-2}
Cl^-	no reaction
HCO_3^-	2.3×10^{-8}
CO_3^{2-}	1.8×10^{-4}

572. Which of the following expressions represents the base dissociation for a solution containing fluorine ions?

A. $K_b = \dfrac{[F^-][OH^-]}{[HF]}$

B. $K_b = \dfrac{[F^-][OH^-]}{[H_2O]}$

C. $K_b = \dfrac{[HF][H_2O]}{[F^-]}$

D. $K_b = \dfrac{[HF][OH^-]}{[F^-]}$

573. When solid KHS is dissolved in pure water, the solution will be:

A. acidic because K_a for HS^- is greater than K_b for HS^-.
B. basic because K_a for HS^- is greater than K_b for HS^-.
C. acidic because K_a for HS^- is less than K_b for HS^-.
D. basic because K_a for HS^- is less than K_b for HS^-.

574. A chemist prepares a 1.0 M solution of KClO. The solution will be:

   A. acidic as ClO^- reacts with water to form hydrogen ions.
   B. acidic as K^+ reacts with water to form hydrogen ions.
   C. basic as ClO^- reacts with water to form hydroxide ions.
   D. basic as K^+ reacts with water to form hydroxide ions.

575. A 1 M solution of which of the following acids will have the lowest pH?

   A. $HC_2H_3O_2$
   B. HF
   C. HClO
   D. HCO_3^-

576. A student made a buffer solution by combining equal volumes of 1 M $HC_2H_3O_2$ and 1 M $NaC_2H_3O_2$. Which of the following expressions should the student use to calculate the pH of the solution?

   A. $-\log\left(5.6 \times 10^{-10}\right)$

   B. $-\log\left(\dfrac{1 \times 10^{-14}}{5.6 \times 10^{-10}}\right)$

   C. $-\log\left(\dfrac{5.6 \times 10^{-10}}{1 \times 10^{-14}}\right)$

   D. $-\log\left(\dfrac{1}{1}\right)$

Questions 577 through 580 are **NOT** based on a descriptive passage.

577. An electron and a proton are projected into a magnetic field at identical speeds. The direction of motion for both particles is perpendicular to the field lines. The electron and proton will experience magnetic forces of:

   A. equal magnitude in the same direction.
   B. different magnitude in different directions.
   C. equal magnitudes in different directions.
   D. different magnitudes in the same direction.

578. What is the approximate pH of a 0.015 M HNO_3 solution?

   A. 0.5
   B. 1.8
   C. 2.3
   D. 3.5

579. When water is added to a buffered solution, the pH of the solution will:

   A. always increase.
   B. always decrease.
   C. always move closer to 7.
   D. not change.

580. A beaker contains 200 ml of a 0.1 M H_2SO_4 solution. Which of the following expressions depicts the relative concentrations of the three species in the beaker?

   A. $[H_2SO_4] > [HSO_4^-] > [H^+]$
   B. $[H^+] > [HSO_4^-] > [H_2SO_4]$
   C. $[H_2SO_4] > [H^+] > [HSO_4^-]$
   D. $[HSO_4^-] > [H^+] > [H_2SO_4]$

STOP. IF YOU FINISH BEFORE TIME IS CALLED, CHECK YOUR WORK. YOU MAY GO BACK TO ANY QUESTION IN THIS TEST BOOKLET.

STOP.

Verbal Reasoning

Time: 20 Minutes
Questions 581–585

...Materialism is frustrating the collective progress of humanity because it, by implication and in total, only allots for the advancement of a few in the long run. So, there is a moral argument against materialism. Materialism may be
5 defined as any hope, aspiration, or love of procuring means that yield benefits at the superficial or physical level, which, in turn, satisfy any individual that obtains them.

Logic speaks against materialism. How much money, or any material mean for that matter, does it take to be rich
10 or, in more general terms, satisfied. Of the myriad answers evoked, all answers must necessarily possess the commonality that it is some amount above and beyond what is needed for survival. How do we designate the magnitude of this marginal amount? It cannot be designated. Unlike the
15 amount that is required for survival, an objective quantity, the marginal amount is subjective and therefore open-ended. A marginal amount cannot be determined and acquired because the interpretations of that amount, in accordance with the breadth of intellectual thought, are infi-
20 nite. Man cannot procure an undefined entity, the marginal amount, and as a result, is precluded from deriving the benefits that stem therefrom.

Economics speaks against materialism. The theory of diminishing marginal utility states that the consumption of
25 successive units of any product yields less and less satisfaction. Materialism is a paradox. The more we get, the less we are getting states the law. So, if this trend of diminishing utility continues, then the acquisition of additional material units moves one farther away from his goal of becoming
30 satisfied with the attainment of material seeing as how more and more is required to supply less and less. One who adopts materialism as his dogma inadvertently distances himself from his end.

Experience speaks against materialism. Materialism is
35 too unwieldy an element to be controlled. This is something inherent to materialism. More often than not, man ends up serving material rather than it serving him. In the pursuit of satisfaction through material means the goal somehow always gets lost. When the pursuit becomes confined to one
40 of material itself, the quest becomes one of a means, not an end, and hence, the end is lost.

It is not possible to correct for materialism by modifying or qualifying it as something else. As discussed above, its flaws are internal, not external. One cannot attain
45 the aims (pleasure/satisfaction) of materialism because materialism itself will not allow it. To correct materialism implies altering its inner structure. Then, one of two things can occur. The alteration will either give rise to a completely new entity or a modified version of the original
50 paradigm of materialism. In the former case, we are, by definition, no longer dealing with materialism and the subject of debate has changed. In the latter case, the possibility of new structural fallacies arising is probable as we are dealing with a modified version of materialism. In seek-
55 ing to rectify those structural fallacies, one of two things must again occur. It is a vicious cycle not unlike the one within which are caught many economists, classical and Keynesians alike, as they endeavor to maintain their platforms.

60 The alternative to materialism is simple, abandoning it without abandoning material itself. Everything then starts to fall into place. This even resolves the fundamental problematic of economics—how to satiate unlimited desires with limited material or resources. Seeing as how we cannot
65 make resources unlimited, the only thing to do is limit our desires. By removing the attachment to material, we curtail desire. Without wanting more, we close the open end. We become content with what we have. We become satisfied.

581. The main purpose of the passage is

    A.   To institute economic reform in the face of globalization
    B.   To convince the reader to abandon materialism
    C.   To show the inherent flaws in materialism
    D.   All of the above

582. What factors does the author believe argue against materialism?

    A.   Politics, psychology, and economics, and morality
    B.   Psychology, logic, and economics
    C.   Experience, logic, morality, and economics*
    D.   Logic, experience, and economics

GO ON TO THE NEXT PAGE.

583. What alternative does the author offer to materialism?

    A. To accept materialism without reservation so as to break the vicious cycle created by Keynesian and classical economists

    B. To leave attachment to material but retain material possession

    C. To renounce all material objects

    D. To modify materialism to generate a new construct that is new and distinct yet still related to the original ideation of materialism

584. Which of the following most naturally and powerfully strengthens a gap in the argument presented in paragraph 2, " Logic speaks against materialism…" (lines 8-18)?

    A. Human desire, like the scope of his determinations of the marginal amount, is infinite.

    B. It is impossible to acquire something that cannot be defined by society.

    C. The magnitude of the marginal amount cannot even be determined individually as a person's psychological perception of what is satisfying is in constant flux.

    D. The argument is well formed and there is no gap in the argument

585. Which of the following is the biggest shortcoming of the argument presented in paragraph 5, "Materialism cannot be corrected…" (lines 42-51),

    A. Not expounding on the internal flaws in materialism.

    B. Not addressing the ramifications of gross conceptual modification of materialism as an idea

    C. The structural fallacies proposed by the author were not defined and the possibility of such fallacies not arising was not addressed.

    D. The argument is sound and has absolutely no shortcomings.

586. If the government were to institute a new federal program to equally distribute societal resources, the author would most likely respond with

    A. Exuberance as it resolves the socioeconomic disparities that the author is primarily occupied with

    B. Reserved approbation because such a program would not address or resolve the individual attachment to material wealth and acquisition

    C. Sadness at the materialistic backlash from the bourgeoning class that would inevitably ensue

    D. Fear because such a move would diminish the validity of the theory of diminishing marginal utility

587. All of the following are examples of an internal flaw of materialism EXCEPT

    A. It helps the rich get richer and this is to the severe disadvantage of the impoverished*

    B. Less pleasure is derived with the acquisition of successive material goods, moving one away from the aim of materialism which is to find pleasure in material goods

    C. Materialism tends to lead one to place greater emphasis on the acquisition of means rather than ends

    D. Materialism's nature and goals are difficult constructs to define, making the aims of materialism impossible to acquire

... A beginning student of *Tahfeezul-Quran* (memorizing the Quran) must complete two lessons a day. The first lesson is termed *Sabaq (pl. Asbaaq)* and consists of a new Arabic text that is to be memorized. In the morning, the student will go to his teacher and repeat the Arabic text after the teacher. The amount of *Sabaq* varies according to the student's ability. If the student makes a mistake in reading the diacritical marks or otherwise errs, then the teacher will correct him. Then the student will return to his place and begin to memorize his *Sabaq*. This involves reading a few words repeatedly until one can reproduce the text without looking into the Quran. We can term these first set of memorized words the first unit. The next few words are similarly repeated until this unit is also memorized. Then the student will repeat the first and second units together. If he can do so without looking in the Quran, he will move on to the next few words, for our purposes termed the 'third unit'. If he cannot, then the first and second units must continually repeated till they can be recited without reference to the Quran. In this manner, subsequent units are added until the entire lesson that the teacher had dispensed is completed.

Most often, however, the student will not start back from the first unit every time he finishes a new unit. For example, by the time the student gets to the twenty-ninth unit, it would simply take too much time to go back and repeat from the first unit every time he completes an additional unit. Instead, the student goes back only fifteen or twenty units. As a consequence, the aggregate set of repeated units shifts forward with every additional unit that is memorized. Then, once the number of beginning units not included in the aggregate set of repeated units becomes substantial, the student will stop and repeat those beginning units again with the current set of repeated units till he can read the entire portion without reference to the Quran. Upon finishing his *Sabaq*, the student must go to his teacher and recite the lesson entirely from memory. The teacher will correct any mistakes.

The second lesson that a neophyte memorizer must recite to his teacher daily is termed *Sabaq-e-Para*. This involves reciting previous lessons (*Asbaaq*) from the *Juz (pl. Ajzaa)* that the student is currently memorizing (The Quran is divided into thirty equal parts. Each one of these parts is called a *Juz*). Different teachers assign varying amounts of *Sabaq-e-Para*. Some teachers require the student to recite all the lessons from the current *Juz* up to the current *Sabaq*. Other teachers will only require the student to go back six to nine *Asbaaq*. In this circumstance, the *Sabaq-e-Para* would shift forward with each new *Sabaq* the student recites leaving the beginning *Asbaaq* of the *Juz* unrevised. When the student finishes the *Juz*, he must recite it from memory to his teacher from beginning to end.

Once a student finishes memorizing his or her first *Juz*, he is no longer a beginner. He will thereon forth have to recite a third lesson everyday called *Amukhta*. This is comprised of revision from *Ajzaa* that the student has already memorized. Depending on the teacher, the student will recite from memory anywhere from one-fourth to two *Ajzaa* of *Amukhta* daily. This ensures that the student does not forget what was previously memorized. From time to time, the student will also undergo formal examinations in which he or she is "spot" tested from that portion of the Quran they have memorized. Upon finally finishing the memorization of the entire Quran, the student will do multiple revisions of the Quran wherein one to ten *Ajzaa* of the Quran are recited daily. Finally, when the teacher perceives that the student is ready, the student is graduated.

588. Which of the following can be directly ascertained from the passage

   I.   Variability in the amount of Sabaq recited depends on teachers' preferences.

  II. The amount of Sabaq-e-Para recited daily depends on the teacher requirements

 III. Teachers assign varying amounts of Amukhta to their students

   A.   I and III
   B.   II only
   C.   II and III
   D.   I, II, and III

589. According to the passage, which of the following is a similarity between *Sabaq-e-Para* and *Amukhta*

   A.   Both require a lot of time to memorize and recite
   B.   Both must be completed daily by the beginning memorizer
   C.   Both can potentially require reciting more than one Juz depending on the teacher
   D.   None of the above

590. "Spot"-tested in line 62 most likely refers to which of the following

   A. Asking the student to recite everything that they have memorized so far

   B. Prompting the student from random points and asking them to recite what comes afterward

   C. Asking the student to recite verses from different *Juz* while looking into the Quran

   D. Request the student to clean any soilage, discoloration, or spots in their Quran to test their reverence and love for the Quran

591. From the passage, one can infer that which of the following characteristics are most integral to the process of memorizing the Quran

   A. Patience and perseverance

   B. Repetition and revision

   C. A teacher who has high standards for *Amukhta* and *Sabaq-e-Para*

   D. Ample time

592. Which of the following statements is INCORRECT:

   A. *Sabaq-e-Para* may consists of six to nine *Asbaaq* daily

   B. Final revision of the Quran consists of revising one to ten *Ajzaa* daily

   C. *Amukhta* consists of one-fourth to two *Ajzaa* daily

   D. *Sabaq* can never be longer than *Sabaq-e-Para*

593. Consider a student who has is on his forty-fifth unit of the fifty units that comprise his current *Sabaq*. He usually repeats about eighteen units previous to the unit he is currently memorizing. Based on the information given in the passage, when he finishes the fiftieth unit, which of the following is most likely true about the first thirty-two units of his current *Sabaq*?

   A. He will recite twenty seven of the units with the next day's *Sabaq* and the remaining five with today's *Sabaq*

   B. He will revise them with today's *Sabaq-e-Para* after reciting the last eighteen units as *Sabaq*

   C. He will join them to the last eighteen units and see if he can recite them all without looking

   D. He will save them to recite them when his *Amukhta* cycles around to include this portion

594. According to the passage, if a teacher only assigns seven *Asbaaq* as *Sabaq-e-Para*, and the student is on the fourteenth *Sabaq* of the *Juz*, then what first becomes of the first seven *Asbaaq* of that *Juz*?

   A. They are recited in *Amukhta*

   B. They are recited once the student finishes the *Juz*

   C. They are never recited again because the *Sabaq-e-Para* shifts forward with each *Sabaq*

   D. The student must rememorize these as *Sabaq*

595. The main theme of the passage would seem to be

   A. To show the reader what is required to memorize the Quran

   B. To show the reader that memorizing the Quran is a difficult and arduous process

   C. To motivate the reader to memorize the Quran

   D. To show the difference between *Sabaq, Sabaq-e-Para,* and *Amukhta*

STOP. IF YOU FINISH BEFORE TIME IS CALLED, CHECK YOUR WORK. YOU MAY GO BACK TO ANY QUESTION IN THIS TEST BOOKLET.

Biological Sciences

Time: 20 Minutes
Questions 596–611

A classical experiment in skeletal muscle physiology is depicted in Figure 1. The gastrocnemius muscle of a frog is attached to a transducer and a current is applied directly to the muscle. Upon electrostimulation, the muscle contracts and the force of the contraction is measured by the transducer. A weight is then applied to the muscle and the experiment is repeated. The results of the experiment are depicted in Figure 2. As the weight increases, the muscle stretches and the diameter of the muscle fiber narrows. This brings the actin and myosin closer together in the sarcomere and allows for increased cross-bridge formation. Therefore, stretch improves the contractility of skeletal muscle.

This length-tension relationship can also be applied cardiac muscle. As venous return to the heart increases, cardiac muscle fibers stretch to accommodate the larger end-diastolic volume. This stretch results in increased cardiac contractility.

Stretching the cardiac muscle is not the only way to improve its contractility. Sympathetic stimulation of the heart increases the strength of contraction by upregulating calcium entry into the cardiac muscle cell. Calcium is important for cardiac muscle contraction as it binds troponin C, allowing the formation of cross-bridges between actin and myosin.

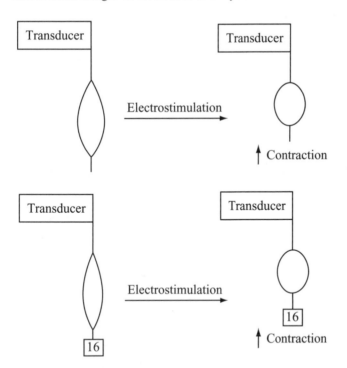

Figure 1 Skeletal Muscle responses to electrostimulation.

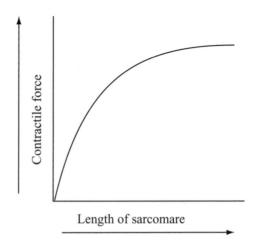

Figure 2 Contractile force as a measure of sarcomere length.

596. As seen in Figure 2, the length-tension relationship is nonlinear; when the muscle fiber is stretched past a certain point, the strength of contraction begins to fall. A reasonable explanation for this is:

    A. when stretched beyond a certain point, the thick and thin filaments do not overlap enough for cross-bridges to form between them

    B. when stretched beyond a certain point, the calcium to troponin C ratio is insufficient

    C. when stretched beyond a certain point, sympathetic stimulation of cardiac muscle decreases

    D. when stretched beyond a certain point, blood flow to cardiac muscle decreases

597. Stoke volume is defined as the average volume of blood pumped in one heartbeat. Stroke volume would most likely be elevated by:

    A. increased parasympathetic stimulation

    B. decreased end-diastolic volume

    C. increased sympathetic stimulation

    D. decreased coronary blood flow

GO ON TO THE NEXT PAGE.

598. The sarcomere is the smallest functional unit of the cardiac muscle cell. Which of the following forms the boundaries of the sarcomere?

A. A bands
B. H zones
C. I bands
D. Z lines

599. Cardiac muscle contractility is controlled primarily by the sympathetic nervous system. Heart rate, on the other hand, is affected by both sympathetic and parasympathetic stimulation. The effects of the two forms of autonomic regulation are best described by which of the following:

A. sympathetic stimulation increases heart rate; parasympathetic stimulation increases heart rate
B. sympathetic stimulation increases heart rate; parasympathetic stimulation decreases heart rate
C. sympathetic stimulation decreases heart rate; parasympathetic stimulation increases heart rate
D. sympathetic stimulation decreases heart rate; parasympathetic stimulation decreases heart rate

600. Dehydration would most likely result in:

A. a decrease in end-diastolic volume and a decrease in myocardial stretch
B. a decrease in end-diastolic volume and an increase in myocardial stretch
C. an increase in end-diastolic volume and an increase in myocardial stretch
D. an increase in end-diastolic volume and a decrease in myocardial stretch

601. The effects of sympathetic stimulation on the heart are mediated through which of the following myocyte structures?

A. sarcolemma
B. nucleus
C. T-tubules
D. sarcoplasmic reticulum

602. Stroke volume, heart rate, and peripheral vascular resistance determine blood pressure. Which of the following vessels are the most influential in affecting intravascular pressure?

A. arteries
B. arterioles
C. veins
D. venules

603. Unlike skeletal muscle, cardiac contraction is governed by involuntary neural stimulation. The pacemaker cells responsible for this automatic contraction are found in the:

A. vagus nerve
B. bundle of His
C. papillary muscle
D. sinoatrial node

The immune system distinguishes self cells from foreign cells via the specificity of glycoproteins, which are expressed on the external surface of cell membranes. These cell surface markers are collectively know as the major histocompatibility complex (MHC). In addition to their role in self cell recognition, MHC molecules play a role in antigen presentation. In an infected cell, the MHC molecule will cradle fragments of the infectious agent and "present" the antigen to T lymphocytes, which will then bind to the MHC molecule. MHC molecules are divided into 2 classes according to their specific role in antigen presentation.

Class I MHC molecules are found on all nucleated cells. An infected, or cancerous, cell of this type will solicit cytotoxic T cells. Upon binding to the Class I MHC molecule, the cytotoxic T cell will release a protein called perforin, which forms pores in the target cell's membrane. The loss of cell membrane integrity results in cellular swelling and lysis.

Class II MHC molecules are found only on a few specialized cell types, including B cells, activated T cells, and macrophages. Macrophages (see figure 1) present antigen to helper T cells through their MHC molecules. Once exposed to antigen, the activated helper Tcells, in turn, activate both cytotoxic T cells and B cells. B cells, stimulated as such, give rise to plasma cells, which secrete antibodies specific to the antigen presented by the macrophage.

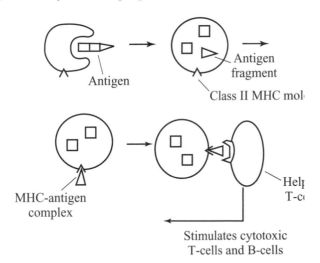

Figure 1

604. Macrophages circulate throughout the blood and engulf foreign matter via phagocytosis. A defect in the production of which of the following types of white blood cells would lead to a shortage of macrophages?

 A.   neutrophils
 B.   basophils
 C.   megakaryocytes
 D.   monocytes

605. Ras is an enzyme required for cell division. Cells which carry an oncogenic allele for Ras, express a constitutively active form of the enzyme and often divide without inhibition. Such a cell is most likely to solicit a response from:

 A.   macrophage
 B.   cytotoxic T cell
 C.   Helper T cell
 D.   Class II MHC molecule

606. A person with defective perforin would have difficulty mounting an immune response against:

 A.   pathogens circulating in the blood
 B.   parasitic protozoans
 C.   cells that display the Class II MHC
 D.   his own infected cells

607. A genetically inherited disorder renders the Class I MHC molecule nonfunctional. Which of the following types of cells would NOT be affected by such a disorder?

 A.   erythrocytes
 B.   endothelial cells
 C.   cardiac muscle cells
 D.   smooth muscle cells

GO ON TO THE NEXT PAGE.

608. According to the information in the passage, which of the following best explains why a person infected with a virus might be unable to produce antibodies?

   I.   Inability of B cells to differentiate into plasma cells
   II. Inability of cytotoxic T cells to secrete perforin
   III. Inability of Helper T cells to bind to Class II MHC molecules
   IV. Inability of the antigen fragment to reach the cell surface

   A.   I & III only
   B.   II & IV only
   C.   I, III, & IV
   D.   I, II, III, & IV

609. Before performing a blood transfusion, donor and recipient blood types must be carefully matched in order to insure compatibility. People with type AB blood are considered "universal recipients", in that they may receive transfusions of any blood type, because:

   A.   Their cells do not present the A or the B antigen
   B.   They do not produce antibodies against the A or the B antigen
   C.   The A and B antibodies that they produce do not attack their own cells
   D.   Their cells present the O as well as the A and B antigens

---

Questions 610 and 611 are **NOT** based on a descriptive passage.

610. Which of the following is NOT an example of innate immunity?

   A.   Phagocytotic cells
   B.   Stomach acid and digestive enzymes
   C.   Memory B cells
   D.   The skin as a barrier to antigens

611. Immunity may be acquired through active or passive means. Which of the following is an example of passive immunity?

   I.   Recovering from an infectious disease by producing antibodies
   II. Artificial injection of antibodies
   III. The passage of maternal antibodies to her developing fetus

   A.   II only
   B.   III only
   C.   II & III
   D.   I, II, & III

STOP. IF YOU FINISH BEFORE TIME IS CALLED, CHECK YOUR WORK. YOU MAY GO BACK TO ANY QUESTION IN THIS TEST BOOKLET.

EXAMINATION 14

Questions 612-658

Physical Sciences

Time: 20 Minutes
Questions 612-627

Passage I (Questions 612-616)

Voltage availability may be modulated via the use of a transformer. Transformers are typically employed in AC circuits, however, there are some applications for transformers in DC circuits. The diagram below shows a typical transformer.

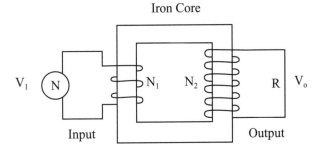

Iron Core

Figure 1 Typical Transformer

Changing the current in the input loop generates a magnetic field in the iron core, which in turn generates current and voltage in the output loop. The relationship between input voltage, V_I, and output voltage, V_O, depends on the relative number of coils of wrapped around the iron core on the input and output sides. The relationship is described by the equation below:

$$V_O = \frac{N_O}{N_I} V_I$$

N_I is the number of coils on the input loop and N_O is the number of coils on the output loop. Current flows in the output loop only when the current in the input loop is changing. Energy is conserved in a transformer, so the input power will be equal to the output power.

A *step-down* transformer is used to change the 24,000 V supplied by a power station to the much smaller 120 V used as household current. Electric power is transferred over long distances at very high voltages and very small currents because this format allows for less power dissipation in transmission lines.

The transformer between a car battery and a spark plug is an example of a *step-up* transformer. This transformer transforms the 12 V provided by a car battery into the 20,000 V required to produce a spark across the spark plug gap. A car uses a DC battery, which necessitates a switch to periodically interrupt the input current. Each of these interruptions result in sudden spikes in the output current and voltage.

612. How much current is required in the input loop of the step-down transformer to provide a house with 200 A of current at a voltage of 120 V?

- **A.** 1 A
- **B.** 2 A
- **C.** 20 A
- **D.** 100 A

613. Which of the following is the correct ratio for the number of input coils to the number of output coils required to step up the voltage from a car battery to a spark plug?

- **A.** $\dfrac{3}{5000}$
- **B.** $\dfrac{1}{1250}$
- **C.** $\dfrac{1250}{1}$
- **D.** $\dfrac{5000}{3}$

614. When the input loop is provided with a constant input voltage of 12 V, the voltage in the output loop will:

- **A.** remain constant at 0 V
- **B.** gradually increase from 0 V to 20,000 V
- **C.** gradually decrease from 20,000 V to 0 V
- **D.** remain constant at 20,000 V.

615. Household electricity consumption is measured in RMS values. If the RMS voltage of a house is 120 V, what is the peak value of the voltage?

- **A.** 140 V
- **B.** 170 V
- **C.** 240 V
- **D.** 280 V

616. When alternating current flows through a step-down transformer, the magnetic field in the iron core:

- **A.** changes direction but maintains a constant magnitude.
- **B.** changes magnitude but maintains a constant direction
- **C.** changes both magnitude and direction
- **D.** maintains constant magnitude and direction

GO ON TO THE NEXT PAGE.

In an experiment, a student measures the concentration of an HCl solution via titration with a standardized solution of NaOH. The NaOH solution is standardized before titration as sodium hydroxide easily absorbs impurities which would cause experimental error. The titrations are performed with the use of a buret and appropriate indicators to signal the endpoints of titration.

Standardization

One liter of distilled water is boiled for five minutes to remove dissolved carbon dioxide. The student dilutes 10.0 ml of a pre-prepared 6 *M* sodium hydroxide solution to approximately 0.1 *M*. The student then titrates 50.0 ml of the approximately 0.1 *M* NaOH solution with a primary standard. In this experiment, the primary standard is 0.145 *M* potassium hydrogen phthalate, $KHC_8H_4O_4$, also known as KHP. The neutralization reaction is shown below:

$$HC_8H_4O_4^- + OH^- \rightarrow H_2O + C_8H_4O_4^{2-}$$

Reaction 1

After standardization with KHP, the concentration of the sodium hydroxide solution is found to be 0.105 *M*.

Titration of an acid of unknown concentration

The standardized NaOH solution is then used to titrate 50.0 ml of a hydrochloric acid solution of unknown concentration. The titration reaches the equivalence point when 24.4 ml of sodium hydroxide solution had been added. The neutralization reaction is shown below:

$$H^+ + OH^- \rightarrow H_2O$$

Reaction 2

617. The hydroxide ion functions as a Bronsted-Lowry base in:

- A. Reaction 1 only.
- B. Reaction 2 only.
- C. Reaction 1 and Reaction 2.
- D. neither Reaction 1 nor Reaction 2.

618. How much distilled water must the student add to the original 6 *M* NaOH solution in order to dilite it to 0.1 *M*?

- A. 50 ml
- B. 60 ml
- C. 590 ml
- D. 600 ml

619. What is the pH of the 0.1 M solution of NaOH?

- A. 1
- B. 2
- C. 7
- D. 13

620. Which of the following titration curves best represents the titration of the unknown HCl solution with the NaOH solution?

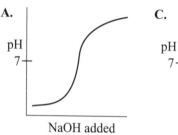

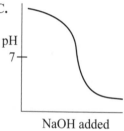

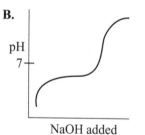

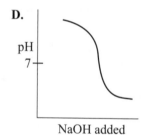

621. Before titrating the unknown HCl solution with the NaOH solution, the student should rinse the buret with

- A. distilled boiled water.
- B. HCl solution.
- C. standardized NaOH solution.
- D. 6 *M* NaOH solution.

GO ON TO THE NEXT PAGE.

622. If the student failed to remove carbon dioxide from water at the start of the experiment, the following reaction occurs.

$$CO_2(aq) + H_2O(l) \rightarrow H_2CO_3(aq)$$

In these conditions, the actual hydroxide concentration in the approximately 0.1 M NaOH solution will be:

A. higher than the expected concentration because hydroxide ions will be neutralized by carbonic acid.
B. lower than the expected concentration because hydroxide ions will be neutralized by carbonic acid.
C. higher than the expected concentration because hydroxide ions will be introduced into the solution by carbonic acid.
D. lower than the expected concentration because hydroxide ions will be introduced into the solution by carbonic acid.

623. Which of the following expressions represents the number of H^+ ions present in the HCl solution?

A. (0.105)(24.4) moles
B. (0.105)(0.0244) moles
C. (0.105)(50.0) moles
D. (0.105)(0.0500) moles

624. The table below describes a few common acid-base indicators:

Indicator	pH range for color change	Acid color	Base color
Methyl violet	0 – 2.0	yellow	violet
Methyl orange	2.9 – 4.0	red	yellow
Bromthymol blue	6.0 – 7.6	yellow	blue
Phenolphthalein	8.3 – 10.0	colorless	pink

Which indicator would be the best choice for the titration of the unknown HCl solution with NaOH?

A. Methyl violet
B. Methyl orange
C. Bromthymol blue
D. Phenolphthalein

Questions 577 through 580 are **NOT** based on a descriptive passage.

625. Three resistors are connected to a voltage source in parallel arrangement. If a fourth resistor is also added in parallel to the others, which of the following would occur?

A. The total resistance of the circuit would decrease and the total current would increase.
B. The total resistance of the circuit would decrease and the total current would decrease.
C. The total resistance of the circuit would increase and the total current would increase.
D. The total resistance of the circuit would increase and the total current would decrease.

626. An electron is projected into a magnetic field as shown in the diagram below. Which of the following best describes the force exerted on the electron by the field?

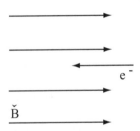

A. The force is directed against the electron's motion.
B. The force is directed upwards.
C. The force is directed out of the page.
D. The force is equal to zero.

627. A 10 V battery is connected to a 10 µF capacitor and the capacitor is allowed to charge fully. The battery is then disconnected while the capacitor is connected to a 100 ohm resistor and allowed to fully discharge over the course of 5 seconds. How much energy was stored in the capacitor?

A. 1×10^{-4} J
B. 5×10^{-4} J
C. 100 J
D. 500 J

STOP. IF YOU FINISH BEFORE TIME IS CALLED, CHECK YOUR WORK. YOU MAY GO BACK TO ANY QUESTION IN THIS TEST BOOKLET.

Verbal Reasoning

Time: 20 Minutes
Questions 628-642

Passage III (Questions 628-634)

Science is interrelated. Some postulate that all of biology is chemistry, and all of chemistry is physics, and all of physics is mathematics. To elaborate, the natural phenomena that biologists describe are predicated, ultimately, on the interactions between various organic molecules, macromolecules, and the like. Enter chemistry. Chemistry characterizes the realm of elemental reactions and interactions. How does iron react to the presence of oxygen? Which element will combine in which configuration under what conditions? However, it cannot be said that this level is not amenable to further reduction. Physics, in its scope, extends beyond characterization. It is more concerned with the laws and principles that govern those descriptions. Instead of answering the question of what a reaction will yield, physics addresses why a reaction will yield what it does. Energy states and relations, entropy, mass properties, elementary particle behavior, natural forces, and multitudinous physical laws all lie within its purview. But even physics is not the most fundamental way of knowing. Mathematics it is that really undergirds the belly of natural or material phenomenon. Without mathematics, science ultimately fails. The stunning order found in natural phenomenon is not the product of random interactions. Chaos theory tends to show that there is an order even to disorder. The seemingly random movements of molecules in any given confined space are not random. There exists a precise mathematical regularity to the reality that we interface with. In this sense, mathematics characterizes all of scientific knowing concerning the natural world.

At this juncture, an objection arises. The previous has paradigm has been step-down in its approach. However, such an approach obscures the possible lack of dependency between types of sciences (or "knowing" for that matter) more than one level removed. Biology may be reduced to chemistry, but it does not necessarily follow that the same reduction can take place from biology to physics. The reason that such an objection can even arise is that the above paradigm cannot fall on the logical model: $A=B$, and $B=C$; therefore $A=C$. The equal signs in the above paradigm are weak if not lacking. The paradigm also cannot fall onto the logical model: if all x is y, and all y is z; therefore all x is z. Each of the sciences previously presented is so vast that it probably cannot be confined in entirety to another science. Notwithstanding, it would seem that the paradigm still holds up reasonably well. Even if we take the two sciences most removed, we are still able to create a reasonable bridge. Biology involves the study of life. Life is, in turn, comprised of matter that is in some state of motion (matter can not be in a zero energy state and be alive). Integration in the fourth dimension, can give the volume of a three dimensional object. Thus, we have a reduction of objective mass to mathematical terms. All mass has motion be it gross, microscopic, molecular, atomic, or subatomic. These motions can be theoretically be characterized mathematically as well with a magnitude and direction. So it is possible to seemingly reduce biology in its entirety to mathematics. It would appear then, that the paradigm holds despite the objection.

The paradigm concurs also with the Western theory of knowledge. The Western theory is more comprehensive as it includes types of knowing hereto unto unaddressed. The Western theory sees human knowledge as an upside down pyramid. At the very tip is mathematics which is acknowledged by this framework as the most precise and definitive way of knowing. Above this are the hard sciences that include physics, chemistry, and biology. The next higher level contains the "soft" sciences like sociology and psychology. At the base of the pyramid lies language with the tacit understanding that anything can ultimately mean almost anything if interpreted as such. All of language carries the capacity to be a metaphor. Each metaphor can in turn be a metaphor for something else. Given this, what remains to be examined is whether or not sufficient reduction is possible between the different levels in this more comprehensive scheme of the Western theory of knowledge.

628. Which of the following is the most significant weakness in the paradigm expounded upon by the author?

- **A.** The possibility that a bridge might not exist between chemistry and mathematics and between biology and physics was not discussed
- **B.** The paradigm does not take language into account
- **C.** The paradigm only takes the hard sciences and mathematics into account
- **D.** All paradigms must fall on the logical models expressed in lines 37-39.

629. Which of the following statements does NOT directly support the overall theme of the passage?

- **A.** Mathematics is a fundamental way of characterizing reality
- **B.** Different sciences yield knowledge of reality at differing levels of perception and depth.
- **C.** Despite possible shortcomings, the paradigm set out in the passage is reasonably valid.
- **D.** Chemistry characterizes the realm of elemental reactions and interactions.

GO ON TO THE NEXT PAGE.

630. In lines 56-57, the author implies that there is a need for further research. Which of the following would best address this need?

A. Explaining chemistry in terms of mathematics
B. Explaining psychology in terms of biology
C. Explaining language in terms of metaphor theory
D. Explaining the hard sciences in terms of soft sciences.

631. The paradigm designated in the passage and the Western theory of knowledge are similar in that:

A. Both place an emphasis on mathematics as a precise way of knowing
B. Both acknowledge that there is ultimately no difference between the different sciences.
C. Both agree that language is more comprehensive in its scope than either chemistry or physics
D. Both are diametrically opposed to the Eastern theory of knowledge.

632. Removing which of the following statements would least affect the overall coherence and stability of the passage?

A. "the above paradigm cannot fall on the logical model: *A* = *B*, and *B* = *C*; therefore *A* = *C*. The equal signs in the previous paradigm are weak if not lacking." (lines 38-40)
B. "Biology involves the study of life. Life is, in turn, comprised of matter that must fundamentally be in some state of motion." (lines 47-49)
C. "such an approach obscures the possible lack of dependency between types of sciences…more than one level removed." (lines 32-34)
D. "The paradigm concurs with the Western theory of knowledge" (line 59)

633. Suppose that the author of the passage was hired as a curriculum director for a local high school. He would like the practically institute his paradigm in the curriculum. Which of the curriculum changes would be most closely be instituted?

A. Tripling class time given to the instruction of mathematics
B. Developing a more integrated scientific curriculum
C. Halving class time devoted to the soft sciences
D. Replacing biology and chemistry with physics

634. From the passage, we can most correctly infer that the author is:

A. a theist arguing the existence of God based on the intelligent design of reality
B. a PhD in mathematics from MIT
C. a humanities professor at Columbia University
D. There is insufficient textual evidence to make this determination.

GO ON TO THE NEXT PAGE.

Colloquial speech is often structurally loose. There is not a strict construction and examination of ideas. There is no crafting of words to embody the precise meaning the speaker wants to convey. There is no evaluation of possible
5 interpretations and reforming of speech to prevent the possibility of any interpretation except that which is congruent with the speaker's intent. On the other hand, in legal writing and formal argumentation, all these factors are thoroughly considered. Legal documents and treatises must
10 employ a highly precise and particular expression style so that both the meaning conveyed, and the meaning understood, are relatively absolute. Such modes of expression are very sophisticated and contemplated and require scholarly attention.

15 To elaborate the aforementioned, let us take the word 'until'. 'Until' is a very important word because it is almost invariably required in circumstances in which a spatial or temporal limit is to be entered on a declarative statement or injunction. The interpretive problematic that arises is
20 whether or not the endpoint (whatever statement follows after the word 'until') is included or excluded from the terms and purview of the primary statement or injunction (that part of the declaration that precedes the word 'until'). If a contract is valid until June 2004, does that mean that the
25 contract expires one second before June starts, June 1st, some day in the middle of June that is not the first or last day of June, or the last day of June. If a property agreement defines the precincts under sale as all area up until the boundary line, is the boundary line included or not. Since
30 there is a possibility of multiple interpretations, scholars develop certain rules in order to set a meaning for a given statement regardless of the intent with which the utterance was made. This is necessary to do in legal cases or formal debates in order to be able to settle on a verdict or achieve
35 closure.

In our case of the word 'until', one scholarly opinion holds that if there is only a simple declaration consisting of a primary statement/injunction and a limit, and there is no direct or indirect indication that the limit is not included,
40 then the entire limit will be included in the purview of the primary statement/injunction. This will be the default interpretation and some level of plausible evidence need be brought to elicit the alternative interpretation (not including the limit). The opinion further holds in order for the word
45 'until' to be used in the context of setting limits two conditions must be met. First, the primary statement/injunction must have the capacity to be extended, temporally or spatially, to a limit. Second, the limit must have the literary and logical capacity to serve as a limit. If either condition is
50 not met, then 'until' will be interpreted as 'in order that' or 'so' depending on the circumstance. Thus in the example that one tells someone, "Light the lamp until the room is lit." In such a statement neither condition is met. Lighting a lamp is a relatively instantaneous act, not one that is gener-
55 ally extended like walking. The room being lit is not primarily appropriate as a limit, as limits are principally relegated to symbols of time and place. By contrast, the room being lit is chiefly a state. In this case, we would set the meaning of this statement as being, "light the lamp in
60 order that the room be lit."

One of the further complex subtleties of legal and formal argumentative expression is that, at least in the scholarly realm, not always is there consensus on the rules that define how something expressed is to be understood or,
65 in another way, how something expressed is assigned a meaning. What was discussed above in the case of 'until' is one approach to assigning meaning. There could reasonably be others as well…

635. Which of the following statements would best support the central theme of the passage?

A. The complexities involved with the word 'until' are best illustration of certain modes of complex expression
B. Everyday talk may be loose but can become sophisticated if the mode of legal expression is used in conversation.
C. Legal and formal argumentative modes of expression are inherently complex and highly sophisticated.
D. Lack of agreement on the "rules" of defining meaning adds to the complex subtleties of legal and formal argumentative expression

636. According the scholarly opinion given in the passage (lines 24-29), which answer choice would be most true regarding the statement: "The book can be kept without a fine until tomorrow."

A. Tomorrow may or may not be included as a limit for keeping the book without a fine.
B. The book may be kept unit the end of tomorrow without having to give a fine.
C. The statement cannot be assessed according to the framework set up in the passage
D. Tomorrow is included in the period exempt from a fine, but the specific time tomorrow is unspecified

637. Which of the following statements would not result in the default interpretation of the word 'until'?

- **A.** Speak to the audience until nine o' clock
- **B.** The house lease will continue until August 23
- **C.** The money must be returned until the bank is satisfied.
- **D.** The new property line continues until the red flag.

638. If someone were to argue that such technicalities are superfluous and merely an intellectual exercise, the author would most likely respond:

- **A.** By stating that such a complex framework is necessary to resolve court cases
- **B.** By agreeing with the objector
- **C.** By recapitulating the sophistication of legal and formal argumentative expression
- **D.** Inventing a new and innovative argument to justify the convolution found in legal texts

639. If you were to discover that the "scholarly opinion" indicated in lines 24-29 was actually the result of a series of leisurely, philosophical discussions that the author (a trained pharmacist) had with his programmer friend, how would the credibility of the passage's thesis be affected?

- **A.** The credibility of the thesis would remain unchanged
- **B.** It would strengthen the credibility of the thesis because it shows the intellectual prowess of the author
- **C.** It would weaken the credibility of the thesis because it would show that the author was dishonest in stating the opinion was a scholarly one.
- **D.** It would weaken the credibility of the thesis because there would be no expert evidence to show that legal and argumentative expression is a sophisticated process

640. According to the passage, which of the following components usually found in legal documents might be lacking in casual conversation?

- **I.** Careful word choice
- **II.** Consideration of how the listener might understand what is being said
- **III.** Circuitous word usage

- **A.** I only
- **B.** II only
- **C.** I and II
- **D.** I, II, and III

641. If a grammarian were to offer an alternative framework for interpreting the word 'until' the author would likely react by

- **A.** Defending the framework given in the passage
- **B.** Accepting the alternative framework in place of the framework expounded upon in the passage in lines 26-42
- **C.** Rejecting the alternative framework since there is a need to set an assigned meaning
- **D.** Regarding the alternative framework as a manifestation of the complexity involved in language expression

Extra question for Passage II test 14

642. According to the passage, under which of the following conditions would the author most likely argue that a verbal agreement is unambiguous?

- **A.** There is an audio recording of the agreement.
- **B.** There is a video recording of the agreement.
- **C.** The exact words used by the agreeing parties is written down as they are spoken.
- **D.** The wording of the agreement was carefully prepared by both parties.

STOP. IF YOU FINISH BEFORE TIME IS CALLED, CHECK YOUR WORK. YOU MAY GO BACK TO ANY QUESTION IN THIS TEST BOOKLET.

STOP.

Biological Sciences

Time: 20 Minutes
Questions 643–658

High blood pressure is a condition which plagues many Americans. Although there are several proposed mechanisms of hypertension, cardiovascular disease is one of the most common. Atheroschlerosis refers to the build up of plaques in blood vessels, and their subsequent loss of elasticity and luminal diameter. As blood volume remains relatively constant, a result of atherosclerosis is increased blood pressure. One of the etiologic agents in atherosclerotic plaques is cholesterol. High cholesterol levels present an increased risk for atherosclerosis and the ensuing increase in blood pressure. Thus, the study of cholesterol and related derivatives remains important for the treatment of cardiovascular disease.

Students in a medical laboratory carry out the reaction in Figure 1, forming cholesteryl acetate. When carried out in acetic acid, the reaction proceeds slowly enough to be followed using thin layer chromatography. The students obtain reaction aliquots at times 0, 15 minutes, and 30 minutes. Each aliquot is then extracted with ether, washed with sodium hydroxide, and dried. The students dissolve the remaining solid in a 1:1 ether:hexane solution (the developing solvent) and spot the solution onto a chromotography plate. Chromatograms A, B, and C below represent the aliquots obtained at the three times, respectively. The chromatographic spots were demarcated under UV light.

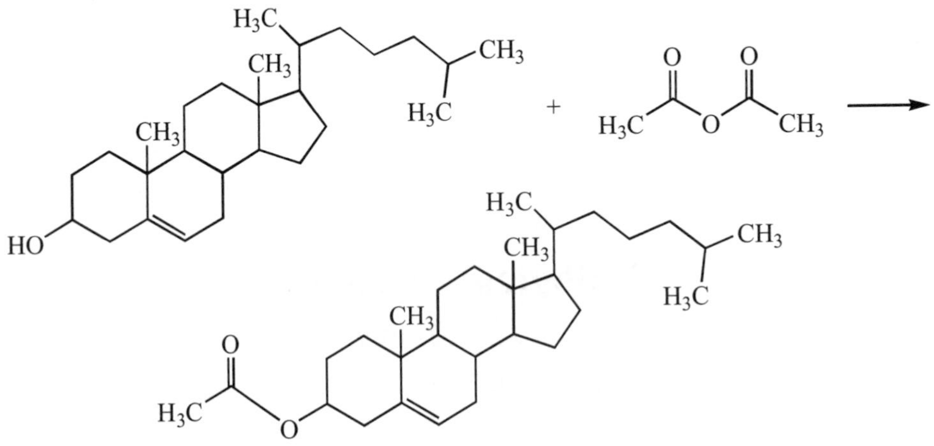

Figure 1

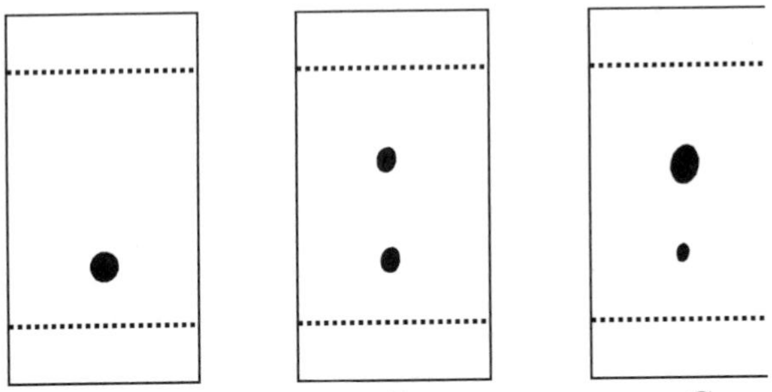

Figure 2

643. Which other reagent could the students have used to form cholesteryl acetate from cholesterol?

   A. NaOH
   B. $NaOCH_3$
   C. CH_3COCl
   D. H_2O

644. Based on the chromatograms, the students should conclude that:

   A. Cholesterol has a larger R_f than cholesteryl acetate.
   B. Cholesterol has a smaller R_f than cholesteryl acetate.
   C. Cholesterol has the same R_f as cholesteryl acetate.
   D. The relationship of the R_f cannot be determined.

GO ON TO THE NEXT PAGE.

645. Which of the following statements regarding cholesteryl acetate is true?

   A. It absorbs energy in the UV portion of the spectrum.
   B. It emits light in the UV portion of the spectrum.
   C. It is a liquid when purified after extraction.
   D. It is more soluble in sodium hydroxide than ether.

646. During aliquot extraction, the ether layer contains:

   A. The ether layer only contains cholesterol.
   B. The ether layer only contains cholesteryl acetate.
   C. The ether layer contains cholesterol and cholesteryl acetate.
   D. The ether layer neither contains cholesterol nor cholesteryl acetate.

647. The students most likely treated the aliquots with sodium hydroxide after the initial extraction in order to:

   A. extract the cholesterol from the ether
   B. extract the cholesteryl acetate from the ether
   C. remove the acetic acid
   D. remove the ether

648. Which of the following solvent systems when used as the developing solvent would increase the Rf value for cholesterol?

   A. 2:1 ether:hexane
   B. 1:1 ether:hexane
   C. 1:2 ether:hexane
   D. 1:3 ether:hexane

649. When the reaction is complete, which of the following separation techniques should the students utilize in order to separate unreacted cholesterol from cholesteryl acetate?

   A. distillation
   B. extraction
   C. recrystallization
   D. column chromatography

Passage VI (Questions 650-656)

Isoamyl acetate is an ester used by the food industry in artificial pear and banana flavoring. Scientists in the Research and Development Department of a major food producer synthesized Isoamyl acetate as shown in the reaction below.

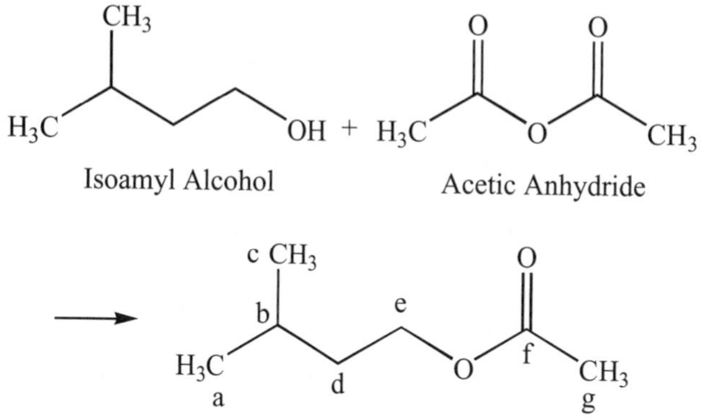

Isoamyl Alcohol   Acetic Anhydride

Figure 1

The scientists refluxed the two reactants by heating the solution and then stopped the reaction with ice. The resulting aqueous solution was extracted with ether and then washed with sodium hydroxide. The scientists then purified the ester via fractional distillation.

A NMR of the final product was obtained. The table below summarizes the data.

Peak	Chemical Shift	Integration	Splitting
1	1.01 ppm	6	doublet
2	1.53 ppm	2	quartet
3	1.83 ppm	1	multiplet
4	2.01 ppm	3	singlet
5	4.08 ppm	2	triplet

Table 1

650. Isoamyl acetate contains six hydrocarbon groups, however, there are only 5 peaks in the nmr spectrum. The most likely explanation for this discrepancy is:

   A. NMR peaks do not appear when the carbons are attached to oxygens
   B. some of the hydrogen signals are too weak to observe
   C. some of the carbon signals are too weak to observe
   D. some of the carbons are chemically equivalent

GO ON TO THE NEXT PAGE.

651. According to the representation of Isoamyl acetate in Figure I, Peak 5 of the NMR spectrum most likely represents the Hydrogens attached to Carbon:

A. g
B. f
C. e
D. d

652. From the NMR spectrum, what can the scientists conclude regarding the relationship between peaks 2 and 4?

A. the hydrogens responsible for peak 4 are more shielded
B. the hydrogens responsible for peak 4 are less shielded
C. the hydrogens responsible for peak 4 are not shielded
D. the hydrogens responsible for peak 2 are equally shielded

653. A laboratory intern notices an additional peak on the NMR spectrum at 0 ppm. Which of the following compounds would produce such a peak?

A. TMS
B. $CDCl_3$
C. D_2O
D. Methane

654. If the scientists followed the synthesis with NMR spectroscopy, the appearance of which peak would be the best indication of product formation?

A. peak 1
B. peak 2
C. peak 4
D. peak 5

655. If the scientists instead followed the reaction with IR Spectroscopy, the appearance of a peak in which range would be the best indication of product formation?

A. $675-1000 \ cm^{-1}$
B. $1680-1740 \ cm^{-1}$
C. $2100-2260 \ cm^{-1}$
D. $3590-3650 \ cm^{-1}$

656. According to the NMR spectrum, which of the following is the most likely explanation of peak 2's splitting?

A. There are 3 hydrogens attached to the carbon.
B. There are 4 hydrogens attached to the neighboring carbons.
C. There are 2 hydrogens attached to the carbon.
D. There are 3 hydrogens attached to the neighboring carbons.

Questions 657 and 658 are **NOT** based on a descriptive passage.

657. Which of the following statements is FALSE regarding spectroscopy?

A. NMR spectroscopy utilizes electromagnetic energy
B. In IR spectroscopy, ionic bonds are oscillated with infrared radiation
C. NMR spectroscopy reveals electron shielding of protons
D. UV spectroscopy delineates conjugated systems

658. Conjugated systems are unique in that they have vacant orbitals close to their highest occupied molecular orital (HOMO) energy levels. These vacant orbitals are called lowest unoccupied molecular orbitals (LUMO). UV photons are able to transiently displance electrons from HOMO to LUMO energy levels. In UV spectroscopy, the longer the chain of conjugated double bonds, the greater the wavelength of absorption. An increase in isolated double bonds, however, does not increase the absorption wavelength. According to this phenomena, which of the following statements is FALSE?

A. 1,3-butadiene will absorb longer wavelengths than 1,4- butadiene
B. 1,3-butadiene will absorb shorter wavelengths than 1,4-butadiene
C. 1,3 butadiene and 1,4-butadiene will absorb equal wavelengths
D. More information is needed to ascertain the relative absorptions of 1,3-butadiene and 1,4-butadiene.

STOP. IF YOU FINISH BEFORE TIME IS CALLED, CHECK YOUR WORK. YOU MAY GO BACK TO ANY QUESTION IN THIS TEST BOOKLET.

EXAMINATION 15

Questions 659–705

Physical Sciences

Time: 20 Minutes

Questions 659–674

When a light beam falls on a thin film covering a reflecting surface, interference will occur between the light that is reflected from the surface of the film, and the light which has refracted into the film and then been reflected from the surface below the film. The nature of interference will depend on the wavelength of the light, the thickness of the film, and the film's index of refraction.

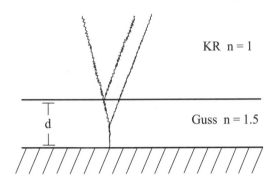

KR n = 1

Guss n = 1.5

d

Figure 1

Light reflected from the surface of the film undergoes a phase change of 180°, while the refracted light does not change phase. Constructive interference will occur in the following conditions:

$$2nd = \left(m + \frac{1}{2}\right)\lambda$$

Total destructive interference occurs when:

$$2nd = m\lambda$$

In both of the above equations, n is the index of refraction of the thin film material, d is the thickness of the film, λ is the wavelength of the light, and m is any integer greater than or equal to zero.

659. Which of the following diagrams represents the reflection of a wave from the surface of the thin glass film shown in Figure 1?

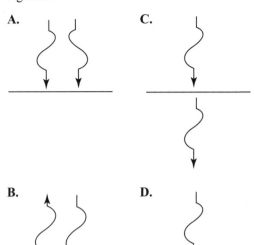

660. If the glass film is 600 nm thick and the light wave is perpendicular to the surface, how much time elapses from the moment the wave enters the glass until it leaves?

A. 2×10^{-15} sec
B. 3×10^{-15} sec
C. 4×10^{-15} sec
D. 6×10^{-15} sec

661. Thin films are often used to reduce the glare of a surface. At what thickness will a glass surface be most effective at reducing glare from a light with a wavelength of 750 nm?

A. 500 nm
B. 600 nm
C. 700 nm
D. 800 nm

662. As light passes from the air into the glass film, the wavelength of the light:

A. increases and the frequency remains the same.
B. increases and the frequency decreases.
C. decreases and the frequency remains the same.
D. decreases and the frequency increases.

GO ON TO THE NEXT PAGE.

663. If a light ray falls on the surface of the glass at an angle of 12° to the normal, what are the angles of reflection and refraction?

A. reflection – 12°, refraction – 16°
B. reflection – 12°, refraction – 8°
C. reflection – 78°, refraction – 74°
D. reflection – 78°, refraction – 78°

664. According to the passage, constructive interference occurs when the reflected light wave and the refracted light wave emerge from the surface of the glass with:

A. a phase difference of 45°.
B. a phase difference of 90°.
C. a phase difference of 180°.
D. no difference in phase.

Passage II (Questions 665–671)

Aluminum, although the most abundant metal found in nature, is not found in its elemental state. Pure aluminum is isolated for commercial purposes by subjecting aluminum oxide, Al_2O_3, to an oxidation-reduction reaction known as the Hall process.

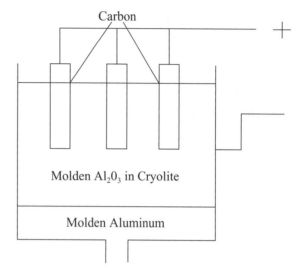

Figure 1 Hall Process

In the Hall process, aluminum oxide is dissolved in molten cryolite, Na_3AlF_6, to produce a liquid that serves as an electrical conductor. Carbon electrodes are connected to the liquid as shown in Figure 1. When the apparatus is connected to a voltage source, an electrolysis reaction takes place. When pure molten aluminum is produced, it sinks to the bottom of the container and can be easily removed through a valve.

The half-reactions of the electrolysis are as follows:

$$C(s) + 2\ O^{2-} \rightarrow CO_2(g) + 4\ e^-$$
$$Al^{3+} + 3\ e^- \rightarrow Al(l)$$

665. Which of the following represents the balanced equation for the Hall process reaction?

A. $Al_2O_3 + C \rightarrow Al + CO_2$
B. $2\ Al_2O_3 + 3\ C \rightarrow 4\ Al + 3\ CO_2$
C. $3\ Al_2O_3 + 3\ C \rightarrow 4\ Al + 4\ CO_2$
D. $2\ Al_2O_3 + 3\ C \rightarrow 3\ Al + 2\ CO_2$

666. Which of the following statements is true regarding the thermodynamics of the Hall process reaction?

   A. It is a spontaneous reaction with positive free-energy change.

   B. It is a spontaneous reaction with negative free-energy change.

   C. It is a non-spontaneous reaction with positive free-energy change.

   D. It is a non-spontaneous reaction with negative free-energy change.

667. Which of the following relationships must be true in order for the Hall process to proceed?

   A. Na^+ must have a greater oxidation potential than Al^{3+}.

   B. Al^{3+} must have a greater oxidation potential than Na^+.

   C. Na^+ must have a greater reduction potential than Al^{3+}.

   D. Al^{3+} must have a greater reduction potential than Na^+.

668. Which of the following reduction-oxidation events take place during the Hall process?

   A. Al^{3+} is oxidized and O^{2-} is reduced.

   B. Al^{3+} is oxidized and C is reduced.

   C. Al^{3+} is reduced and O^{2-} is oxidized.

   D. Al^{3+} is reduced and C is oxidized.

669. In Figure 1, bubbles may be observed at the:

   A. anode, where oxidation is taking place.

   B. cathode, where oxidation is taking place.

   C. anode, where reduction is taking place.

   D. cathode, where reductionis taking place.

670. If 5.0 moles of electrons are transferred during the reaction, what is the mass of pure aluminum produced?

   A. 16 g.

   B. 27 g

   C. 36 g

   D. 45 g

---

671. An object is placed 12 cm in front of a concave mirror with a focal length of 8 cm. The image formed will be:

   A. virtual and larger than the object.
   B. virtual and smaller than the object.
   C. real and larger than the object.
   D. real and smaller than the object.

672. The eye adjusts focus using ciliary muscles which modulate lens curvature, as shown below. Compared to the lens A, lens B has:

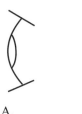 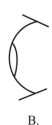

   A.   B.

   A. longer focal length and less power.
   B. longer focal length and greater power.
   C. shorter focal length and less power.
   D. shorter focal length and greater power.

673. The reduction potentials for two half-reactions are shown below.

$$Ag^+ + e \rightarrow Ag(s) \qquad E° = 0.80\ V$$

$$Zn^{2+} + 2e \rightarrow Zn(s) \qquad E° = -0.76\ V$$

What is the standard potential for the following reaction?

$$Zn^{2+} + 2\ Ag \rightarrow Zn + 2\ Ag^+$$

   A. −1.56 V
   B. −0.04 V
   C. 0.04 V
   D. 0.08 V

674. The following reaction provides the emf for a galvanic cell.

$$Fe(s) + Cu^{2+}(aq) \rightarrow Fe^{2+}(aq) + Cu(s)$$

If the concentration of $Cu^{2+}(aq)$ is increased, which of the following describes the effect on the cell?

   A. The voltage and the equilibrium constant would increase.
   B. The voltage and the equilibrium constant would decrease
   C. The voltage would increase and the equilibrium constant would decrease.
   D. The voltage would increase and the equilibrium constant would remain the same.

STOP. IF YOU FINISH BEFORE TIME IS CALLED, CHECK YOUR WORK. YOU MAY GO BACK TO ANY QUESTION IN THIS TEST BOOKLET.

STOP.

Verbal Reasoning

Time: 20 Minutes
Questions 675–689

Frankenstein met with mixed reviews when first published 1818. We must understand that the mores and conventions of the nineteenth century were a far cry from those of today. Religiously, the world was at the tail end of the
5 age of reason. Romanticism was the up and coming ideology of the day. Politically, the French Revolution was still fresh in everybody's minds. More than a passing incidence of political turmoil and upheaval, the revolution showed the world that the proletariat was a class to be reckoned with.
10 Despotism was soon to give way to democracy. Technologically, the early 1800's heralded the Industrial Revolution and years of great advances. Until the Industrial Revolution, the family would work as a unit on the farm. Industrialism started to fragment the family unit. Young
15 girls and boys would leave home earlier, and even if they did not, they would seldom have the opportunity to work at the side of family members. The world was in a period of transitions that both influenced and were influenced by the writers like Shelly. This socio-historic context bore upon
20 and, perhaps to some degree, raised the theme of individual isolation and the caution against the reckless pursuit of knowledge that we find in *Frankenstein*.

The first criticism, one done by *The Endinburgh Magazine and Literary Miscellany*, dates back to the same
25 year that *Frankenstein* was published. It grudgingly acknowledges the "beauty and power" of Shelly's writing. Notwithstanding this slight praise, the criticism reproaches Shelly for her impious material. At a time in history in which religious orthodoxy was much more pervasive than it
30 is today, the attribution of the ability to create life to anyone other than God did in fact border on impiety. At the same time, the changing trends of the day were creating a readership that was demanding more and more exciting material in the fictional pieces that they read. Frankenstein was
35 catering to that trend. In this light, the criticism cedes that some of the morbid exaggerations and dark irregularities found in the novel can be excused.

The second criticism was done by Elizabeth Nitche. It is contemporary criticism. Nitche criticizes Shelly for her
40 idealization, sentimentality, and grandiloquent style. In the bigger picture, however, Nitche sees Shelly as writer "full of merits." In her criticism, Nitche analyzes Shelly's structure and style, noting the use of allusions, irony, and word usage.

45 The next landmark criticism was done by M.A. Goldberg in 1959. Goldberg deals with the structure, motifs, and themes of Frankenstein. He concentrates in his criticism on the constant symbolic references to the Genesis story and the recurring element of isolation that we find in
50 the novel. Goldberg ends his analysis by arguing that concept of loneliness that Shelly tried to convey in her novel

was a message to society at large. It was not just Shelly speaking of her own isolation, as Nitche would argue.

The last criticism is that of Kingsley Amis's. It is more
55 recent than any of the above essays on Frankenstein. Amis asserts that themes found in Frankenstein have set the precedent for, and so, found their way into numerous modern works. These themes are three in number: 1) the existence of a half human, half non-human entity, 2) artificial
60 creation, and 3) the need to take moral responsibility when undertaking scientific endeavors.

675. Which of the following statements would most completely depict the author's belief about the relationship between life and art ?

   A.   social and historical context shape the art produced in a given era
   B.   Art influences the social environment in which it exists
   C.   There is no interaction between life and art
   D.   Life and art influence each other

676. The criticism published in the *Endinburgh Magazine and Literary Miscellany* is most likely dated:

   A.   1859
   B.   1818
   C.   Late nineteenth century
   D.   There is not enough information to ascertain the date

677. Which of the following types of thematic literature would be most readily accepted, and thus most popular, if published in 1820?

A. A controversial horror novel
B. An analysis of the Industrial Revolution
C. A run-of-the-mill romantic love story
D. A novel promoting atheism

678. Which of the following INCORRECTLY pairs a criticism with a perspective on Frankenstein

A. *Endinburgh Magazine and Literary Miscellany*—marginally heretic
B. Elizabeth Nitche—overly expressive syntax
C. Goldberg—social commentary
D. Kingsley Amis—futuristic science fiction

679. Given only the information in the passage, the first two criticisms are most alike in that they:

A. Give attention to the style in which Frankenstein was written
B. Analyze the future ramifications of Frankenstein on other literature
C. Critique Shelly for her shortcomings as a writer
D. Analyze the coherence of Shelly's ideas expressed in Frankenstein.

680. The criticism written by Elizabeth Nitche was most likely published during which time period

A. 1800-1815
B. 1945-1960
C. 1970-1985
D. The time period cannot be inferred from the given information

681. In the above passage, the word "criticism" most closely refers to which of the following?

A. Scholarly Analysis and study
B. Effort to uncover the shortcomings in Shelly's Frankenstein
C. Thematic commentary
D. Disapproval and disparagement of Shelly for her inclusion of "impious" content

682. Suppose Shelly had written another book about a scientist cloning a human being. Based upon the passage, which of the following might object to this book on moral grounds?

I.   Endinburgh Magazine and Literary Miscellany
II.   Elizabeth Nitche
III. M.A. Goldberg
IV.   Kingsley Amis

A. I only
B. IV only
C. I and IV only
D. I, II, III, and IV

GO ON TO THE NEXT PAGE.

In one sense, *The Issa Valley* (1955) is a simple story of a young boy named Thomas living in the rural town of Gine, Lithuania and his experiences as he grows into a young man. More fundamentally, however, *The Issa Valley*
5 is a commentary on Christianity, paganism, and Nature, on the innocence of youth and the hypocrisy of adulthood. Nobel laureate Czeslaw Milosz deals with these issues by questioning the premises on which they are based and explores how they are interwoven with both human
10 emotions and cognitions.

The protagonist of *The Issa Valley*, Thomas, is made the voice of truth. Thomas is instructed under the guidance of one Joseph the Black, a nationalist revolutionary and proponent of liberation ideology. Thomas's early erudition
15 is borne out in his persisting and enduring hate for hypocrisy. For example, Thomas is discomforted by the "tedious proprieties" of social decorum. Later in the story, in the culmination of an epiphany, Thomas punishes himself for certain sins. He cannot accede to the fact that
20 another has died for his sins, while he believes that he himself is responsible for his deeds. To deny this conscious belief, to Thomas, is tantamount to being untrue to oneself, and this, in the story, is the pinnacle of hypocrisy. Through Thomas, Milosz underscores the roles of truth and sincerity
25 in achieving true knowledge and union with the natural world.

Milosz devotes a considerable amount of time to the discussion of Christianity, which at times becomes a more global argument on religion. In Gine, where the story takes
30 place, Christianity is an essential aspect of societal existence that permeates the fabric of social life. Christianity, however, does not exist in a vacuum. It is a religion that is in constant discourse with the pagan values of society, not to mention human emotions/perceptions and world happen-
35 ings. In its own capacity, Christianity serves for the people of Gine the role of answering life's problems, of providing structure and affiliation in one's life, of providing hope in the face of adversity. Notwithstanding this extant role, Milosz somewhat subtly asks the reader grapple with what
40 he deems are the many failings, shortcomings, and discrepancies in the religion itself and in those who follow it. In *The Issa Valley*, a recurring motif is that of the hypocrisy of Christians and of the Church. In one passage, Thomas sarcastically states that God "clearly favors hypocrites"
45 when observing the pious air that people assume on Sunday at Church and the vicious sins and evils they commit outside the Church at other times.

Christianity in Gine does not exist in a vacuum, as there are heavy overtones of pagan values and beliefs in
50 community life. The evaluation and attitude of the author toward the pagan aspects of society is neither overtly positive or negative—pagan values simply exist. Milosz,

however, does discuss the psychology that underlies paganism. He notes that any evidence contrary to pagan beliefs is
55 readily reconciled in the minds of the proletariat by creating myths or imaginative theories. Milosz argues that the need for such pagan beliefs is grounded in the need to ascertain signs from the other world, the need to connect with the divine, and the need to make mythical what may
60 merely be mundane. We also learn that pagan beliefs have a certain logic to them. In this way, paganism is just one mode amongst many in which man tries to make sense of the world around him.

Historically, Nature is a major element of pagan
65 beliefs, and if there is anything extolled in *The Issa Valley*, then it is Nature. The book begins with, and is filled with rich, beautiful descriptions of nature. In fact, nature is described in so much detail that one feels, at once, that it is of the greatest importance to Milosz. In one passage, there
70 is a wooden figure of Christ, seemingly forgotten, overgrown with moss implying the author's preference for Nature over Christianity. For Thomas, nature is his reprieve, his recourse from hypocrisy…

683. Given the information in the passage, which of the following would be most plausible inference regarding *The Issa Valley?*

   A. It is loaded with bright, colorful, and detailed imagery of lakes and forests
   B. It is loaded with crass, obscene anathemas hurled at Christendom
   C. It is filled with praise and justification for pagan practices
   D. It includes themes of coming to grips with the unpredictable nature of the world

684. According to the passage, which of the following locales would Czeslaw Milosz most prefer?

   A. The capital city of Lithuania
   B. Vatican City
   C. Walden Pond
   D. The comfort of his home

262

685. According to the passage, Christianity and paganism are most similar in that:

  A. Their constituents are hypocrites
  B. They give birth to many legends and myths
  C. They make superordinary the mundane existence of everyday Lithuanian life
  D. They offer their constituents a way to make sense of and/or deal with the world

686. If one had to predict based on the information given in the passage, Thomas might most likely grow up to be a:

  A. Political revolutionary
  B. Recluse in the forest
  C. Protestant priest
  D. Painter

687. If Milosz were to discover that he had erred in his perception of the hypocrisy of Christians, how might his view change?

  A. His antagonistic views would only be slightly softened
  B. He would hold a neutral view of Christianity
  C. He would become a weak proponent of the Christian faith
  D. His views would remain unchanged

688. In which way does Thomas feel that accepting Christ as his savior is hypocritical?

  A. It is tantamount to not taking responsibility for one's actions
  B. It goes against his personal belief system
  C. It requires that one place less emphasis on the natural world
  D. It creates a dichotomy within him consisting of both pagan and Christian values

689. According to the passage, what approach does Milosz take in exploring issues of Christianity, paganism, and Nature?

  I. He analyzes the basics tenets and workings of all three
  II. He sees how individuals existentially experience all three
  III. He makes implicit judgments on the inherent worth of all three

  A. I only
  B. II only
  C. I and II only
  D. I, II, and III

STOP. IF YOU FINISH BEFORE TIME IS CALLED, CHECK YOUR WORK. YOU MAY GO BACK TO ANY QUESTION IN THIS TEST BOOKLET.

STOP.

Biological Sciences

Time: 20 Minutes

Questions 690–705

While space travel is both mentally and emotionally challenging, maneuvering through a gravity-free environment is physically effortless. Gravity is a force seldomly considered as "muscle-building", despite the fact that on Earth, organisms are incessantly working against gravitational force. The muscles used to combat the pull of gravity include the gastrocnemius muscles of the calves, the quadriceps, and the vast musculature of the back and neck. With the continued disuse experienced in the weightlessness of space, these muscles rapidly atrophy or waste, posing serious health risks for astronauts who remain in space for prolonged periods of time. A flight as short as 5 days can result in up to 20% loss of muscle mass.

To investigate the cellular mechanisms underlying muscle atrophy in space, an experiment was conducted to examine the relationship between oxygen consumption (absolute max VO_2) and muscle function. Oxygen intake increases with greater work loads that requires recruitment of additional muscle fibers. Astronauts were subjected to cardiovascular exercise pre-flight, in-flight and post-flight on an ergometer, and maximum oxygen intake was measured. Muscle testing was performed at each of these intervals to assess how well each astronaut could contract his calf muscle before tiring. Finally, a biopsy or tissue sample was taken from each crew member's semitendinous muscle to assay for changes that occurred on the cellular level.

These cellular studies allowed researchers to determine whether declines in performance were due to the deleterious effects of hypogravity alone, or neural and cardiovascular factors. Both fast-twitch and slow-twitch muscle fibers were examined.

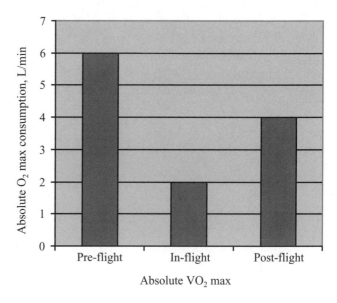

Figure 2

690. Fast twitch muscle fibers depend on energy produced by the anaerobic breakdown of glycogen, while slow twitch fibers rely mostly on aerobic processes. The efficiency of which fiber type will most likely be decreased in-flight?

A. Fast twitch fibers, because of their increased dependence on anaerobic energy sources
B. Slow twitch fibers, because of their increased dependence on anaerobic energy sources
C. Fast twitch fibers, because of their increased usage in space
D. Slow twitch fibers, because of their increased usage in space

691. The length of a sarcomere is critical because it determines the maximal contractility of a muscle. This is because:

A. Sarcomere length maximizes the surface area to which potassium is exposed to
B. Sarcomere length maximizes the number of myofibrils recruited
C. The length of a sarcomere must allow for maximum overlap between thick and thin filaments
D. The length of a sarcomere must allow for minimum overlap between thick and thin filaments

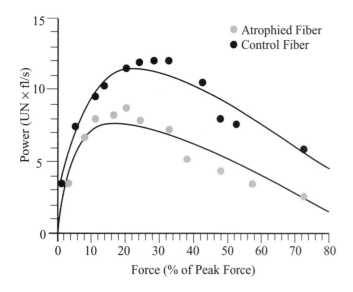

Figure 1

692. The semitendinous muscle is only employed in voluntary movement. Which of the following would most likely be seen on a biopsy of the semitendinous?

   I. striations
  II. mononucleated cells
 III. a system of T-tubules

  A. I only
  B. I and III only
  C. II and III only
  D. I, II and III

693. Muscle contraction is *directly* dependent on the presence of an ion in the blood. Levels of this ion are controlled by which of the following hormones?

  A. Thyroid hormone
  B. Cortisol
  C. Epinephrine
  D. Calcitonin

694. After a prolonged flight in space, which of the following muscles would incur the LEAST amount of atrophy?

  A. biceps
  B. semitendinous
  C. gastrocnemius
  D. heart

695. Excess stretch on cardiac muscle can lead to enlargement of the heart, a condition commonly seen in those with high blood pressure. Excess stretch on skeletal muscle will result in which of the following?

  A. Hypertrophy of skeletal muscle cells
  B. Hyperplasia of skeletal muscle cells
  C. Rupture of skeletal muscle
  D. No effect—skeletal muscle is of fixed length with minimal room for stretch

696. Skeletal muscle differs from cardiac muscle in all of the following ways EXCEPT:

  A. Cardiac muscle cells are mononucleated
  B. Cardiac muscle cells are connected by intercalated disks
  C. Cardiac muscle cells are microscopically striated
  D. Cardiac muscle depends on sodium-calcium channels

697. The force of contraction of a muscle can be increased by all of the following except:

  A. Recruitment of additional motor units
  B. Increasing the size of action potentials
  C. Increasing the amount of calcium released from the sarcoplasmic reticulum
  D. Increasing the size of individual muscle cells (hypertrophy)

Lethal mutations, although relatively rare, are a significant concern for many Americans. There are three ways in which mutations may can be inherited in the genome.

(1) An autosomal recessive genetic disorder will be fatal only if the individual's genotype is homozygous recessive. Fatal sex-linked disorders on the other hand will only affect hemizygous males. Tay-Sachs is an example of an autosomal recessive disorder in which affected individuals lack a functional enzyme that breaks down lipids in the brain. Build-up of sphingolipids results in progressive CNS damage, and premature death within 2-3 years.

(2) A dominant lethal disorder is fatal in both homozygous dominant as well as heterozygous individuals. However, a dominant lethal disorder may only be passed on if affected individuals survive until reproductive age. One such disorder is Huntington's Disease, a neurodegerative disorder which is first symptomatic in the fourth decade of life.

(3) Genetic mutations of incomplete dominance affect both heteroqygotes and individuals homozygous for the disease allele. Heterozygotes are often affected to a leser degree. In achondroplastic dwarfism, heterozygotes exhibit dwarfism while homozygosity results in fetal death.

The pedigree below depicts three generations of a family with a genetic disorder.

Square = Male

Circle = Female

Filled = Phenotypically affected

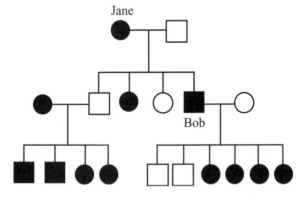

Figure 1

698. Pseudohypertropic muscular dystrophy is a genetic disorder that results in gradual muscular deterioration and subsequent death. If the disorder only affects males of unaffected parents, the most likely pattern of inheritance for pseudohypertrophic muscular dystrophy is:

A. Autosomal dominant
B. Autosomal recessive
C. Sex-linked dominant
D. Sex-linked recessive

699. A man heterozygous for achondroplasia and a woman have a child who dies in utero. The woman's genotype is most likely:

I.   Homozygous for achondroplasia
II. Heterozygous for achondroplasia
III. Homozygous normal
IV. A dwarf

A. I & II
B. II & IV
C. I, II, & IV
D. I, II, III, & IV

700. Colorblindness is a sex-linked, recessive disorder. A colorblind man heterozygous for Huntington's mates with a woman who is a carrier of the colorblind trait and is also heterozygous for Huntington's. What percentage of their children will have both Huntington's and colorblindness?

A. 25%
B. 37.5%
C. 50%
D. 75%

701. What is the most likely type of inheritance for the disease shown in the pedigree above?

A. Autosomal dominant
B. Autosomal recessive
C. Sex-linked dominant
D. Sex-linked recessive

702. If Bob mates with a woman who was heterozygous for the disease, what percentage of their sons would be affected?

A. 25%
B. 50%
C. 75%
D. 100%

703. Huntington's disease has been associated with certain DNA repeat-sequences on Chromosome 4. The length of these sequences increases with each successive generation, resulting in earlier disease manifestation. If individuals became symptomatic at the age of 8, Huntington's chorea would most likely:

A. Be regarded as a more serious disorder, as the nervous system is more vulnerable in children
B. No longer be sexually transmitted
C. Eventually cease to exist in nature
D. Become a pediatric disorder

Questions 704 through 705 are **NOT** based on a descriptive passage.

704. Hemophilia is rarely observed in females because:

I. Females require 2 defective X chromosomes to be affected, whereas males only require one.
II. Excessive bleeding from menstruation results in death of females that survive until puberty
III. The blood clotting mechanism in females is enhanced by their higher levels of estrogen and progesterone

A. I only
B. I & II
C. I & III
D. I, II, & III

705. A geneticist hypothesizes that an inherited disorder of cell metabolism is due to a defective mitochondrial gene. Which of the following findings would support such a hypothesis?

A. The mothers, but not the fathers, invariably have the same disorder
B. The disorder is found to be autosomal dominant
C. The fathers, but not the mothers, invariably have the same disorder
D. The disorder is found to be autosomal recessive

STOP. IF YOU FINISH BEFORE TIME IS CALLED, CHECK YOUR WORK. YOU MAY GO BACK TO ANY QUESTION IN THIS TEST BOOKLET.

EXAMINATION 16

Questions 706–751

Physical Sciences
Time: 20 Minutes
Questions 706–721

The apparent size of an object depends on the distance from which it is viewed. A small object held close may appear larger than a large object in the distance. The eye bases its perception of the actual size of an object on the angular size of the object. Angular size can be approximated by the ratio $\frac{h}{d}$, where h is the actual size of the object and d is the distance from which it is perceived. The simplest way to increase the angular size of an object is to move it closer to the eye. This method is limited, however, by the eye's inability to focus properly on objects that are closer than 25 cm.

A magnifying glass functions on an object close to the eye by creating an image at a distance of 25 cm or greater, while maintaining the angular size at, or near, the original ratio.

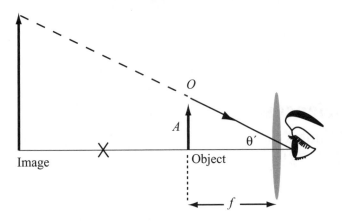

Figure 1 Lens Diagram

Typically, an object is placed within the focal length of a converging lens so that the image appears a distance of –25 cm behind the lens. As this is the closest point at which the eye may perceive the image clearly, this arrangement will provide maximum magnification. Maximum magnification is given by the formula:

$$M = 1 + \frac{25}{f}$$

where M is the angular magnification and f is the focal length of the lens in cm.

The eye is more relaxed when focused at greater distances. If an object is placed at the focal point of the lens, the image will be of infinite size and will appear at infinity. Also, for an object at the focal point of a lens, the angular size of the image is the same as the angular size of the object. When perceiving an image at infinity, the eye experiences less strain, but the magnification is reduced. For an object placed at the focal point of a magnifying glass, the magnification is given by the formula:

$$M = \frac{25}{f}$$

where M is the angular magnification and f is the focal length of the lens in cm.

706. At what distance from a magnifying glass, with a 12.50 cm radius of curvature, should an object be placed order to achieve the maximum magnification of the image?

A. 4.0 cm
B. 4.5 cm
C. 5.0 cm
D. 5.5 cm

707. As an object moves closer to the focal point, the image will grow larger and move farther away from the viewer. The viewer achieves a clear image with the largest possible magnification when the image is located (neglect the eye-lens distance):

A. less than 25 cm from the lens.
B. exactly 25 cm from the lens.
C. more than 25 cm from the lens but not at infinity.
D. at infinity.

708. The image formed by a magnifying glass is:

A. virtual and upright.
B. virtual and inverted.
C. real and upright.
D. real and inverted.

709. An object with a height of 2 cm is placed at the focal point of a magnifying glass with a focal length of 6 cm. What is the angular size of the image formed?

A. $\dfrac{1}{12}$

B. $\dfrac{1}{6}$

C. $\dfrac{1}{3}$

D. $\dfrac{1}{1}$

710. At what range of magnification does a magnifying glass with a focal length of 5 cm produce clearly visible images?

A. $1 < M < 5$
B. $1 < M < 6$
C. $5 < M < 6$
D. $6 < M < 25$

711. A coin with a diameter of 2 cm is viewed from a distance of 1 meter, without any magnification. At what distance must a plate with a diameter of 30 cm be placed in order for the eye to perceive the same angular size for both objects?

A. 6 m
B. 15 m
C. 30 m
D. 60 m

Passage II (Questions 712-717)

One of the most familiar, and noisome, corrosion reactions is the conversion of iron to rust. The reaction takes place on the surfaces of solid iron which are in contact with both air and water.

In the formation of rust, iron undergoes the half-reaction below.

$$Fe(s) \rightarrow Fe^{2+} + 2\ e^- \qquad E^\circ = 0.44 \text{ V}$$

Reaction 1

The electrons move through the metal until they reach a region where oxygen and water are both readily available. At this point the electrons combine with oxygen gas as shown below.

$$O_2(g) + 4\ H^+ + 4\ e^- \rightarrow 2\ H_2O(l) \qquad E^\circ = 1.23 \text{ V}$$

Reaction 2

The hydrogen ions required for Reaction 2 are supplied by the water present at the reaction site. Water also provides mobile ions which serve to complete the electric circuit required for an oxidation-reduction reaction.

Hydrated iron(III) oxide, or rust, is formed in a second oxidation-reduction reaction:

$$2\ Fe^{2+}(aq) + O_2(g) + (1 + x)H_2O(l) \rightarrow$$
$$Fe_2O_3 \cdot xH_2O(s) + 2\ H^+(aq)$$

Reaction 3

Iron is often coated with tin or zinc in an attempt to prevent rust formation. The reduction potentials for the two metals are shown below.

$$Sn^{2+} + 2e^- \rightarrow Sn(s) \qquad E^\circ = -0.14 \text{ V}$$

$$Zn^{2+} + 2e^- \rightarrow Zn(s) \qquad E^\circ = -0.76 \text{ V}$$

712. Which of the following statements best describes electron movement in Reaction 3?

A. Fe^{2+} is oxidized and O_2 is reduced.
B. Fe^{2+} is reduced and O_2 is oxidized.
C. Fe^{2+} is oxidized and H_2O is reduced.
D. Fe^{2+} is reduced and H_2O is oxidized.

713. If 4 moles of $H_2O(l)$ are consumed in Reaction 3, what will be the formula of the hydrated iron (III) oxide formed in Reaction 3?

A. $Fe_2O_3 \cdot H_2O$
B. $Fe_2O_3 \cdot 1\ H_2O$
C. $Fe_2O_3 \cdot 2\ H_2O$
D. $Fe_2O_3 \cdot 3\ H_2O$

714. What is the standard reaction emf when Reaction 1 and Reaction 2 are combined?

A. 0.35 V
B. 0.79 V
C. 1.67 V
D. 2.11 V

715. In an experiment two iron bars are partially immersed in water. Iron bar A is placed in fresh water and iron bar B is placed in salt water. Which bar will most likely rust first?

A. Bar A, because fresh water is a better conductor than salt water.
B. Bar A, because fresh water is a better insulator than salt water.
C. Bar B, because salt water is a better conductor than fresh water.
D. Bar B, because salt water is a better insulator than fresh water.

716. Solid iron is LEAST likely to be oxidized when placed in contact with an aqueous solution at pH:

A. 2
B. 5
C. 7
D. 10

717. Which of the following lists presents iron, tin, and zinc metals in order of increasing corrosion reactivity?

A. Sn, Fe, Zn
B. Zn, Fe, Sn
C. Fe, Sn, Zn
D. Zn, Sn, Fe

718. Light from distant stars undergoes a Doppler shift before reaching Earth, as the stars and Earth are constantly moving apart from one another. Compared to the light emitted at the source star, the light observed on Earth will have a lower:

A. frequency.
B. speed.
C. index of refraction.
D. wavelength.

719. Which of the following scenarios best demonstrates light dispersion?

A. White light is broken up into colors by a prism.
B. Shadows appear blurry around the edges.
C. Light enters a diamond and cannot escape.
D. Cancellation occurs when two light rays are combined.

720. What is the oxidation state of chlorine in potassium perchlorate, $KClO_4$?

A. -1
B. $+1$
C. $+5$
D. $+7$

721. A reversible oxidation-reduction reaction has a standard free energy change of -340 kJ. Which of the following is true for the reaction?

A. $E° < 0$ and $K_{eq} < 1$
B. $E° < 0$ and $K_{eq} > 1$
C. $E° > 0$ and $K_{eq} < 1$
D. $E° > 0$ and $K_{eq} > 1$

STOP. IF YOU FINISH BEFORE TIME IS CALLED, CHECK YOUR WORK. YOU MAY GO BACK TO ANY QUESTION IN THIS TEST BOOKLET.

GO ON TO THE NEXT PAGE.

Verbal Reasoning
Time: 20 Minutes
Questions 722–736

Personology, the scientific attempt to understand the whole person, is perhaps different from other sciences. In other fields, as time advances and research continues, our perceptive depth of the given field matures. In personology,
5 this may not necessarily be true. The understanding of persons has an inherent complexity that is almost commensurate to the intricacy of man himself, making the quest for understanding personality no simple task. Consequently, the modern quest to understand man has spawned multifar-
10 ious and variegated theories, propositions, and algorithms. McAdams comprehensively compartmentalizes these multitudinous conceptions into four broad categories.

In McAdams' scheme, one group of personality psychologists has tried to understand man in the context of the
15 unconscious motives and desires. It is these veiled entities that determine who a person is. Approaches that fall into this category not only explore hidden wishes and conflicts but biological determinants as well. Many are familiar with the Freudian psychoanalytic theory that well exemplifies
20 this category of approaches.

The next set of approaches concentrates on behavior. Theories that fall into this category seek to define the person in terms of how a person given certain traits interacts with a specific set of environmental conditions. How do dif-
25 ferent types of people react to different set circumstances? What effect do a certain set of environmental conditions have on the way one observably behaves? These are the type of questions addressed by this second set of approaches. Bandura's social learning theory and the Big 5
30 traits theory fall into this category.

The third category of approaches places an emphasis on the cognition and understanding of the person. These approaches look at the constructs and perceptions that comprise the way an individual views the world and himself.
35 These approaches state that the person's subjective perception defines the individual and his behavior. Existentialism and Maslow's theory of self-actualization typify this category.

The final cluster of approaches has in common the
40 tendency to analyze the person in terms of the socio-historic context in which he or she exists. These types of models also concentrate on the individual's past experiences in an attempt to understand the present person. The person is studied not as a snap shot of who he or she is at the current
45 moment, but rather as an ongoing narrative that has a past, present, and future.

722. Bandura's theory of social learning can be best categorized as:

A.   A theory that emphasizes the role of society on the way one learns
B.   A theory that interprets human behavior in terms of the learned social consequences of one's behavior in given situations
C.   A theory that is fundamentally different from the Big 5 traits theory
D.   A theory that looks at how past social interactions influence the way one perceives the world

723. The attempt understand the person in terms of a human story is most consistent with which category of approaches?

A.   The first category
B.   The second category
C.   The third category
D.   The fourth category

724. According to the passage, there is most probably a diverse range of methods to understand humans because:

A.   Humans have unconscious, conscious, behavioral, and social aspects
B.   Human are inherently complex
C.   Our methods of scientifically studying personality are not yet mature
D.   Man is the product of his social context, a context that has too many variables to ever be fully understood

725. Which of the following assertions would most weaken the main idea of this passage?

A. Ultimately, we can achieve a reasonable understanding of personality

B. Existentialism is not appropriately classified in this scheme because there are significant differences between it and the other approaches of the third category

C. There are many theories whose approach to understanding man does not fall into any of the four categories listed.

D. McAdams created this classification during a time of great turmoil

726. According to the author, in which following ways are all the modern approaches of personology most similar?

A. Each of the modern approaches looks at multiple aspects of the person

B. Modern approaches all address the central role of the intellect in understanding man

C. Modern approaches all concur that man is a complex entity that is difficult to study

D. Modern approaches may not be more accurate in understanding man than earlier approaches.

727. A man goes to work and is reprimanded by his boss for a mistake that he did not commit. He keeps quiet, but feels perturbed and uneasy the rest of the day. When he gets home, he kicks the dog and yells at his wife for not having supper ready. He has a short fuse for the rest of the evening but cannot seem to understand why he is acting as such. Which of the following approaches would be the most appropriate to study and explain this man's behavior?

A. Bandura's social learning theory

B. Maslow's theory of self actualization

C. Erik Erickson's theory of life stages

D. Freudian theory of conflict sublimation

728. A young college student falls passionately in love with a colleague and they marry. Growing up, the student's parents had been exacting and very strict. The student is now in a stage in his life where people generally feel the need to belong. The young bride finds her new husband very clingy and controlling. Which of the following theories stated in the passage would take all these factors into account when analyzing the student's personality?

A. Big 5 traits theory

B. Behaviorist theory

C. Existentialism

D. No such theory was mentioned in the passage

GO ON TO THE NEXT PAGE.

The Congress consists of two branches or chambers, the House of Representatives and the Senate. The Congress is the legislative branch of the United States government. Laws start out as bills in either the Senate or the House.
5 Though theoretically anyone can formulate or write a bill, only a member of Congress can introduce it to the chamber. Once a bill is introduced, the bill is referred to committee. The committee, which itself consists of bipartisan Congress members, will convene and evaluate the bill. They may
10 require further information about the bill in which case they will call committee action. The committee may also make amendments to the bill during markup sessions. Eventually the committee will vote on the bill. If the bill is reported favorably, a committee report will be drafted. In the Senate,
15 the bill then moves directly to the chamber floor for debate. In the House, the report will first go through the rules committee, which will set regulations regarding how long the bill may be debated and other such issues. Once on the floor, Congressional members will debate the various issues
20 raised by the bill. They will take into account financial ramifications, impact on other legislation, and other issues during the debate.

Following debate on the floor, the chamber in which the bill was introduced will vote on the bill. If it is passed,
25 then it will be referred to other chamber. If the second chamber also passes the bill, then the vote will be considered "enrolled" and sent to the president. In the case that the second chamber passes a modified version of the bill that was passed in the original chamber, the bill will move to
30 conference committee. In conference, members from both chambers will negotiate and reconcile any disagreements about the bill. The bill that comes out the conference committee is sent back to both the Senate and the House for a re-vote. The bill that comes out of conference is final; no
35 further amendments are allowed. If both chambers approve the conference report, the bill is sent to the president for his signature. The president is given only ten days to review the bill and either sign the bill into law, or to veto it. If he takes no action, the bill will automatically be passed. Also, if the
40 Congress adjourns before the president signs the bill during the ten-day presidential review period, then the bill will be considered to have been pocket vetoed. If the president does issue a formal veto, the bill will go back to the chamber in which it originated. A two-thirds vote is required to over-
45 ride the veto. If this is obtained, then the bill will again be sent to the other chamber. This chamber must also gather a two-thirds vote to override the veto. If both chambers override the veto, then the bill becomes law.

On Capitol Hill, legislative change occurs as the end
50 sum of much deliberation, contestation, and investigation. Beyond what occurs in the actual Congressional sessions, there is a lot of research, debate, and discussion that goes on in the offices of Congress members. Congressional staff, which consist of personal and committee staffers such as
55 L.A.'s and Congressional fellows, will educate, brief, and advice Congress members on the scores of issues they are required to debate and adjudicate on. Lobbyists will sometimes also meet with Congressmen but more often they create influence at the level of Congressional staff.
60 Legislation is final product of the complex interplay between all these factors.

729. The term *Congressional staff* most accurately refers to:

A. Senators and Congressmen
B. Members of congressional committees and subcommittees
C. The president's cabinet
D. L.A.'s, fellows, and press secretaries

730. Consider a case in which a group of Senators are in almost complete agreement on a bill that has come out of conference. However, they would like to make some minor changes to the bill. Which of the following courses of action are at their disposal?

A. Start all the way at the beginning of the legislative process by introducing their desired changes in the form of a new bill.
B. Filibuster to prevent the passage of the bill in vote unless their changes are incorporated into the bill
C. Make the changes to the bill and resubmit the bill to the conference committee
D. Use lobbying power to convince Congressmen of the importance to incorporate the desired changes into the bill

GO ON TO THE NEXT PAGE.

731. The president's party holds majority in both the House and the Senate. Consider the situation in which a bill has gone out of Congress to the president. For political reasons, the president would like the bill to die without issuing a formal veto. Which of the following actions might the President take to achieve this end?

   A.   Wait for the ten-day presidential review period to pass

   B.   As party members in Congress to create a movement for Congress to adjourn

   C.   The president has no options. He must issue a formal veto to stifle the passage of the bill into law.

   D.   The president will put pressure on the minority leader in Congress to get a 2/3 consensus for a veto

732. Some Congressmen want to ensure that the president does not veto a health care reform bill. They forward the president the bill, so that he may review it ahead of time, while the bill is still in consideration at the congressional level. With this goal in mind, the most effective stage to forward the bill to the president would be:

   A.   As soon as the bill is introduced

   B.   During committee action

   C.   During conference committee

   D.   Soon after a pocket veto

733. The term "reported favorably" in line 13 most likely refers to:

   A.   The complete consensus of both chambers

   B.   That the bill is mostly agreed upon by committee but may be subsequently modified

   C.   That the bill was passed into law by majority vote

   D.   The media presents the bill positively during reporting

734. A tobacco company spent millions of dollars lobbying over the past six fiscal years. This year they decide to evaluate the efficacy of their lobbying efforts. Based on the passage, which of the following is most likely the biggest obstacle to the tobacco company's lobbying platform?

   A.   Financial constraints due to new tax laws concerning the sale of tobacco

   B.   Changing constituency of Congress members

   C.   Changing constituency of Congress staff members

   D.   Inability to find enough time to convince Congress

735. Which of the following statements is TRUE?

   A.   A bill is first deliberated upon by committee before is debated on the floor

   B.   Anyone can introduce a bill to Congress but only a Congressman can draft a bill

   C.   A bill will be considered "enrolled" so long as it is passed by one chamber of Congress

   D.   A three-fifths vote is required to override a presidential veto.

STOP. IF YOU FINISH BEFORE TIME IS CALLED, CHECK YOUR WORK. YOU MAY GO BACK TO ANY QUESTION IN THIS TEST BOOKLET.

STOP.

Biological Sciences

Time: 20 Minutes
Questions 736–752

Bone consists of inorganic hydroxyapatite deposited on an organic matrix known as osteoid. Hydroxyapatite is comprised of inorganic calcium phosphates, and serves as the main storage for calcium in the body. Osteoid primarily contains proteoglycans and collagen. Mature bone has three types of cells: osteoblasts, osteoclasts, and osteocytes. Osteoblasts and osteocytes maintain and form bone while osteoclasts are responsible for bone resorption.

Bone is constantly remodeled and replaced; an estimated 500 mg of calcium enters and leaves bone per day. Control of calcium flux to and from bone affects serum calcium concentrations and is tightly regulated by three hormones: parathyroid hormone (PTH), calcitonin, and vitamin D metabolites.

PTH is released and acts primarily on bone and kidney to increase serum calcium and decrease serum phosphate concentrations. Calcitonin acts primarily on bone to decrease serum calcium and phosphate concentrations. Vitamin D3 acts primarily on the small intestine to increase calcium absorption from the diet. Parathyroid hormone enhances the activity of vitamin D3 and vice versa.

A reduction in overall bone mass is a condition known as osteoporosis, and is characterized by an equal loss of both organic and inorganic bone matrix. Osteomalacia, called rickets in children, is a disease in which there is inadequate mineralization of bone matrix. Osteomalacia/rickets is characterized by a ratio of mineral to organic bone material that is lower than normal.

Hormone Change	Effect on Serum $[Ca^{2+}]$	Effect on Serum $[PO_4^{3-}]$	Effect on Kidney	Effect on Bone	Effect on GI Tract
↑ PTH	↑	↓	↑ Ca^{2+} Reabsorption, ↓ PO_4^{3-} Reabsorption	↑ Bone Resorption	Synergistic with ↑ Vitamin D3
↑ Calcitonin	↓	↓	↓ Ca^{2+} Reabsorption, ↓ PO_4^{3-} Reabsorption	↓ Bone Resorption	No effect
↑ Vitamin D3	↑	↑	↑ Ca^{2+} Reabsorption, ↑ PO_4^{3-} Reabsorption	Synergistic with ↑ PTH	↑ Absorption of Ca^{2+} and PO_4^{3-}
↓ PTH	↓	↑	↓ Ca^{2+} Reabsorption, ↑ PO_4^{3-} Reabsorption	↓ Bone Resorption	Synergistic with ↓ Vitamin D3
↓ Calcitonin	↑	↑	↑ Ca^{2+} Reabsorption, ↑ PO_4^{3-} Reabsorption	↑ Bone Resorption	No effect
↓ Vitamin D3	↓	↓	↓ Ca^{2+} Reabsorption, ↓ PO_4^{3-} Reabsorption	Synergistic with ↓ PTH	↓ Absorption of Ca^{2+} and PO_4^{3-}

Table 1 Effects of Hormone Changes on Effector Organs and Serum Levels of Ca^{2+} and PO_4^{3-}.

736. It is well known that a deficiency in vitamin D activity causes osteomalacia. Given the composition of bone, what other vitamin deficiency would be expected to cause bone abnormalities?

   A. Vitamin A
   B. Vitamin C
   C. Vitamin B_{12}
   D. Vitamin E

737. Active osteoblasts producing osteoid have extensive rough ER and golgi complex, and are cuboidal in shape. Inactive osteoblasts appear flat in appearance. According to the passage and accompanying table, what hormone profile would you expect if osteoblasts appeared flat in appearance?

   A. ↑ PTH, ↓ Calcitonin
   B. ↓ PTH, ↑ Calcitonin
   C. ↑ PTH, ↑ Calcitonin
   D. ↓ PTH, ↓ Calcitonin

738. Osteoporosis is common in post-menopausal women. Hormone replacement therapy using estrogen was, until recently, a common treatment to combat osteoporosis in women. What effect is hormone replacement therapy with estrogen likely having in post-menopausal women?

- **A.** decreasing Ca^{2+} and PO_4^{3-} reabsorption in the kidney
- **B.** stimulating osteoclasts activity
- **C.** lowering the ratio of mineral to organic bone material
- **D.** increasing Ca^{2+} and PO_4^{3-} reabsorption in the kidney

739. As a fat-soluble vitamin, vitamin D is retained by the body. Excessive intake of vitamin D over long periods of time causes symptoms of vitamin D intoxication. A primary symptom of vitamin D intoxication is calcification of soft tissue such as the kidney (kidney stone formation). What is the likely composition of kidney stones under conditions of vitamin D intoxication?

- **A.** collagen
- **B.** vitamin D
- **C.** calcium phosphate
- **D.** proteoglycans

740. Paget's disease is a condition characterized first be excessive bone resorption and later by excessive bone formation. In the late stage of Paget's disease, osteoclast activity is reduced. What hormone treatment may beneficial in late stage Paget's disease?

- **A.** PTH
- **B.** calcitonin
- **C.** PTH + calcitonin
- **D.** Vitamin D

741. Osteosarcoma is a common type of bone cancer and most commonly develops in teenage boys. A prevalent symptom of osteosarcoma is weakened bones commonly leading to fracture. The most common cell type that has become a malignant neoplasm in osteosarcoma is osteoblasts. The bone composition of an individual with osteosarcoma is most likely to resemble which disease?

- **A.** osteoporosis
- **B.** scurvy
- **C.** sickle cell anemia
- **D.** rickets

742. Glucocorticoid administration for the treatment of various pathologies has many deleterious side effects. One side effect is glucocorticoid-induced osteoporosis, which is due to inhibition of protein synthesis by osteoblasts and an increase in secretion of a particular hormone. Secretion of which hormone is likely increased with glucocorticoid administration?

- **A.** Calcitonin
- **B.** PTH + calcitonin
- **C.** PTH
- **D.** Vitamin D

743. Osteoblasts are commonly located on the surface of bone. Osteocytes are osteoblasts that have been engulfed by mineralized bone and no longer reside on the bone surface. In addition to location, osteoblasts can be differentiated from osteocytes by morphology. Osteoblasts are either cuboidal or flat in shape, while osteocytes are spider-shaped. Which hormone(s) affecting bone and serum calcium levels is/are synthesized and secreted by the thyroid gland?

- **A.** PTH
- **B.** Calcitonin
- **C.** PTH + Calcitonin
- **D.** Vitamin D

GO ON TO THE NEXT PAGE.

Passage VI (Questions 744-750)

A population is said to be in equilibrium when its genetic structure does not change between generations. In order for this to be true, there are several necessary caveats, such as completely random mating. The factors necessary for population equilibrium rarely exist in reality as most populations are in constant flux. However, for the purposes of statistical analysis of allelic prevalence in a certain population, and for assessment of phenotypic probability, it is important to consider the theoretical situation in which a gene pool is stable. The Hardy-Weinberg equation allows for such calculations.

In the Southern Caribbean, there are two distinct populations of sand lizards, each living on a separate island. Assuming both populations are in a state of Hardy-Weinberg equilibrium, researchers may calculate allelic frequency for a gene coding for skin texture. In these lizards, there is a dominant allele (S) for smooth skin and a recessive allele (s) for scaly skin. On Island 1, the frequency of allele s was 0.4. On Island 2, only 1 in 100 lizards had scaly skin.

744. Which of the following population characteristics is NOT necessarily true of a gene pool of a stable population?

   A.   Large population size
   B.   No migration in or out of the population
   C.   Regular, random mutation
   D.   None of the above

745. Which of the following statements most accurately describes genetic drift?

   A.   The natural adaptation of a species to its environment
   B.   A random mutation that is made common in a population due to selective mating
   C.   A change in one population from another population of the same species due to geographic isolation
   D.   A change in allelic frequency due to a small population size

746. A certain gene has three possible alleles, A, B, and C. Nine percent of a population is homozygous for the A gene while sixteen percent is homozygous for the B gene. What is the frequency of the C gene in the population?

   A.   0.09
   B.   0.75
   C.   0.25
   D.   0.30

747. What percent of the lizard population on Island 2 is heterozygous?

   A.   10%
   B.   9%
   C.   90%
   D.   18%

748. In a population of 10,000 lizards on Island 1, how many would be expected to have smooth skin?

   A.   8400
   B.   3600
   C.   4800
   D.   48

749. Which of the following factors could account for the different frequencies of each allele observed on the two different islands?

   A.   The temperature of one island favors scaly skin more than the other.
   B.   Scales allow lizards to hide from certain predators. Island 1 is inhabited by such a predator, but Island 2 is not.
   C.   Several years prior, a group of lizards managed to move from Island 2 to Island 1. A higher proportion of lizards with scales than were present on Island 2 emigrated.
   D.   All of the above.

750. A female lizard that is heterozygous for smooth skin mates with a male lizard that is also heterozygous. What is the percent chance that their first child will have scaly skin?

   A.   10%
   B.   16%
   C.   25%
   D.   None of the above.

GO ON TO THE NEXT PAGE.

751. A population of bears in Northern California is almost completely wiped out by an earthquake. A small group of bears survive, all from the same clan/family, and most of which share similar characteristics. Which of the following phenomena accurately describes the ensuing shift in the gene pool?

   A.   Bottlenecking
   B.   Divergent Evolution
   C.   Isolationist Evolution
   D.   Natural Selection

STOP. IF YOU FINISH BEFORE TIME IS CALLED, CHECK YOUR WORK. YOU MAY GO BACK TO ANY QUESTION IN THIS TEST BOOKLET.

STOP.

EXPLANATIONS 01

Answers to Questions 1–47

ANSWERS TO EXAMINATION 1

PHYSICAL SCIENCES	VERBAL REASONING	BIOLOGICAL SCIENCES
1. A ✓	17. C ✓	32. D ✗
2. B ✓	18. B ✗	33. A ✗
3. B ✓	19. C ✓	34. C ✓
4. D ✓	20. A ✓	35. A ✗
5. D ✓	21. D ✓	36. D ✓
6. A ✓	22. B ✗	37. D ✗
7. A ✓	23. B ✗	38. A ✓
8. A ✓	24. C ✗	39. B ✓
9. B ✓	25. D ✗	40. A ✓
10. D ✗	26. A ✓	41. C ✓
11. C ✓	27. B ✗	42. B ✓
12. B ✓	28. C ✗	43. A ✗
13. A ✓	29. D ✓	44. A ✓
14. D ✓	30. B ✓	45. D ✓
15. B ✓	31. D ✓	46. C ✓
16. B ✓		47. B ✗

Examination 01: Physical Sciences

Passage I (Questions 1-7)

1. **A is correct.** Object 1 starts with an initial velocity of 20 m/s. The velocity immediately starts to decrease at the rate of -10 m/s^2, or g. After 2 seconds, at peak height, the velocity is equal to 0, and then the velocity becomes negative as the object starts to fall. After 4 seconds, the velocity is -20 m/s as the object returns to its initial height.

2. **B is correct.** The velocity of Object 2 is always positive, so the displacement is always increasing. Another way to think about this one is to remember that the displacement is given by the area under the velocity curve. As you go from left to right on the graph for Object 2, the area continues to increase during the entire 4 seconds.

3. **B is correct.** The acceleration is equal to the slope of the velocity graph. The slope of the graph for Object 3 is constant at -10 m/s^2 for the first 2 seconds, and then becomes 10 m/s^2 for the next 2 seconds. So the acceleration graph will be a horizontal line below the x-axis for the first 2 seconds and then another horizontal line above the x-axis for the next 2 seconds.

4. **D is correct.** Speed is the magnitude of the velocity vector. During the first 2 seconds, the speed decreases as the velocity goes to zero. For the next 2 seconds, the velocity becomes increasingly negative, so its magnitude is increasing. Thus the speed decreases for the first 2 seconds, then increases for the next 2 seconds.

5. **D is correct.** As acceleration is equal to the slope of the velocity curve, one can extrapolate from the graph that the acceleration of Object 4 is 5 m/s^2. Then the equation, $d = (1/2)at^2$, can be employed to calculate the displacement for each time period. Alternatively, one can find the area under the curve (which is just the area of a triangle) for each time period.

6. **A is correct.** The shorter the time intervals between measurements, the more accurate the students' approximations of instantaneous velocity will be. If the acceleration is constant, the velocity graph will show a straight line, which is much easier to approximate than the curved velocity graph that would be generated by a varying acceleration.

7. **A is correct.** The graph for Object 1 is the only one that dips below the x-axis, so it's the only one that goes forward and then backward, ending up where it started. If you think of displacement as the area under the velocity curve, you can see that the positive and negative areas on the graph for Object 1 will cancel each other out.

Passage II (Questions 8-13)

8. **A is correct.** The velocity components across and down the river form the right triangle shown below. The Pythagorean theorem gives the resultant vector.

$$8^2 + 15^2 = 17^2$$

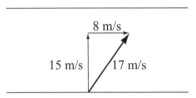

9. **B is correct.** Use the 30-60-90 triangle shown below to find that the Westward component of the canoe's velocity is 3 m/s. Then add the vectors pointing to the East and West. (8 m/s E) + (-3 m/s W) = 5 m/s to the East.

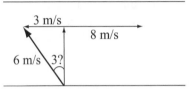

10. **D is correct.** The canoe travels at 6 m/s and the current flows at 8 m/s, so no matter how far the canoe is angled to the West, there will always be some motion to the East and the canoe will always be taken some distance down the river.

11. **C is correct.** This is similar to projectile motion. The time it takes to cross the river depends only on the velocity directed to the North. The current will move the boat farther down the river, but it will have no effect on the time of the crossing. So the boat should be pointed directly across the river to maximize the velocity in that direction.

12. **B is correct.** The time depends only on the Northward speed and the distance straight across the river.

    $t = d/v = (1800 \text{ m})/(15 \text{ m/s}) = 120 \text{ sec} = 2 \text{ minutes.}$

13. **A is correct.** Since the Northward velocity and the Westward velocity due to the current are constant, the resultant velocity is also constant. When velocity is constant, the acceleration must be equal to zero.

Independent Questions (Questions 14-16)

14. **D is correct.** In projectile motion, the horizontal component of velocity is proportional to the cosine of the angle of elevation. As the sine of the angle increases, the cosine must decrease, and so will the horizontal speed. The vertical component of velocity is proportional to the sine of the angle of elevation, so when the sine increases,

so does the vertical speed.

15. **B is correct.** If the velocity and acceleration vectors are in opposite directions, the automobile is decelerating. In other words, the automobile's velocity is approaching zero and it must be slowing down.

16. **B is correct.** Projectile B has greater mass, so it will have greater weight, and thus, greater force due to gravity. All projectiles accelerate downward at 9.8 m/s^2 by gravity, irrespective of their mass, so the accelerations will be equal.

Examination 01: Verbal Reasoning

Passage III (Questions 17-23)

17. Suppose that a study found that contrary to popular belief, the majority of people have little or no experience with copiers and printers, but instead patronize commercial printers and copiers for these services. Which of the following statements is an assumption of the author related to this study that would be called into question?

    A. Smaller publishers should choose their printing services wisely.
    WRONG: This is not an assumption of the author's that would be called into question. The above statement is actually the author's thesis, and, though the supposition does weaken the author's thesis, it is not strong enough to completely call it into question.

    B. One of the differences between offset and digital printing is visual.
    WRONG: This assumption would not be called into question by the supposition. Experience with printers and copiers is a distinct topic from the differences between offset and digital printing.

    C. The experience of changing a toner cartridge is common to us all.
    CORRECT: This is an assumption of the author's that would be called into question by the supposition. "Outside of the publishing world, the majority of us are familiar with digital style printers …[because] We have all had to change toner cartridges" (lines 13-16).

    D. Most people own their own copiers or printers.
    WRONG: Although this statement contradicts the results of the study, it is not an assumption of the author's.

18. According to information in the passage, the loss of pages would be likely to occur later in the life of a book, when:

    A. bound with the use of high speed rollers and cutters.

WRONG: This is not the point when, "later in the life of the book" the loss of pages would be likely. This answer is not specific enough. It is either the heat from the printing, the application of the adhesive, or the binding with no regard for the grain of the paper which can cause pages to fall out.

II. the pages have been dried out and part of the pages are sealed.
CORRECT: This is the point when, "later in the life of the book" the loss of pages would be likely.

III. the book is smaller than 8 1/2 × 11 inches.
WRONG: This is not the point when, "later in the life of the book" the loss of pages would be likely. Though the author provides that "problems are exacerbated if the book is smaller than the common 8 1/2 × 11 inches" (lines 54-55), he expands upon this idea in the second to last paragraph to explain that this is because there is a higher likelihood that the printer may disregard the potential problems with the grain of the paper.

A. I only

B. II only
CORRECT: See the above answer explanations.

C. III only

D. II and III only

19. Which of the following conclusions can most reasonably be drawn from the author's description of printing companies, printers, and his advice to publishers?

    A. Digital printers, though less expensive, are not worth using in the long run.
    WRONG: This is not the most reasonable conclusion as its clear that the author feels there is a place for digital printers in the publishing business. He suggests, however, that one must remain aware of the advantages and disadvantages. This suggested awareness is one of the reasons the author recommends, "use an older established printer who has recently acquired a digital printing capability" (lines 72-73). A long-established printer would presumably be better able to handle the problems associated with digital printing.

    B. Older established publishers should seek out printers who use offset presses.
    WRONG: This conclusion does not support the arguments presented in the passage. It is nonsensical in that older established printers would most likely use offset presses.

    C. Older establisher printers would be less likely to ignore paper grain, even if they were using digital printers.
    CORRECT: This is the most reasonable conclusion, and also one of the reasons the author recom-

mends, "use an older established printer who has recently acquired a digital printing capability" (lines 72-73). A long-established printer would presumably be better able to handle the problems associated with digital printing.

D. A publisher would be well advised to avoid using digital printing altogether.
   WRONG: This is not the most reasonable conclusion. It is clear that the author feels there is a place for digital printers in the publishing business. He only suggests, however, that one remain aware of the advantages and disadvantages.

20. If the hypothesis of the passage is correct, one would generally expect that, in the printing business:

A. a printer who has only used high-speed digital presses has not been in business as long as an offset printer.
   CORRECT: The author conveys that offset printers have been around quite a bit longer than digital printers. Therefore, "generally" this answer would be an expected finding.

B. the grain of the paper is one of the most important characteristics of the binding process to be aware of.
   WRONG: There is no indication from the passage that paper grain is one of the "most important characteristics".

C. digital style printers and presses are by far the most prevalent in existence today.
   WRONG: There is no support for this answer in the passage.

D. a recently acquired digital printing capability indicates that the printer will be better established in the practice.
   WRONG: This answer is based upon the final sentence of the passage, "use an older established printer who has recently acquired a digital printing capability" (lines 72-73). However, the answer is misleading because it does not also provide that the printer who "recently acquired digital printing" had been using offset printing prior to this acquisition. However, a novice printer may have recently acquired digital capability.

21. What is the intended relevance of the comment, "Loupes have been largely relegated to the stereotypical squinting diamond merchant, and with them, the skills to detect such minor visual variations" (lines 8-10), to the rest of the passage?

A. To explain how difficult it is to acquire the skills necessary to distinguish one style of printing from another
   WRONG: This is not the intended relevance of the

comment to the rest of the passage. The comment does not have so much to do with the "acquisition" of skills, but the "loss" of skills. There is no implication of how difficult the skills are to acquire in any event.

B. To provide a framework from which to understand the more arcane areas of offset printing
   WRONG: This is not the intended relevance of the comment to the rest of the passage. The statement was not made in order to explore certain areas of printing, but rather to support the author's argument of decreased attention and awareness of the changes in the printing industry. Note that this answer is very vague. Generally, unless a vague answer is appropriate, it should be avoided.

C. To express the subtleties in the flaws of diamonds and other gemstones
   WRONG: This is not the intended relevance of the comment to the rest of the passage. The author makes no attempt to discuss aspects of the jewel industry.

D. To indicate that there is less attention paid to minute visual detail than there has been in the past
   CORRECT: This is the intended relevance of the comment to the rest of the passage. The referenced comment highlights a change over time, which is reflected in this answer choice. Keep in mind the author's main purpose of raising awareness of the differences between digital and offset modalities.

22. Suppose that the author was unaware of a new adhesive, which is permeable to air and moisture, that had been introduced into the perfect binding process. Which of the following *changes* in the author's advice would be most appropriate?

A. Since the heat from digital printing would not cause curling, the only difference between offset and digital press would be the almost imperceptible visual differences.
   WRONG: This would not be the most appropriate change in the advice of the author. The author additionally seems to feel that "digital printers are notorious for ignoring paper grain" (line 67) and implies that there is a lack of experience with many digital printers (lines 69-74).

B. The author's advice to smaller publishers would still be valid, though his reasoning regarding why the paper was curling would have to be changed.
   CORRECT: This would be the most appropriate change in the advice of the author.

C. Because curling of the pages later in the life of a book would not be a problem, a publisher would only have to ensure that digital printers were

aware of the ramifications of paper grain.
WRONG: This would not be the most appropriate change in the advice of the author. This answer overlooks the author's insistence of subtle, yet visually apparent, differences between digital and offset printing.

D. There would no longer be a strong argument supporting the use of offset printers over digital printers.
WRONG: This would not be the most appropriate change in the advice of the author. This is not true.

23. The author's primary purpose in addressing his audience is to:

A. Consider the effects of newer technology on smaller publishing businesses as a whole.
WRONG: The author does not discuss the effects of digital printing on the publishing industry as a whole, and thus this cannot be the author's primary purpose in the passage. Note, that this answer is inappropriately broad.

B. Clarify the advantages and disadvantages of one form of printing over another.
CORRECT: The passage presents the pros and cons of digital printing in order to raise awareness in the audience regarding the advantages and disadvantages of the two techniques. Note that the author is neither for nor against digital printing as opposed to offset printing. He simply believes that the smaller publishers ignore some of the important differences between the two.

C. Question the need for the newer digital presses in the printing industry.
WRONG: It is not apparent that this is the author's primary purpose in the passage. The author acknowledges that the newer digital printing has its place and it at the very least, provides less expensive options to publishers.

D. Justify the use of the older, better established businesses and offset printers.
WRONG: It is not apparent that this is the author's primary purpose in the passage. The author acknowledges that the newer digital printing has its place and it at least, less expensive.

Passage IV (Questions 24-31)

24. Which of the following statements, if true, would most directly *challenge* the ideas of the author?

A. Canine identification is actually not required in East Germany.

WRONG: This statement does not most directly challenge the ideas of the author. The author's question in line 2 was metaphorical, and might just as well have been Communist China, or Russia.

B. Puppies that don't pass their Schutzhund trials are neutered.
WRONG: The passage states, "If the animal fails its Schutzhund trials it is illegal to breed that German Shepherd. Puppies which the breeders believe lack the proper conformation, are destroyed in order that they don't breed…" (lines 56-9) Whether the puppies are neutered or destroyed, the fact that they are not bred remains constant. This statement does not contradict the author's arguments.

C. Most American 'dog lovers' have a good understanding of the conformation characteristics of their particular breed.
CORRECT: This statement most directly challenges the ideas of the author. "To most American dog lovers, having papers would also seem to convey something more …" (lines 8-9), which the author clearly disagrees with. If American dog lovers were well aware of conformation standards, then the author would be largely refuted.

D. The Schutzhund competitions have become increasingly lax in their standards.
WRONG: This statement does not most directly challenge the ideas of the author. How lax is lax? In what way? This answer is ambiguous. They may or may not still be stricter than the 'dog lovers' and 'puppy farms' that the author is railing against. This is not the best answer.

25. Elsewhere, the author of the passage states that far too many people in so-called 'free societies' place trust in well-known organizations that is unwarranted by the results of these organizations' performance. This statement most directly supports the passage assertion that:

A. the West German Schutzhund trials are a model which the United States should be following.
WRONG: This passage assertion is not directly supported by the statement. It does not closely follow the tenets of the statement and is not as appropriate an answer as Answer D.

B. it should be illegal to breed dogs within the United States unless they have passed a Schutzhund trial.
WRONG: This is not a clear passage assertion.

C. purebred breeding within the United States has proven disastrous for dogs.
WRONG: This passage assertion is not directly supported by the statement. The "well-known or-

ganization" aspect of the statement is missing from this assertion.

D. reliance upon a purebred status from the AKC has resulted in inbreeding.
CORRECT: This passage assertion is directly supported by the statement.

26. For which of the following conclusions does the passage offer the *most* support?

A. In West Germany, the German Shepherd breed benefits from the Schutzhund trials.
CORRECT: The passage offers the most support for this conclusion.

B. It is the desire of the AKC that as many dog owners as possible register their dogs as purebreds.
WRONG: The passage does not offer the most support for this conclusion.

C. It is the goal of the AKC to ruin breeds of dogs within the United States.
WRONG: The passage does not offer the most support for this conclusion. This is not a passage conclusion.

D. The goals of the Schutzhund trials and the AKC are diametrically opposed to one another.
WRONG: The passage does not offer the most support for this conclusion. It is not at all clear that this is an accurate conclusion.

27. On the basis of the passage, one can most reasonably infer that careful judging has the capacity to distinguish:

A. between who should and who should not be breeding dogs.
WRONG: This is not the most reasonable inference.

B. which animals will contribute most to the future of a given breed.
CORRECT: This is the most reasonable inference based upon passage information. This is what the author believes Schutzhund trials do.

C. whether or not 'papers' should be conferred upon a given dog.
WRONG: This is not the most reasonable inference.

D. why a certain dog might or might not be able to pass a Schutzhund competition.
WRONG: This is not the most reasonable inference. This idea is not supported by the passage.

28. Implicit in the passage is the assumption that:

A. most people love dogs.
WRONG: This assumption is not implicit in the passage. The generalities in the passage are about people who love their dogs.

B. whoever is reading the passage must love dogs as much as the author.
WRONG: This assumption is not implicit in the passage.

C. anyone who doesn't agree with the author is stupid.
CORRECT: This assumption is implicit in the passage. Particularly in the first and second paragraph, the author's sarcastic and derogatory way of referring to people who believe what he doesn't would lead one to this assumption. For instance, he refers to others as sometimes "poorly educated", and "dolts".

D. an animal's purebred status nothing.
WRONG: This assumption is not implicit in the passage. Beware particularly aware of unequivocal statements in an answer unless they are supported within a passage. Although, not to the same degree as in Answer C. Obviously the purebred status must be of some relevance because it seems that only German Shepherds are bred to other German Shepherds by the author's vaunted West German breeders.

29. According to the passage, the Conformation area of Schutzhund (lines 34-53) focuses primarily on which of the following aspects of a German Shepherd?

A. Will the dog be able to perpetuate the breed?
WRONG: This is not the primary aspect that is focused upon during Conformation trials. Whether the dog should be bred is considered in light of the trial results. All dogs with functioning reproductive systems will be able to breed.

B. Should the dog be disqualified for hip displasia?
WRONG: This is not the primary aspect that is focused upon during Conformation trials. Dysplasia is mentioned as only one example of many disqualifying characteristics.

C. Can the dog obey the rules of the Schutzhund competition?
WRONG: This is not the primary aspect that is focused upon during Conformation trials. A dog cannot be expected to understand and obey rules per say. This answer does not make much sense.

D. Does the dog meet the standards for physical perfection?
CORRECT: This is the primary aspect that is focused upon during Conformation trials (lines 34-43).

30. In the past, some breakaway chapters of the AKC have placed stricter limits on their certification of an animal for breeding purposes than those now used by the parent association. Given this information, the author could best clarify his argument with the stipulation that:

A. his argument applies to both the present and future.
WRONG: This stipulation is not an appropriate clarification of the passage given the additional information. This answer is vague and not really pertinent to the additional information provided.

B. The passage addresses only certain parts of the AKC.
CORRECT: This stipulation is an appropriate clarification of the passage given the additional information; such as the "parent association", and perhaps, other chapters of the AKC.

C. The passage addresses only these breakaway chapters.
WRONG: This stipulation is not an appropriate clarification of the passage given the additional information. The "breakaway chapters" is apparently whom it would not apply to.

D. his argument applies to certifications in West Germany.
WRONG: This stipulation is not an appropriate clarification of the passage given the additional information. The author's arguments still apply to the "parent association" and the other "chapters" of the AKC to whom his arguments are relevant.

31. Of the following statements, which would most *weaken* the purpose of the Schutzhund trials?

A. Strict adherents to AKC breeding guidelines produce dogs that are very sound, both structurally, and temperamentally.
WRONG: This statement would not weaken the purpose of the Schutzhund trials. This begs the question, "Is everyone a strict adherent?" The author states that he is referring to "poorly educated" breeders.

B. The Schutzhund trials invariably produce the soundest animals for perpetuation of the breed.
WRONG: This statement would strengthen the purpose of the Schutzhund trials.

C. Euthanizing dogs who have failed the trials is inhumane.
WRONG: This statement would not weaken the purpose of the Schutzhund trials, as they are intended to identify superior members of the breed. The practice of euthanasia is a tangential issue.

D. National sanctioning of the trials results in bribery and unfair judging.
CORRECT: This statement would most weaken the purpose of the Schutzhund trials. This could mean that the results were not choosing the most qualified dogs for breeding, resulting in detrimental effects similar to those alleged by the author to be occurring in the U.S

Passage V (Questions 32-38)

32. **D is correct.** The student should be familiar with the absorption mechanisms for carbohydrates, proteins, and lipids. Galactose (not fructose!) and proteins (amino acids, dipeptides, and tripeptides) are transported via Na-dependent cotransport, while lipids are absorbed as micelles. Fatty acids are component molecules of lipids, along with glycerol, and are thus transported within micelles. Bile acids are reabsorbed via Na-dependent transport, however, this information is not necessary to answer correctly.

33. **A is correct.** This question touches on mechanisms of enzyme regulation, including activation. Pancreatic peptidases must be tightly controlled to prevent degradation of human proteins. Thus they are only activated once in the intestinal lumen by brush border enzymes. Pepsin is the frequently sited example of pH-dependent activation. The pancreas secretes HCO_3 to neutralize gastric acidity, thus ideally there is no significant change of pH within the intestinal lumen. Temperature does not change and peptidases do not require cofactors.

34. **C is correct.** This question addresses the common misconception that bile acids are absorbed with micelles. Bile acids function to stabilize micelle formation, however only lipid components are absorbed, which include choices A, B, and D. Bile acids may be excreted or reabsorbed via Na-dependent transport.

35. **B is correct.** In order to answer this question correctly, the student must be remember that proteins, unlike carbohydrates, do not have to be hydrolyzed to single subunits (i.e. monosaccharide or amino acid) in order to be absorbed. Amino acids, dipeptides, and tripeptides are all transported across intestinal cell membranes via carriers. Sucrose must first be digested, as alluded in the passage, before absorption. Sucrose is not absorbed via a carrier—its component monosaccharides are. Fructose, unlike glucose and galactose, is absorbed via facilitated diffusion and thus requires a carrier protein.

36. **D is correct.** Competitive inhibition should be suspected when the passage clues the reader with the phrase "directly inhibits" and compares acarbose's binding affinity to that of the substrate. This notion should be confirmed upon examining the graph: as the concentration of substrate is increased, the reaction rate becomes closer and closer to the reaction rate in the absence of acarbose. In other words, when more substrate is around, it outcompetes acarbose for the same binding side. Although, Vmax and K_M are not tested directly on the MCAT, the student should be familiar with enzyme kinetics and how they are affected by inhibition.

37. D is correct. Acarbose directly blocks the substrate binding site, thereby reducing the amount of enzyme that is available to bind substrate. Acarbose directly blocks a productive reaction from proceeding, decreasing the observed rate as a consequence of there being less functioning enzyme available. Acarbose is acting as a competitive inhibitor, which is an irreversible type of inhibition. Answer choice B is incorrect as competitive inhibitors are not irreversible and do not inactivate active site residues. The enzyme kinetics graph is meant to show the reaction rate as a function of substrate concentration, not acarbose (inhibitor) concentration. Choices A and C are phenomena that may be seen in either non-competitive inhibition or allosteric regulation.

38. A is correct. This one may require a bit of thinking. If the glucosidase is blocked, polysaccharides will not be digested, and subsequently not absorbed (only monosaccharides can be absorbed). Thus they will be excreted. The passage mentions lactase as another enzyme that digests saccharides (lactose). Without lactase, lactose cannot be digested into monosaccharides, and thus will not be absorbed but excreted as well. Bile acid deficiency will result in fat malabsorption (steatorrhea) and intrinsic factor deficiency will result in vitamin B12 malabsorption (pernicious anemia). Cholera affects ion channels in the intestinal mucosa.

39. B is correct. The answer is in the *y*-axis of the graph. An enzyme that hydrolyses bonds is a hydrolase. Although the six categories of enzymes need not be memorized, the student should be familiar with enzyme nomenclature and kinases. Oxidoreductases catalyze oxidation/reduction reactions. Lyases are also more commonly known as synthetases, or synthases.

Passage VI (Questions 40-46)

40. A is correct. Citrate levels will increase if the flux of glycolysis exceeds the flux of the Krebs cycle under aerobic conditions. As mentioned in the passage, the pyruvate formed in glycolysis is converted to acetyl CoA, which then combines with oxaloacetate to form Citrate. As shown in the diagram, Citrate down regulates an upstream reaction, in this case the formation of Fructose-1,6-bisphosphate. This is the definition of negative feedback. The other answer choices are false..

41. C is correct. Along with the enzymes and glucose, NAD^+, ATP, ADP, and Pi are required for glycolysis to proceed. FAD^+ is involved in the Krebs cycle and oxidative phosphorylation, and NADH is a product of glycolysis and the Krebs cycle.

42. B is correct. Glycolysis, although often referred to as anaerobic respiration, is also a requisite for aerobic respiration. The reaction series takes place in the presence or absence of oxygen. The fate of pyruvate, however, is determined by oxygen availability: fermentation or aerobic respiration.

43. B is correct. Glucose phosphorylation results in a charged molecule, thus creating a barrier for the molecule to recross the cell membrane. Once a cell has glucose, it wants to hold on to the source of energy. The other answer choices are false.

44. A is correct. Glucagon levels would be upregulated as the body mobilizes glucose stores into the bloodstream. According to the passage, when glucose levels are low, the body preferentially allocates glucose for the brain. This is accomplished by upregulation of gluconeogenesis to supply the body (primarily the brain) with glucose. Glycolysis will be directly proportional to the metabolic rate, and only indirectly proportional to blood sugar level. In other words, there is a basal level of glycolysis that will be maintained, mostly via gluconeogenesis and the glycogenolysis.

45. D is correct. By definition, allosteric regulation involves enzyme binding at a site other than the active site. Once bound, an allosteric regulator can affect enzyme activity by changing the conformation of the enzyme, which usually results in an increase or decrease of the enzyme affinity for substrate at the active site. Covalent modification is often a reversible process that can be either inhibitory or activating, and zymogen activation is usually achieved by cleavage or phosphorylation.

46. C is correct. Diffusion of a solute up its concentration gradient without energy input, in some form, does not happen. All other answer choices release energy, and thus have a negative free energy change.

Independent Question (Question 47)

47. B is correct. Aerobic respiration cannot take place as erythrocytes lack mitochondria. RBCs must meet their energy needs with glycolysis.

EXPLANATIONS 02

Answers to Questions 48–94

ANSWERS TO EXAMINATION 2

PHYSICAL SCIENCES	VERBAL REASONING	BIOLOGICAL SCIENCES
48. C	64. B	79. B
49. C	65. C	80. D
50. D	66. B	81. C
51. B	67. B	82. B
52. D	68. D	83. D
53. C	69. D	84. D
54. D	70. C	85. C
55. D	71. A	86. D
56. A	72. D	87. A
57. B	73. C	88. B
58. C	74. D	89. B
59. C	75. C	90. A
60. A	76. D	91. B
61. B	77. B	92. C
62. D	78. D	93. C
63. A		94. B

Passage I (Questions 48-55)

48. C is correct. As all three projectiles are launched at the same speed and projectile C attains the highest height, thus projectile C must have had the greatest angle of elevation. If this relationship is not intuitive, the height equation can be used to see that a projectile's height is a function of the launch angle. The greatest angle will have the greatest value for sine, which will produce the greatest value for height.

49. C is correct. As the angle of elevation increases from zero, the horizontal distance will increase until the angle reaches 45°. At 45°, the horizontal distance is at a maximum. From 45° to 90°, the distance will decrease until it returns to zero at 90° elevation. The distance equation may be employed to demonstrate this phenomena with real values.

50. D is correct. Plug the values into the horizontal distance formula given in the passage.

$$d = \frac{2v^2}{g}\sin(90-x)\sin x = \frac{2(50)^2}{10}\sin 45° =$$

$$\frac{2(50)^2}{10}(0.7)(0.7) = 250 \text{ m}$$

51. B is correct. After 2.5 seconds, the projectile is at its peak height, and the vertical component of velocity is zero. As the horizontal component of velocity is constant throughout the flight, the speed (or magnitude of velocity) will be at a minimum when there is no vertical velocity to take into account.

52. D is correct. The height of the projectile (95 m) can be found on the graph, and subsequently plugged into the equation provided.

$$h = \frac{(v\sin x)^2}{2g}$$

$$95 = \frac{50^2(\sin x)^2}{20}$$

$$\sin x = \sqrt{\frac{(20)(95)}{(50)^2}} = \sqrt{\frac{1900}{2500}} = \sqrt{\frac{19}{25}}$$

53. C is correct. The passage tells you that the two projectiles had the same initial speed. From the horizontal distance equation, the sines of the two angles will be identical if the two angles add up to 90°. Choice A may seem correct when considering only the equation. However, the graph shows that the two projectiles rose to different heights, so they must have different angles of elevation.

54. D is correct. Use $d = vt$. The graph shows a time of 5 seconds for projectile A.

$$v = d/t = (125 \text{ m})/(5 \text{ sec}) = 25 \text{ m/s}.$$

55. D is correct. The acceleration for any projectile is equal to the acceleration due to gravity, 10 m/s² downward. Note that there is no horizontal acceleration in projectile motion as horizontal velocity remains constant.

Passage II (Questions 56-60)

56. A is correct. To convert 60 m/s to km/hr, you need to multiply by (3600 sec/1 hour) and then multiply by (1 km/1000 m).

57. B is correct. Use the formula for distance when acceleration, intial speed and final speed are known. (the time-independent equation)

$$v_f^2 - v_o^2 = 2ad$$

$$3600 - 0 = (2)(3)\,d$$

$$d = (3600)/(6) = 600 \text{ m}$$

58. C is correct. The 12 km and 16 km distances form the legs of a 3-4-5 right triangle. The total horizontal displacement forms the hypotenuse of the triangle, which is equal to 20 km.

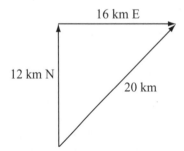

59. C is correct. The time from rest until cruising altitude is found by adding the time spent on the runway and the time spent in the air reaching cruising altitude.

Runway time = (runway final speed)/(runway acceleration) = (60 m/s)/(3 m/s2)= 20 sec

Air time = (height)/(vertical speed) = (2250 m)/(9 m/s) = 250 sec

$$250 \text{ sec} + 20 \text{ sec} = 270 \text{ sec}.$$

60. A is correct. The passage states that the plane has a horizontal acceleration, however, the plane is climbing at a constant velocity and thus lacks vertical acceleration.

Independent Questions (Questions 61-63)

61. B is correct. Use the time-independent equation.

$$v_f^2 = v_o^2 + 2ad$$

$$v_f^2 = 0 = (2)(10)(3) = 60$$

The square root of 60 is closest to 8.

62. D is correct. First use $d = vt$ to find the radius of the Earth's orbit.

$$d = vt = (3 \times 10^8 \text{ m/s})(500 \text{ sec}) = 1.5 \times 10^{11} \text{ m/s}$$

In one year, the Earth travels once around the circle, so the circumference will yield the distance traveled.

$$C = 2\pi r = (2)(3.14)(1.5 \times 10^{11} \text{ m/s}) = \text{about } 9 \times 10^{11} \text{ m/s}$$

63. A is correct. The velocity of the box is constant, so the acceleration must be equal to zero.

Examination 02: Verbal Reasoning

Passage III (Questions 64-69)

64. Which of the following assertions did the author NOT provide support for in the passage?

A. Some people in Denmark, Germany, Sweden, and the U.S are wearing surgical facemasks.
WRONG: This is not one of the author's assertions. Therefore, the question of support provided in the passage is moot.

B. It is a fact that many bacteria and germs are actually helpful to human life.
CORRECT: This is one of the author's assertions and there is no support provided for this assertion in the passage. "Beyond the well-known fact that many of these organisms are actually helpful and necessary to human life … " (lines 17-19).

C. Having pets that bring dirt into your home might make you healthier.
WRONG: This is one of the author's assertions, however, there is support provided for this assertion within the passage.

D. Anti-bacterial soaps, in particular, are not good for us.
WRONG: This is arguably not one of the author's assertions to the inclusion of "in particular" in this answer stem. There is no support for this assertion within the passage. This is not the best answer.

65. Which of the following conclusions can justifiably be drawn from the experience of the "grad-student-now-associate-professor" (lines 42-43) mentioned in the passage?

A. Frequently, a seemingly failed study can provide valuable insights when analyzed from a different perspective.
WRONG: This is not a conclusion that can justifiably be drawn from the experience. Although valuable insights may be found with new perspective in any study, a failed study producing new insight is a rarity. Additionally, though the results of the studies were unexpected, it is questionable whether they can be described as "failed". This is not the best answer.

B. A researcher who does not have preconceived notions of what he will find from the data may do a better job.
WRONG: This is not a conclusion that can justifiably be drawn from the experience. This generalization is too broad to be the best of the answer choices, though the use of the 'softener' "may" makes this answer choice seem attractive.

C. Important information may be gained from a study that does not support its initial hypothesis.
CORRECT: This is a conclusion that can justifiably be drawn from the experience. Here again the use of the 'softener' "may" makes this answer choice appropriate for a wider variety of situations. Additionally, the answer choice is appropriate and applicable to the passage itself.

D. It is possible that the "grad student" got his associate professor position because of his findings from the first study.
WRONG: This is not a conclusion that can justifiably be drawn from the experience. There is no support for this conclusion.

66. The author's referral to the *first* "rather bland study" in lines 20-31 contains the unstated assumption that:

A. all of the children in the control group had indoor pets.
WRONG: This is not an *unstated* assumption in the author's referral. This is clearly explained in the body of the passage and it is not true. "… a commonality among most of them [the students in the control group] was the presence of a household pet; either an 'inside' cat or a dog." (lines 27-29).

B. the children with allergies did not have household pets.
CORRECT: This is an unstated assumption in the first study.

C. the homes were not as clean as the owners might have wanted them to be.
WRONG: This is not an unstated assumption in the author's referral. The statement that, "The domiciles with pets were not nearly so clean as those without, despite the best efforts of the person re-

302

sponsible for cleaning the home." (lines 37-40), does not mean that all the owners wanted cleaner homes, as indicated by this answer choice. This is not the best answer.

D. the young graduate student had been one of the children in the control group.
WRONG: This is not an unstated assumption in the author's referral.

67. The statement that pets were bringing "dirt, bacteria and germs into a household" (line 36), is NOT supported by information in the passage regarding:

A. the types of owners of these pets.
WRONG: The author mentions that the traffic of dirt was not under complete control of the owners. Regardless of the cleanliness of the owner, a pet can bring in dirt and pathogens.

B. the fact that the pets were 'inside' cats and dogs.
CORRECT: This information does not support the above statement. The pets are described as "a household pet; either an 'inside' cat or a dog" (lines 28-29). If they were an "inside" pet, how then, would they be bringing the dirt into the household?

C. the original goals of the study.
WRONG: The goals of the study were never changed, only the interpretation of the findings. Futhermore, the goals of the study do not support or refute the above statement.

D. the cleanliness of children themselves.
WRONG: There is no information in the passage concerning the cleanliness of the children themselves.

68. A critic asks the author, "Suppose it were possible to raise a child in an absolutely germ-free environment, and this resulted in an adult who was free of allergies and relatively impervious to infectious diseases. How would this affect your recommendations to parents?" Which of the following responses would best allow the author to maintain his thesis:

A. "Though this might be physically healthy, it would pose serious social and developmental problems for the child."
WRONG: This response introduces new information which is based upon pure speculation. The author would have a stronger response if he addressed the question with respect to immunology.

B. "The supposition is flawed and I stand by my thesis."
WRONG: The author fails to address the question and instead refutes the supposition. Not that the answer is rather extreme.

C. It is important to find options that are available to people from all walks of life all over the world."
WRONG: Althought this may be a true statement, it is peripheral to the immunologic basis of the question. Note that this choice is broad and vague.

D. "Since the supposition is not feasible at present, it is currently the best practice to allow child some exposure to germs and bacteria."
CORRECT: This is the author's most likely response to the supposition. Here the author places his argument in the context of present day research and technologies, which should form the basis his recommendations for parents.

69. The author would most likely agree with which of the following statements?

A. If the trend towards using 'anti-bacterials' continues, we will all soon be forced to wear surgical masks.
WRONG: The author does not comment on the ramifications of using anti-bacterials. Rather, the author mentions the masks to further his argument of people becoming overly preoccupied with cleanliness.

B. Being exposed to antigens at an early age can only be beneficial to children.
WRONG: This assertion is not most clearly a thesis presented by the author. The inclusion of the word "only" immediately brings this answer choice into question. Additionally, the author does not assert that there are not germs or bacteria that are harmful.

C. Advertisements are not usually meant to be accurate health advisements.
WRONG: Although this statement may be true, it is not the best answer as it is peripheral to the author's thesis. The reference to advertisements was meant to support the presence of a trend, not to call into question their intent.

D. Increasing incidences of atopic disorders are probably the result of our houses being too clean.
CORRECT: This statement is a thesis presented by the author himself.

70. The author's purpose in referencing the "business-attired local populace nonchalantly sporting surgical facemasks" (lines 8-10), is to suggest that:

A. wearing these facemasks has become fashionable in certain parts of the world.
WRONG: This is not the author's apparent point in making the reference.

B. the 'better-educated' are not taking chances with their health.
WRONG: This is not the author's apparent point in

making the reference. The author's point would usually tend to further the thesis. This answer does not since it is probably that the author believes that the wearing of these surgical masks is frivolous.

C. people have begun acting in an unreasonable manner.
CORRECT: This is the author's apparent point in making the reference. It is clear from his tone that the author believes that the preoccupation with germs is silly and unnecessary.

D. surgical facemasks alone will not protect you from germs and bacteria.
WRONG: This is not the author's apparent point in making the reference. This may or may not be true.

Passage II (Questions 71-78)

71. According to the passage, handmade details with respect to furniture is characteristic of:

I. Arts and Crafts
CORRECT: This is a characteristic of handmade details with respect to furniture. There are many indirect allusions to the fact that Arts and Crafts furniture was handmade. The most specific being, "… Arts and Crafts adherence to a medieval kind of handcraft …" (lines 39-40).

II. L.&J.G. Stickley
WRONG: This is not a characteristic of handmade details with respect to furniture. Beginning with the second paragraph there is recurring information that Stickley furniture was not exclusively handmade, even though they had "firmly established" this idea "symbolically". Further, I is certainly one of the correct choices and therefore "II only" would not be a good choice. There are no "I and II only" options for the correct answer.

III. European sophistication.
WRONG: This is not a characteristic of handmade details with respect to furniture. In the first paragraph a distinction is made between Stickely and Limbert's "European sophistication". Be weary of selecting answer choices that closely approximate some words or phrases that you remember from the passage.

A. I only
CORRECT: See the above answer explanations.

B. II only

C. III only

D. I and III only

72. In line 12, the use of the phrase *second geneneration* indicates which of the following characteristics of L.&J.G. Stickley's ideas:
The phrase refers to "Many ideas used by L.&J.G. Stickley were "second generation" having been interpreted earlier by Gustav Stickley from such British designers as C.F.A. Voysey and H.M. Baillie Scott" (lines 11-15).

A. European.
WRONG: This phrase is used only to some degree in this sense. This is the second most likely of the answers, but it does not embody the sense of the phrase as completely as Answer D.

B. poorly crafted.
WRONG: This phrase is not used in this sense. None of the furniture in the passage is poorly crafted.

C. finely crafted.
WRONG: This phrase is not used in this sense. This is not at all the sense of the phrase.

D. unoriginal.
CORRECT: This phrase is used in this sense. The sentence prior to the one containing the phrase "second generation" gives additional clues. "The catalog's claim that this was "entirely American" furniture may have been an overstatement. Many ideas used by L.&J.G. Stickley were "second generation" …" (lines 10-12).

73. On the basis of the passage, it is reasonable to conclude that:

A. the Stickleys were the forefathers of the Arts and Crafts furniture movement.
WRONG: There is no passage information which would support this idea. You may have knowledge outside of the scope of the passage which would lead you to this answer.

B. the Stickleys were not interested in producing consistently high-quality furniture.
WRONG: Although some of their advertising and public statements may have been disingenuous or exaggerated, there is no support in the passage for this answer choice.

C. the Stickley's catalog claims were often self-serving.
CORRECT: This is a reasonable conclusion on the basis of the passage. At least twice in the passage, examples of "overstatement[s]" are mentioned regarding Stickley's catalog claims (lines 10-11, and 54-57, for instance).

D. the Stickleys usually used fumed quarter sawn oak.
WRONG: This is not a reasonable conclusion on the basis of the passage. There were a number of finishes that the Stickleys used on their furniture.

74. The author implies that, for a furniture company, production of strictly hand-made furniture is NOT:

A. an antique vestige.
WRONG: The author does not imply this. Despite the author's use of this word (thought not in the context of 'handmade'), this answer is nonsensical.

B. possible.
WRONG: Certainly, making furniture by hand is literally "possible". Whether such operations are conducive to longevity is questionable. This is an extreme answer.

C. without risks.
WRONG: Although this may be a true statement, the author does not imply that such operations are risky as much as they are impractical. Choice D is a better answer for this reason.

D. practical.
CORRECT: The author states that there are clear "advantages of adapting to machine production" (lines 51-52) with respect to a company's "longevity". Tangential to the discussion of the furniture are allusions to the changing tastes of the consumers buying the furniture. This is indicated by the Stickley's changing emphasis in its claims, from handmade to more scientific methods of production.

75. According to the author, L.&J.G. Stickley was not only able to evolve to changing production methods, but also a relatively successful company. If both of these assertions are true, which of the following statements is true?

Notice first that this type of question is restricting you to the information within the question itself. It would not have been necessary to have read the passage to answer this question correctly. Remember that the statement "If A then B" leads only to "If not B then not A". It does not lead logically to "If B then A". Finally, you may not "like" any of the answer choices available. Don't waste *any* time fretting over this, but choose the best answer available. You can rest assured that the test's creators have.

A. If a company was able to evolve to changing production methods, then it would probably be successful.
WRONG: This conclusion is not the most reasonable based upon the premises given. See the notice following the question above.

B. If the Stickley company had not evolved to changing production methods then it would not have been successful.
WRONG: This conclusion is not the most reasonable based upon the premises given. See the notice following the question above.

C. If a company was not able to evolve to changing production methods, then it was not the Stickley company.
CORRECT: This conclusion is the most reasonable based upon the premises given. This answer is the only "If not B, then not A".

D. If a company was not able to evolve to changing production methods, then it was probably not successful.
WRONG: This conclusion is not the most reasonable based upon the premises given. See the notice following the question above.

76. The passage states that Stickley furniture could often be identified by the most obvious details of joinery. Which of the following assertions is NOT clearly consistent with above statement?

A. "loose wedge pinned mortise and tenon joints… appeared in non-functional situations"
WRONG: This information is completely unrelated to the statement, and thus cannot be inconsistent.

B. L&J.G. Stickley began a a philosophical evolution in Arts and Crafts beginning in Britain.
WRONG: This information is completely unrelated to the statement, and thus cannot be inconsistent. The answer choice also lacks any support in the passage.

C. The Stickley's employed trademark use of four interlocking pieces of wood for furniture legs.
WRONG: This information is consistent with the assertion. If Stickely consistently used the four interlocking pieces of wood to the extent that they became a 'trademark', then that would be a detail that would help in identification of Stickley pieces.

D. the construction often varying from one piece to the next.
CORRECT: This information is not clearly consistent with assertion. If the construction of the Stickley pieces varied, then it is difficult to see how they could have been identified by that construction.

77. The author of the passage would be most likely to agree with which of the following ideas expressed by other furniture craft historians?

A. The Stickleys were the originators of using four interlocking pieces for furniture legs.
WRONG: The author would not be most likely to agree with this idea. This may or may not have been true. Though this production technique was a Stickley trademark, we are informed that it became so because of Stickley's extensive use of the technique. We are not told that Stickley was the originator.

B. Many of the claims made by the Stickley company have been embellished.

CORRECT: The author would be most likely to agree with this idea. This idea is returned to at least twice in the passage, with the author's reference to an "overstatement".

C. The Stickley company was driven to make money and succeed at all costs.

WRONG: The author would not be most likely to agree with this idea. This may or may not have been true. Be weary of such an extreme answer.

D. Limbert and Stickley were on par with one another regarding their level of craftsmanship.

WRONG: The author would not be most likely to agree with this idea. The contrast between Limbert and Stickley in the first paragraph was based upon "sophistication", which may, or may not have included craftsmanship.

78. Elsewhere, the author of the passage states that the Stickley's name became synonymous with the finest of painstakingly handmade furniture. This statement most directly supports the passage assertion that:

A. the Stickley's name became almost a trademark for the Arts and Crafts movement's emphasis on handcrafted quality.

WRONG: This is not a passage assertion, whether it supports the statement or not.

B. Stickley furniture can be identified by the more obvious handmade details of its joinery.

WRONG: This is a passage assertion, but it does not strongly support the statement.

C. the Stickleys were later able to make furniture by more modern machine methods, yet fool the consumer into thinking the furniture was actually handmade.

WRONG: It is questionable whether this is an accurate passage assertion or not, since the author does not provide any evidence that the Stickleys were trying to "fool" anybody. Additionally, it does not necessarily support the statement.

D. the Stickleys were later able to make furniture by more modern machine methods, yet still have it perceived as having the original handmade quality.

CORRECT: This is a passage assertion, and, it is the only answer choice which comes close to supporting the statement. Again, look for the best answer choice according to the test makers.

Examination 02: Biological Sciences

Passage V (Questions 79-84)

79. B is correct. One ATP is used in the conversion from Glycerol to DHAP, and subsequently 2 ATP are produced in glycolysis. Thus, the process yields 1 ATP per molecule of glycerol. Notice however that eventually, the pathway will stall due to a shortage of NAD^+: one mole of NAD^+ is reduced to convert glycerol to DHAP. Another mole is used later in the glycocitic pathway for a total of two moles. However, homolactic fermentation only regenerates one mole of NAD^+ per mole of lactic acid, and thus the cell will eventually run out of NAD^+. The question did not, however, ask for the eventual circumstance.

80. D is correct. Lactic acid, water, and heat are byproducts of lactic acid fermentation.

81. C is correct. The converstion of glycerol to DHAP involves the tranformation of one ATP → ADP and one NAD → NADH. During the rest of glycolysis, another NAD is converted to NADH and 2 ATP's are produced. During the Krebs cycle, 1 ATP is produced (in the form of GTP), and 4 NADH (one from the conversion of pyruvate to acetyl coA) and 1 $FADH_2$ are made. This is total 6 NADH, 1 $FADH_2$, and 2 ATP. Each NADH makes 3 ATP and $FADH_2$ makes 2 ATP.

82. B is correct. The addition of inhibitor Y to the medium will stop the conversion of succinic acid to fumaric acid. Although a small amount of Succinic acid will build up, no more than all the other intermediates in the pathway ahead of this reaction step. The more significant result is that the Krebs cycle will stall, and subsequently, the conversion of pyruvate to acetyl-CoA. Glycolysis, however, will be unaffected—thus, there will be a buildup of pyruvate much greater than that of any other pathway intermediate.

83. D is correct. Answer choice A can be eliminated as it describes an enzyme that is not inhibited by addiction of compound W, which is contrary to the question stem. Answer choice C can be eliminated on the same grounds, as it describes an enzyme that actually increases its rate and efficiency of substrate utilization in the presence of compound W; in this case W would be described as an allosteric activator which is contrary to the question stem. Answer choice B can be eliminated as it describes a competitive inhibitor. Competitive inhibitors bind to the active site of the enzyme in lieu of the substrate and increase the apparent K_m without affecting the apparent V_{max}. Inhibitor W is a strict non-competitive inhibitor.

84. D is correct. The equilibrium constant of the ketose-aldose isomerization is [GAP]/[DHAP]. A ketone is much more stable than an aldehyde because the increased electronegativity of the carbonyl carbon is dispersed throughout the molecule. Thus, the K value must be less than one. The choices B and D are both less than 1, but B (0.8) would mean that the stability of DHAP is only slightly higher than that of GAP. In actuality, DHAP is much more stable and thus the answer is D.

Passage VI (Questions 85-91)

85. **C is correct.** The passage states that lactic acid fermentation is used to regenerate NAD^+ in the absence of oxygen. NAD^+ is a required substrate for glycolysis.

86. **D is correct.** The most obvious effect of the drug was to increase the rate of fermentation in the setting of low NADH. In order for this to occur, the drug must act as a substitute for NADH.

87. **A is correct.** The electron transport chain harvests the energy carried by NADH, and in the process, regenerates NAD^+.

88. **B is correct.** The liver is the only organ with the enzymes necessary to convert lactic acid into pyruvate. More importantly, the liver is responsible for the neutralization of all body toxins, usually via chemical modification which is followed by renal excretion.

89. **B is correct.** According to the passage, alcohol fermentation does not produce any ATP, so the only ATP produced are those from converting glucose to pyruvate. 2 ATP are used in this reaction, while 4 are produced, giving a net of 2 ATP.

90. **A is correct.** ATP stores within a muscle are depleted within a few seconds of exertion, so ATP must be regenerated using a fast source, readily available source of fuel. Lactic acid and pyruvate are readily available, however, lactic acid cannot be used to produce ATP and pyruvate requires oxygen. The fastest form of available energy is glucose, either free or released from glycogen stores.

91. **B is correct.** Fermentation does not produce ATP, however, it does regenerate NAD^+ in order for glycolysis to proceed. Thus, it is indirectly related to ATP production. Low ATP is a driver for glycolysis, while low NAD^+ is a driver for fermentation.

Independent Questions (Questions 92-94)

92. **C is correct.** Since the pH is low, the body removes excess H^+ from the blood in order to raise the pH. Thus, the reaction will run from right to left, producing extra carbon dioxide that is then exhaled.

93 **C is correct.** Ammonia is potentially toxic to cells and must be combined with carbon dioxide to form urea, which is then excreted in the urine.

94. **B is correct.** The concentration gradient of H^+ across the inner mitochondrial membrane drives ATP synthetase to form ATP from ADP (secondary active transport).

EXPLANATIONS 03

Answers to Questions 95–141

ANSWERS TO EXAMINATION 3

PHYSICAL SCIENCES	VERBAL REASONING	BIOLOGICAL SCIENCES
95. C	111. C	126. A
96. B	112. B	127. D
97. A	113. B	128. D
98. C	114. B	129. B
99. D	115. D	130. B
100. B	116. B	131. A
101. C	117. A	132. D
102. A	118. D	133. C
103. B	119. B	134. A
104. D	120. C	135. D
105. B	121. B	136. B
106. C	122. B	137. B
107. B	123. C	138. D
108. C	124. D	139. D
109. A	125. A	140. C
110. D		141. A

Passage I (Questions 95-110)

95. C is correct. Aluminum has a nuclear charge of 13. It has 3 valence electrons, so 10 electrons reside in lower numbered shells, shielding the valence electrons. $13 - 10 = 3$. As the passage states, this is a very rough estimate. In reality, overlap of shells prevents shielding by electron in lower shells from being as effective as this calculation suggests.

96. B is correct. According to the passage, only the principal energy level affects the energy for a single electron atom, so a change in the subshell will make no difference. "For atoms or ions with a single electron, the energy of the electron is determined only by the principal quantum number n."

97. A is correct. Both H and He$^+$ have single electrons. He$^+$ has a nuclear charge of 2 and H has a nuclear charge of 1. According to the formula in the passage, the greater the nuclear charge, Z, the greater the change in energy E for a given electron jump.

98. C is correct. If visible light appears, then the change must be part of the Balmer series, moving from principle energy levels 4 or 3($n = 3$ or 4) to the second principal energy level ($n = 2$).

99. D is correct. If a photon is emitted, then the atom must be releasing energy. Energy is released when an electron moves to a lower energy level because the atom becomes more stable.

100. B is correct. Use the formula from the passage.

$$E_n = -R_H\left(\frac{Z^2}{n^2}\right)\left(\frac{1}{n_i^2} - \frac{1}{n_f^2}\right)$$

$$= -2.18 \times 10^{-18} \text{ J}\left(\frac{2^2}{2^2}\right) = -2.18 \times 10^{-18} \text{ J}$$

101. C is correct. Hydrogen has a smaller nuclear charge, which will exert less of a pull on the single electron, so hydrogen will have a larger radius. The smaller nuclear charge will also make it easier to remove hydrogen's single electron, so it will have a lower ionization energy.

Passage II (Questions 102-110)

102. A is correct. The forward motion of the tractor depends on the force of static friction between its tires and the ground. If the maximum force of static friction on the crate is greater than the maximum force of static friction on the tractor, the tractor tires will slip and the crate will not move.

103. B is correct. As long as the tires do not slip, the surfaces of the tires and the ground do not slide across each other. As a new surface of the tire is constantly coming into contact with a new surface on the ground, static, rather than kinetic friction is responsible. The crate, however is being dragged along the ground, with the same surface sliding along the ground. Here the friction is kinetic.

104. D is correct. The sum of the forces on the crate must be equal to ma. The free body diagram below shows the forces.

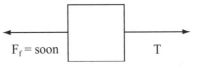

$$T - F_f = ma$$
$$T = F_f + ma = 500 + (500)(0.6) = 500 + 300 = 800 \text{ N}$$

105. B is correct. As long as the tires do not slip, the circular motion of the tires will translate directly into the straight line motion of the tractor. First, revolutions per minute must be converted to meters per second. An important point to keep in mind is that 1 revolution is $2\pi r$ meters. Also don't forget that if the diameter is 2 m, then the radius is 1 m.

$$\left(\frac{30 \text{ rev}}{\text{min}}\right)\left(\frac{(2)\pi(1) \text{ m}}{\text{rev}}\right)\left(\frac{1 \text{ min}}{60 \text{ sec}}\right) = \pi \text{ m/s} = 3 \text{ m/s}$$

106. C is correct. This is Newton's third law. The speed and acceleration of the tractor are irrelevant as the crate will always exert a reciprocal force. In order to envision the crate's acceleration, it must be considered as an isolated system.

107. B is correct. The 1000 N force must be exactly enough to overcome the force of static friction, which is equal to the product of the coefficient of static friction and the normal force. In this case, the normal force is equal to the weight of the crate.

$$1000 = \mu \, mg = \mu(500)(10) = 5000 \, \mu$$
$$\mu = (1000)/(5000) = 0.2$$

Independent Questions (Questions 108-110)

108. C is correct. Sodium nitrate, $NaNO_3$, contains covalent bonds between N and O, and ionic bonds between Na$^+$ and NO_3^-.

109. A is correct. The weight of the block is constant and equal to mg and it always acts downward, so it will not be changed when the angle changes. The normal force acts opposite the component of the weight that's perpendicular to the surface of the plane. As the angle is increased, this component gets smaller, so the normal force will decrease.

110. D is correct. The formula for centripetal force is $F = mv^2/r$. If the speed is doubled and all else remains the same, then the force must be quadrupled to maintain the path.

Examination 03: Verbal Reasoning

Passage III (Questions 111-118)

111. The contention that the tensions and anxieties of adolescence "are imposed by society in advanced countries, because society's timetables are not synchronized with man's natural growth timetable" (lines 61-63) can most justifiably be interpreted as support for the idea that:

A. in most other countries, adolescents experience less tension and anxiety.
WRONG: This idea is tempting, however it requires a leap of logic that is one step beyond the justifiably supported Answer C.

B. a long childhood is necessary to acquire information and skills.
WRONG: This idea is another one of the author's contentions, but is unrelated to the discrepancy between natural and societal growth timetables.

C. in less advanced countries, these timetables are better synchronized.
CORRECT: This idea is most justifiably supported by the contention. This is all that can be supported.

D. in less advanced countries, society is less concerned about adolescent appearances.
WRONG: Although many may consider this statement true, it is unrelated to the discrepancy between natural and societal growth timetables.

112. The author most likely mentions, "The slow-growing boy's difficulties are heaped on top of the problems that affect both boys and girls in the early years of adolescence." (lines 35-37) in order to:

A. demonstrate the strength of his theories regarding a girl's difficulties.
WRONG: This is not the most likely reason for the author's mentioning the quote in the question. The passage is primarily about boys, not girls.

B. support the claim that a boy's problems are more acute than a girl's.
CORRECT: This is the most likely reason for the author's mentioning the quote in the question. The passage is not only primarily about boys, but the author does believe that a boy's problems are more acute (line 19-20).

C. illustrate the persistence of beliefs that conflict with the author's theories.
WRONG: This is not the most likely reason for the author's mentioning the quote in the question. There is no counterpoint to the author's arguments or efforts on his part to refute them.

D. provide an example of a girl's problems to maintain parity in the passage.
WRONG: This is not the most likely reason for the author's mentioning the quote in the question. The second aspect of this answer is very vague. This is not the best answer.

113. Which of the following statements would most likely be supported by the author of the passage?

A. A late-maturing girl would be more self-critical of herself than a normally maturing boy.
WRONG: The author, in fact, presents the opposite argument in the passage.

B. Both late-maturing and normally maturing adolescents perceive the former as dissatisfied with themselves.
CORRECT: The author himself delineates how, "Late-maturing boys' dissatisfactions with themselves are reflected both in the opinions of their classmates and in their own responses to psychological tests" (lines 20-23). Since their "classmates" are not included in the "late-maturing" category, we may assume that they are either early-maturing or normally maturing.

C. Boys are much more concerned about their appearances than are girls.
WRONG: The author presents an equivalent amount of information to support both male and female preoccupation with appearance. Be weary of the third person use of 'he'—the introduction of the passage is referring to all adolescents, male and female.

D. In other societies adolescence does not present much of a problem.
WRONG: There is no information in the passage to support this answer choice. Although the author discusses American adolescents, he does not mention whether this phenomena is present or absent in other societies.

114. What is the author's most likely response to the argument that adolescents focus too much on how they look instead of whom they are?

Please be aware that the prefacing words to these answer choices are of much less importance than the accompanying clausal justification. In other words, you could believe that the author "accepts" the standard story, and yet find that the premise following the word

"Acceptance" (as in this case) is inappropriate reasoning.

A. Acceptance: adolescents prize physical beauty too highly.
WRONG: This would not be the author's most likely response to the "standard story". In fact, the author admits that, "Good looks, however defined, are valued virtually everywhere— so the adolescent measures his worth as a person, and his chances of success, by the degree to which he meets society's standards of attractiveness." (lines 2-6).

B. Neutral: physical beauty is valued almost everywhere.
CORRECT: This would be the author's most likely response to the above argument. In fact, the author admits that, "Good looks, however defined, are valued virtually everywhere" (line 2).

C. Revisionist: this focus is not a cause of concern for the average adolescent.
WRONG: The author actually presents the opposite argument in the passage: the imbalance in focus (physical vs. personality) is a cause of concern for the average adolescent.

D. Skepticism: it is who a person is that is most important.
WRONG: Although this may seem like an appropriately politically correct answer choice, the author does not address the relative importance of one's inner qualities. Instead, he recognizes the reality of the importance of external characteristics—at least in the adolescent world.

115. If the author's primary criterion for "intelligence" were applied to different animals in a given situation, which of the following animals would be most intelligent?

In order to answer this question you must have gleaned the author's criterion. "…the capacity to learn, to substitute flexible thinking for the rigidities of instinct, is a basic measure of intelligence in man or any other species" (lines 67-70).

A. A chimpanzee that moves next to its food dish because it knows the exact time it will be fed by its keeper
WRONG: This animal would not be the most intelligent, given this situation, based upon the author's primary criterion for judging "intelligence". The above Pavlovian response to a food stimulus is not an example of "substituting flexible thinking for the rigidities of instinct". In fact, such a response is quite instinctual.

B. A mother cat that quickly adapts to nursing orphaned baby skunks
WRONG: This animal would not be the most intelligent, given this situation, based upon the au-

thor's primary criterion for judging "intelligence". Nursing is instinctual, particularly when that "mother" cat may already be nursing. The cat did not make a conscious decision (in this case, to help out another species) that countered her natural instinct.

C. A dog that learns to whine in order to be let outside its master's home
WRONG: The dog's whining is a natural instinct. There is not adaptive mechanism demonstrated.

D. A rat that learns to use a can for a raft in order to obtain food
CORRECT: This animal would be the most intelligent, given this situation, based upon the author's primary criterion for judging "intelligence". "…the capacity to learn, to substitute flexible thinking for the rigidities of instinct, is a basic measure of intelligence in man or any other species" (lines 67-70). Here the rat is adapting by using a manmade product in a non-instinctual manner to obtain food. Such an action show that the rat has learned to deal with its environment.

116. The main idea of the passage is that, in advanced countries:

A. adolescents are not advancing at a satisfactory rate.
WRONG: This is not the main idea of the passage. What does "advancing" mean? If anything, the author feels that adolescents are pressured to mature (psychologically) too rapidly.

B. adolescence, particularly in boys, is a difficult time.
CORRECT: This is the main idea of the passage. The passage is on adolescence, most specifically male adolescence, and the difficulties therein.

C. adolescents deserve more nurturing societies.
WRONG: This is not the main idea of the passage. There are no suggestions offered in the passage to ameliorate the current situation.

D. adolescence is a difficult period for both boys and girls.
WRONG: This is not the main idea of the passage. The author admits adolescence is difficult for both boys and girls, however, he spends a great deal of time highlighting that it is more difficult for boys—especially late-maturing boys (lines 19-20).

117. Suppose later child development research reveals that the problems encountered by adolescent boys, as presented in the passage, are unique from those encountered by their female counterparts. Which of the following *changes* in the passage would be most appropriate?

A. A distinction regarding which gender was concerned about appearance.

CORRECT: This change would be most appropriate as the author describes preoccupation with appearance as a commonality between male and female adolescents. If none of the male concerns overlap those of females, and males are presented in the passage as appearance-sensitive, then the females must not be.

B. The beliefs of Margaret Mead should be expunged.
WRONG: Margaret Mead's opinion on 'going steady' is the only belief presented in the passasge. Her opinion does not concern the distinct problems of male and female adolescents. Rather, her beliefs reflect on parent-teenager dynamics, an unrelated topic.

C. There should be more emphasis placed on the adolescence of girls.
WRONG: That adolescent girls have separate concerns from teenage boys does not dictate the emphasis of their struggles in the passage. Just because their problems are different does not mean the girls deserve more of the author's attention in the passage.

D. Late-maturing girls should no longer be viewed as more self-critical.
WRONG: The author does not believe late-maturing girls are more self critical to begin with. That they should no longer be viewed as such is a nonsensical assertion.

118. Which of the following statements is NOT supported by the passage?

A. Boys are concerned with being too short or felt ugly.
WRONG: This statement does not challenge any of the assertions made in the passage.

B. Boys and girls worry about their height.
WRONG: This statement does not challenge any of the assertions made in the passage.

C. Boys and girls worry about being overweight.
WRONG: This statement does not challenge any of the assertions made in the passage.

D. Girls worry about having bad skin.
CORRECT: The author describes adolescent boys being concerned about their skin, not girls (line 12).

Passage IV (Questions 119-125)

119. Assume that the United Nations was interested in implementing a program to subsidize sub-Saharan nations in an effort to strengthen their economic standing in the world. Based on the information provided in the passage, which of the following programs would the author consider most helpful?

A. A program designed to decrease urban unemployment rates by creating farming jobs for metropolitan youth
WRONG: Most inhabitants of sub-Saharan Africa are already involved in farming (line 29). This program would only perpetuate the status quo rather than ameliorate the economic standing of sub-Saharan nations.

B. A program designed to increase literacy and provide technical training to villagers
CORRECT: This is the best answer. The author feels that the inability of sub-Saharan nations to compete in the world market is due to a lack of an educated or technically trained class. Such a class would help these countries shift from exporting raw materials to manufactured goods via catalyzing industrialization and in doing so close the import-export gap (lines 42-46).

C. A program designed to increase agricultural production, especially cash crops
WRONG: African countries already rely largely on cash crops to generate income (lines 47-48). Such a program would only perpetuate the status quo rather than ameliorate the economic standing of sub-Saharan nations.

D. A program designed to promote family planning and close the "1% gap" (line 60)
WRONG: Although the 1% gap is presented as one of the problems facing sub-Saharan Africa, closing this gap is not presented as a solution that would lead to economic development and stability. The author believes this desired endpoint should instead be pursued with the industrialization of these nations (lines 42-46).

120. Which of the following statements regarding foreign familiarity with sub-Saharan lands is most consistent with the information in the passage?

A. The Western world was completely oblivious to sub-Saharan Africa up until the twentieth century
WRONG: The Western world was not *completely* oblivious to sub-Saharan Africa. In fact, the passage indicates that European penetration into inland sub-Saharan Africa had already begun in the mid-nineteenth century (lines 8-10)

B. European familiarity with African lands was based only on commercial interests
WRONG: There is no support for this answer in the passage.

C. Though the lowland coastal areas of sub-Saharan were known to traders, highland, tropic areas of the interior remained unfamiliar territory for some time
CORRECT: Though the passage did not indicate the geographic topography of sub-Saharan Africa, the fact that traders were familiar with coastal African before its interior regions is consistent with the information in the passage (lines 6-10).

D. Familiarity with sub-Saharan Africa increased in the Western world after colonial independence, due to an increase of raw materials from African countries
WRONG: Though the passage does state that sub-Saharan nations largely export raw materials. The passage does not state that such exports grew after independence or that familiarity with the region increased after independence.

121. "The lack of utilization of resources developed during the colonial era, resources that became available to African nations post-colonially, was due to none other than the mismanagement of those resources by African aristocracy. Therefore, the post-colonial dilapidation of sub-Saharan nations can be blamed on none but the African people themselves." This statement would most likely illicit which of the following responses from the author?

A. Strong agreement because the author feels that elitism was a true obstacle to accessing and utilizing the infrastructure left by colonial nations
WRONG: The author does agree that elitism was an obstacle to utilizing the infrastructure left by colonial nations. However, he would not agree that the blame lies completely on the post-colonial exploitation of resources by African aristocracy. The author feels that the abrupt withdrawal of colonial governing nations from the area is also to be blamed for the lack of utilization of the infrastructure left by colonial nations (lines 22-24).

B. Partial disagreement because the author feels that colonizing nations are also partly responsible for the post-colonial state of affairs
CORRECT: This is the best answer. The author would not agree that the blame lies completely on the post-colonial exploitation of resources by African aristocracy. The author feels that the abrupt withdrawal of colonial governing nations from the area is also to be blamed for the lack of utilization of the infrastructure left by colonial nations (lines 22-24).

C. Strong opposition because the author feels that the colonizing nations were entirely responsible for the post-colonial decline of sub-Saharan nations.
WRONG: This is not true because the author cites local elitism by indigenous African as a factor contributing to the lack of utilization of the infrastructure left by colonial nations (lines 22-24).

D. Partial agreement because the author agrees that sub-Saharan nations are in a dilapidated state post-colonially
WRONG: The author does see the current situation of sub-Saharan nations as "precarious" (line 37). However, this answer choice does not address the author's response as completely as answer choice B. This answer choice does not embody the author's reaction to the assertion that resources were misappropriated post-colonially and that such misappropriation was due to exploitation by African elitists themselves.

122. The author would most likely agree with which of the following statements?

A. Inhabitants of sub-Saharan Africa are, for the most part, very much alike
WRONG: The author states in line 1 that sub-Saharan African is "socially complex."

B. The origins of sub-Saharan culture and history antedate the discovery of the New World in the fifteenth century.
CORRECT: The author states that the history of sub-Saharan Africa is as old as human civilization itself (lines 2-3). Thus the origins of sub-Saharan culture and history antedate the discover of New World in the 1400's.

C. Sub-Saharan countries are only now steadily developing into industrialized nations
WRONG: There is no support for this answer in the passage.

D. If there were better transportation links available, sub-Saharan nations would easily modernize
WRONG: Though transportation is cited as an obstacle, it is clearly not the only obstacle to growth. Drought and illiteracy are also major hindrances (lines 41-42). Without resolving these and other issues it would seem to be an oversimplification to state that if there were better transportation links available, sub-Saharan nations would very easily modernize.

123. According to the passage, which of the following scenarios is NOT characteristic of sub-Saharan inhabitants or sub-Saharan living

A. A large joint family engaged in growing corn

WRONG: This statement would characterize sub-Saharan inhabitants or sub-Saharan living. Family structure in sub-Saharan Africa is based on the model of an extended family (line 33). Also, most sub-Saharan Africans are subsistence farmers (line 29),

B. A group of village people offering devotional services to a tree

WRONG: This statement would characterize sub-Saharan inhabitants or sub-Saharan living. Sub-Saharan Africans ascribe religious or spiritual value to their natural surroundings and environment (lines 29-31).

C. An illiterate group of people living in crowded city quarters with poor sanitary conditions

CORRECT: This statement would not characterize sub-Saharan inhabitants or sub-Saharan living. Though most inhabitants of this area are illiterate (lines 41-42), they mostly occupy rural areas not urban areas (line 39).

D. A group of farm workers that are severely emaciated and have several health problems

WRONG: Food shortage and poverty are recognized problems in the area (37-41). Public heath status is also in substandard (lines 49-50). This statement would characterize sub-Saharan inhabitants or sub-Saharan living.

124. Which of the following statements best conveys the main idea of the passage?

A. There is a need for greater awareness of the history and current state affairs of sub-Saharan nations in the West

WRONG: This is not the main idea. The fact that there is not or was not a greater familiarity with this region is the Western world serves more as an introductory prelude than a main idea of the passage (line 1-2, 5).

B. The subsistence farmers of sub-Saharan African have been repeatedly marginalized due to various political and historical factors.

WRONG: Though it is true that sub-Saharan African farmers have been repeatedly marginalized (lines 12-14, 47-48), this is not the main idea of the passage. The passage touches on many other historical and contemporary problems that have afflicted the sub-Saharan region.

C. Colonialism has grossly retarded the growth of sub-Saharan nations

WRONG: Though the author may agree with this statement, this is not the principle idea of the passage. The discussion on colonialism is just a part of a larger presentation of the historical and contemporary problems that have afflicted the sub-Saharan region.

D. The sub-Saharan region has been historically wrought with problems and faces many challenges today

CORRECT: This is the overriding theme of the passage. The passage delineates the historical and contemporary problems that have afflicted the sub-Saharan region.

125. The author would be most likely present which of the following statements in an address to the United Nations Hearing Committee?

A. We must implement controls and policies to remove the remnants of colonial control in the region

CORRECT: The author does not make very many qualitative statements in the passage. However, in lines 25- 26, he takes a stand against the legacy of colonialism by qualifying that legacy as "disparate and unjustifiable." In the rest of the passage, the author lays out various problems, however, his emphasis is placed on the legacy of colonialism in the area.

B. Stiffer tariff regulations need to be in place to close the import-export gap

WRONG: This is not the best answer. Though the import-export gap is cited as a problem, the author does not make a **direct** value judgment or statement of action indicating that this gap needs to be bridged. Though we can infer that author agrees that this gap needs to be bridged, he does not emphasize this problem as does he the legacy of colonialism in the area. Concerning this legacy, the author states that it comprises "disparate and unjustifiable [influence]" in the area (lines 25-26). The strength and clarity with which this type of value judgment is made is simply not found in the author's discussion of the import-export gap.

C. There is an undeniable need to create better health care facilities to stave off a pandemic public health crisis

WRONG: This is no the best answer. Though public health is cited as a problem, the author does not make a **direct** value judgment or statement of action indicating that public health conditions need to be changed. Though we can infer that author agrees that the impending public health crisis needs to be addressed, the author does not use the type of language describing this problem as does he concerning the legacy of colonialism in the area. Concerning this legacy, the author states that it comprises "disparate and unjustifiable [influence]" in the area (lines 25-26). The strength and clarity with which this type of value judgment is made is simply not found in the author's discussion of public health.

D. We must overcome donor fatigue and pump heavy aid into African nations

WRONG: Though poverty is cited as a problem, the author does not make a **direct** value judgment or statement of action indicating that the indigent condition of these nations needs to be changed. Though we can infer that author agrees that the problem of poverty needs to be dealt with, the author does not use the type of language describing this problem as does he concerning the legacy of colonialism in the area. Concerning this legacy, the author states that it comprises "disparate and unjustifiable [influence]" in the area (lines 25-26). The strength and clarity with which this type of value judgment is made is simply not found in the author's discussion of poverty which seems more a statement of fact.

Examination 03: Biological Sciences

Passage V (Questions 126-133)

126. **A is correct.** Anticancer drugs that cause hair loss and a decrease in immune activity target rapidly proliferating cells. According to the passage, the drug curtails the growth of cancerous cell, and thus must be increasing the activity of tumor-suppressor genes. If the drug suppressed oncogenic activity, it would *prevent* cancerous growth instead.

127. **D is correct.** Choices A-C are all examples of highly regenerative tissues. Skeletal muscle, however, is terminally differentiated and rarely undergoes mitosis.

128. **D is correct.** A lysosome functions to digest phagocytosed materials, while mitochondria function primarily in energy production. The endoplasmic reticulum cleaves proteins, not mRNA. mRNA splicing (and most other processing) occurs in the nucleus.

129. **B is correct.** DNA is replicated in the S phase, in between the phases of cellular growh, G1 and G2. Mitosis occurs during the M phase.

130. **B is correct.** The modified tRNAs will still allow translation to occur, however, the resulting proteins will be completely different, and most likely dysfunctional. Without effective translation, the cancerous cell will not be able to produce proteins vital to cellular function and reproduction, and will most likely undergo apoptosis.

131. **A is correct.** Microtubules (spindle fibers) pull the chromosomes away from the middle of the cell (the metaphase plate). Without this separation, sister chromatids remain associated and mitosis cannot continue through anaphase or telophase.

132. **D is correct.** Adenine is needed to duplicate the DNA prior to mitosis. Histones are needed to package the DNA into discrete chromosomes. Ribose is the sugar backbone to DNA and is needed when duplicating the DNA. Beta oxidation is used to oxidize fats, and is not required for mitosis.

Passage VI (Questions 133-141)

133. **C is correct.** A mutation which affects an exon/intron splice junction would result in exclusion of that exon from the processed mRNA and affect the size of mRNA on a blot. D is wrong because introns are excluded from processed mRNA (Note that only processed mRNA is allowed to leave the nucleus). A and B are wrong because these mutations would affect the resultant protein instead of the mRNA.

134. **A is correct.** In lymphoma research, one is looking for mutations in genes specific to lymphocytes. All human cells (except mature erythrocytes and gametes) have the same DNA, so what distinguishes one cell type from the other is the unique combination of genes that are expressed from cell to cell. Choice B is thus not plausible. C is incorrect because this technique is used with every type of tissue. The passage mentions blood as the source of cell sampling only because blood cells are easiest to obtain from patients. The fact that answer choice D reads "The mRNA is most stable in lymphocytes and thus easier to examine" is obviously a strong and incorrect statement. MCAT students should be aware to look out for these kinds of statements. This alone justifies why this statement is incorrect, let alone the fact that this is not true scientifically.

135. **D is correct.** A less intense band will result from lower levels of mRNA transcripts, or decreased gene transcription. Missense (the exchange of an amino acid) and nonsense (premature stop codon) mutations are only detected in the resultant protein. Small deletions/insertions in the coding region would not affect the mRNA size significantly to be detected on a blot so C is wrong. Only small deletions/insertions in noncoding DNA could affect regulatory regions which control transcription, and thus mRNA levels.

136. **B is correct.** The agarose gel electrophoresis separates nucleic acids based on their size and secondary structure would affect how the nucleic acids migrate through the agarose. A is wrong because hybridization favors specific binding over nonspecific—This is how the probe displaces the blocking agent in RNA fragments that contain the sequences complementary to the probe DNA. RNA transfer and cross-linking is done in the absence of formaldehyde (after it has been washed off), and thus must not be affected by secondary structure.

137. **B is correct.** A strong band corresponds to high desmoglien 2 expression, as measured by the levels of

mRNA, and vice versa. The absence of a band, indicating a lack of desmoglien 2 expression would be most likely in tissues lacking epithelium, such as brain and skeletal muscle. Skin, oral mucosa, and heart tissues encounter frequent stress and will have high level of expression. Bladder epithelial cells experience slightly less stress and will show a weaker band on Northern Blot.

138. D is correct. The Northern blot had to work otherwise the control band would not be detected either (only the patient's lanes are empty). The deletion in Choice A would likely affect the regulatory region and may result in the inability to express gene X. Chromosomal rearrangement could also affect a chromosomal locus containing X, resulting in nonexpression. A deletion of the gene would also explain the lack of mRNA.

139. D is correct. A, B, and C would all result in exclusion of exon(s) and thus a smaller mRNA transcript. Smaller molecules will travel further, resulting in a longer migration for a band on a blot. Ribosome binding is important for translation and not transcription, and would not affect the length of the mRNA transcript.

Independent Questions (Questions 140-141)

140. C is correct. The quick rate of HIV mutation is mentioned in the question stem. Triple cocktail therapy is Medicine's response to patients quickly becoming resistant to single drug antiretroviral therapy. Opportunistic infections are treated prophylatically with separate medications, usually antibiotics, or antifungal medication, in addition to triple cocktail therapy.

141. A is correct. The virus most likely mutated to become resistant once it was exposed to the drug. As this resistance was noted, the patient was taken off the drug. In the absence of the drug, the virus no longer has selection pressure to maintain its resistance and mutates back to the wild type (which is always the most stable). Such a process is defined as backward mutation. Mutation away from the wild type, such as developing resistance, is termed forward mutation. Missence and Nonsense mutations are less likely to affect drug resistance as the majority of viral proteins are translated from the original RNA genome (or its complement). RNA polymerase, and reverse transcriptase are much more accurate than DNA polymerase.

EXPLANATIONS 04

Answers to Questions 142-188

ANSWERS TO EXAMINATION 4

PHYSICAL SCIENCES	VERBAL REASONING	BIOLOGICAL SCIENCES
142. B	158. B	173. A
143. B	159. A	174. D
144. C	160. C	175. C
145. B	161. D	176. B
146. A	162. B	177. A
147. D	163. D	178. D
148. B	164. D	179. C
149. D	165. B	180. B
150. B	166. B	181. D
151. C	167. A	182. C
152. D	168. C	183. D
153. C	169. A	184. C
154. A	170. D	185. B
155. A	171. C	186. B
156. D	172. D	187. B
157. A		188. A

Passage I (Questions 142-147)

142. **B is correct.** The torque from each set of spheres is equal to the product of the force and the lever arm. In this case, the lever arm is the distance between the center of the bar and the end, or 20 cm.

$$\text{Torque} = (1 \times 10^{-7} \text{ N})(0.2 \text{ m}) = 2 \times 10^{-8} \text{ Nm}$$

There are two gravitational forces acting, so we need to double the torque to 4×10^{-8} Nm.

143. **B is correct.** The distance r is measured from the center of mass of the sphere, which would be at the geometrical center if the spheres were of uniform density. If the spheres are not of uniform density, the center of mass could be elsewhere. The mass M and gravitational constant G will not be affected by variations in the density of a sphere.

144. **C is correct.** The passage states that the wire acts according to Hooke's law, so the greater the displacement of the wire from its rest position, the greater the force (or torque) it will exert. In this case, the displacement corresponds to the angle of rotation.

145. **B is correct.** Each gravitational force is tripled, so the net force is also tripled. Note that the mass m of the small balls was not changed.

146. **A is correct.** Force varies with the inverse square of distance. Choice A represents the basic graph for inverse relationships. Choice B depicts a linear relationship. Choice C does not depict the correct relationship between force and distance at small and large values of r. Choice D demonstrates a direct relationship rather than an inverse one.

147. **D is correct.** The distance r is calculated from the centers of of the spheres. Adding the radii of the spheres to the distance between them yields 16cm, or 0.16m. (12 + 3 + 1 = 16).

Passage II (Questions 148-154)

148. **B is correct.** Phosphorous has 5 valence electrons. It uses 3 of them to form single bonds with chlorine atoms and the other 2 remain a lone pair. Since it has four electron pairs, its hybridization is sp^3 and its shape is tetrahedral. A central atom with tetrahedral structure and a single lone electron pair will form a trigonal pyramidal molecule. Alternatively, if you know that NH_3 has a trigonal pyramidal structure, you can deduce that PCl_3 will be the same as the valence electron relationships are identical.

149. **D is correct.** Reaction 5 is a double replacement reaction because both the anions and cations in the reactants trade places in the products.

150. **B is correct.** To form PCl_5, phosphorous uses its $3d$ orbitals to form dsp^3 hybrids. Nitrogen has only two shells, so it has no d orbitals available for bonding.

151. **C is correct.** Reaction 4 requires 2 moles of O_2 for every mole of PH_3. If there are 50 grams of each, then there is more than 1 mole of PH_3 (MM = 34) and less than 2 moles of O_2 (MM = 32). Thus, oxygen is the limiting reactant, and there will be some phosphine left after the reaction runs to completion.

152. **D is correct.** Percent yield is found by dividing actual yield by expected yield. From the balanced equation, 20 moles of phosphoric acid should be produced, however, only 18 are produced. 18/20 = 0.9 = 90%

153. **C is correct.** The balanced equation for Reaction 2 reveals that 5 moles of oxygen are needed for every mole of phosphorous. Each mole of oxygen takes up 22.4 liters, so we need (5)(22.4) = 112 liters of oxygen. However, since oxygen makes up only 20% of air, we need (5)(112) = 560 liters of air to get all the oxygen we need.

154. **A is correct.** As phosphorous and hydrogen are non-metals with unequal electronegativities, they must form polar covalent bonds. Non-polar covalent bonds are formed between atoms with equal electronegativities. Coordinate covalent bonds are formed when one atom donates an electron pair to another atom. Hydrogen bonding occurs only between a hydrogen atom on one molecule and a small, highly electronegative atom (F, O, N) on a separate molecule.

Independent Questions (Questions 155-157)

155. **A is correct.** If the spring is stretched by 2 cm when a 0.4 kg block is added, then it will stretch half as much when a 0.2 kg block is added, so the total length will be 11 cm. Be careful here, the 0.5 kg block doesn't give you any information about the spring or its spring constant.

156. **D is correct.** In centripetal motion, the magnitudes of the velocity and acceleration are constant, but as the object moves around the circle, the directions of both vectors are constantly changing. If the direction of a vector is changing, then the vector is changing.

157. **A is correct.** Sulfur's valence electrons are in the third shell, with a full 3s orbital and 4 electrons in the p subshell.

Passage III (Questions 158-164)

158. The word *institution* (line 58) is used to communicate:

    A. a building.
    WRONG: Although the other examples provided in the sentence are buildings, the author is trying to convey the painting's permanence, familiariy, and symbolism by using these examples. She is not suggesting that the painting has become a building.

    B. a tradition.
    CORRECT: The author is trying to convey the sense of something that is established and that everyone is familiar with—a tradition. This is also the best answer choice.

    C. a famous painting.
    WRONG: The Mona Lisa is a famous painting, but this is not what is has in common with the others institutional examples: The White House, etcetera.

    D. an anomaly.
    WRONG: Although the author may believe the Mona Lisa to be an anomaly on several fronts, this is not the aspect of the painting she is highlighting here.

159. What is the author's response to the story about the children playing in the neighborhood 'haunted house', who come running home to tell their parents that they had seen the figure in the painted portrait on the wall *moving*?

    A. The children had likely been staring at the painting too long, and expected it to move.
    CORRECT: This is likely to be the author's response to the story. "Any object stared at to the point of strain will appear to change in one way or another, especially if we expect it to" (lines 20-22).

    B. The figure in the painting was probably the person whom the children felt was haunting the house.
    WRONG: This is not likely to be the author's response to the story. There is nothing in the passage to support this answer.

    C. If the children had been looking at the figure for a long time, it would begin to move.
    WRONG: This answer is not as complete as Answer A. The expectation of movement is "especially" significant. "Any object stared at to the point of strain will appear to change in one way or another, *especially if we expect it to*" (lines 20-22).

    D. The children had probably expected the painting to move because it had been 'staring' at them.

WRONG: This is not likely to be the author's response to the story. This answer implies that the picture was animated in some way. The answer uses bits and pieces from the passage to make it an attractive choice, but it is using the information incorrectly.

160. According to the passage, one drawback of an art object's being "too famous for too long" (line 8) is that it can:

    A. lead to mischaracterization.
    WRONG: Although many may agree with this idea, it is not a drawback presented in the passage.

    B. become stale.
    WRONG: Although many may agree with this idea, it is not a drawback presented in the passage.

    C. preclude original ideas.
    CORRECT: This is a drawback which is implied in the passage. "Familiar legends and conjectures have accumulated around it to the point where it is impossible to see it with a fresh vision. We never see it for the first time; it has always been around" (lines 8-12).

    D. inhibit criticism.
    WRONG: Not only is this idea not presented in the passage, but the author herself participates in criticism of the painting.

161. Assume that a later, revised series of paintings by Leonardo da Vinci is discovered. Which of the following characteristics of the discovered paintings would most *compromise* the author's analysis?

    A. portrayed a slowly aging Mona Lisa.
    WRONG: The author actually does not believe Mona Lisa to be a symbol of timeless mysteries (line 48), so this discovery would strengthen her opinion.

    B. pictured the Mona Lisa smiling brightly.
    WRONG: Although the author comments that the smile some witness may be an illusion, she does not make any assertions about Mona Lisa's capability to smile in another painting.

    C. showed other examples of portraits where the eyes "follow you around the room".
    WRONG: The author acknowledges that this effect is found in many paintings, and thus this finding would not compromise her analysis.

    D. proved that the Mona Lisa background was a real landscape.
    CORRECT: This is the single characteristic that would most compromise the author's analysis. Though prefacing the information with "If ...", the author spends the entire second to last paragraph

on the significance of the landscape in the background, *as if the artist created it himself.* "Leonardo has *invented* a landscape half *fantastic* and half logical, where both time and place are mysterious" (lines 51-52).

162. The main idea of the passage is that:

- **A.** perfection may be in the eye of the beholder.
  WRONG: Although the author mentions the subjectivity inherent in perfection, this is not the main idea of the passage.

- **B.** if possible, art should always be viewed firsthand.
  CORRECT: This is a reasonable conclusion based upon the passage. The author mourns that, "Familiar legends and conjectures have accumulated around [the painting] to the point where it is impossible to see it with a fresh vision" (lines 8-10). In the final paragraph it seems as if she is going so far as to say that we should not indulge in any art education lest it ruin seeing an original, in-person, with a fresh perspective.

- **C.** interpretation of famous paintings is becoming increasingly difficult.
  WRONG: Although the author presents an example of 'should not be', she does not suggest that criticism of famous work is difficult, or that interpretation must be original to be good.

- **D.** fame frequently hurts an artist more than it helps him.
  WRONG: This is not a reasonable conclusion based upon the passage. There is no evidence that fame hurt da Vinci.

163. If the author's primary criterion for judging the standard of "*perfection*" of a picture were applied to directions, which of the following directions would be *most* perfect?

- **A.** Walk east for 720 centimeters, then turn right and go 62 centimeters.
  WRONG: These directions would not be most perfect. "… then turn right", but how *much* right? This is ambiguous.

- **B.** Move at a brisk pace north by northeast for 7 minutes, then turn sharply left and continue for 52 seconds.
  WRONG: These directions would not be most perfect. Move "north … then turn sharply left", but how far left? Exactly what direction?

- **C.** Run quickly 270 degrees for 1/2 mile, then turn left and walk for 129 feet.
  WRONG: These directions would not be most perfect. "… then turn left", but how far left? Which direction are you really headed in?

- **D.** Walk 352 degrees for 62 meters, then turn 20 degrees and continue for 5 meters.
  CORRECT: These directions would be most perfect, because they are the least "ambiguous". "If such a standard [as perfection] could exist, it is difficult to see how so ambiguous a picture as the Mona Lisa could represent it anyway" (lines 26-28). In this answer the directions cannot be misinterpreted with assumptions that a "right turn" would lead in a certain direction. Compass headings and distances are the only reliable directions. Degrees are more specific (less ambiguous) than "north", "south", directions. This is the only set of instructions that will guarantee that a person will get exactly from point A to point B.

164. The author's argument that the Mona Lisa "has always been around" and "is no longer a picture", depends on the acceptance of which of the following premises?

- **A.** It can be conclusively proven that it was a da Vinci painting.
  WRONG: The author's argument does not depend on the acceptance of this premise.

- **B.** The picture can be dated by the fashions which the Mona Lisa is wearing.
  WRONG: The author's argument does not depend on the acceptance of this premise.

- **C.** The painting has been recreated innumerable times in photographs.
  WRONG: The author's argument does not depend on the acceptance of this premise.

- **D.** Almost anyone can recognize and envision the painting.
  CORRECT: The author's argument depends on the acceptance of this premise. Here the author is arguing that the picture has "become ubiquitous" (line 62), and "an institution" (line 63). This answer and premise are critical to his arguments regarding the painting.

Passage II (Questions 165-172)

165. The claim that during the second six months of the experiment the children in Orphanage A gained less than the children in Orphanage B necessitates which of the following conclusions?

- **A.** The children of Orphanage A weighed less than the Children in Orphanage B.
  WRONG: This conclusion is not necessitated by the claim. The passage does not compare actual weights, but "growth rates", or the rates of weight gain.

B. The proffered dietary supplements were insufficient to override the emotional stress.

CORRECT: This conclusion is necessitated by the claim. During the *second* six months, the children of Orphanage A were offered the dietary supplements yet they failed to gain as much weight as the children in Orphanage B. We know from the passage that there is "a clear connection between emotional states and growth" (lines 8-9), and that the headmistress was with the children of Orphanage A during the second six months causing them emotional distress.

C. The children of Orphanage A were not eating their supplemented meals.

WRONG: While this conclusion is entirely possible, it is not necessitated by the claim.

D. Emotional sustenance is even more important than nutrition to growth.

WRONG: This conclusion is not necessitated by the claim. Though the passage provides that there is a connection between emotional state and growth, it reallyonly shows us that emotional distress retards growth. It does not tell us that a warm, cheerful, and wonderful headmistress would have caused a growth spurt in the children. In particular we don't know that emotional sustenance is "more important". The study conditions do not include poor nutrition and high states of emotional support.

166. According to the Passage, which of the following statements must be true?

A. During the first six-month period the headmistress's favorite children were at Orphanage A.

WRONG: Passage information does not indicate that this must be true.

B. The headmistress probably did not favor her "pets" with much extra food.

CORRECT: According to the passage, her favored children gained more weight once they were receiving the dietary supplements. Additionally, this answer includes the qualifiers "probably" and "much", which leaves open the possibility that she gave them some extra food on occasion.

C. At least some of the headmistress's favorite children were girls.

WRONG: Passage information does not indicate that this must be true.

D. Without the food supplements, the "teacher's pets" would not have weighed more than the Orphanage A children.

WRONG: Passage information does not indicate that this must be true. Again, the passage is comparing "growth rates" and "rates" of weight gain, not the actual weights of the children themselves.

167. Which of the following statements, if true, would most WEAKEN the author's contention that there is "a link between emotional state and the rate of growth" (line 66)?

A. Children were not allowed to eat while being rebuked by the headmistress.

CORRECT: If true, this statement would most weaken the author's contention. This answer eliminates the possibility that the children were receiving dietary supplementation. Remember, "What was worse, she chose mealtimes to administer public (and often unjustified) rebukes" (lines 62-64),—the same time that the children received the supplemental food.

B. The headmistress's favorite children were often given extra food.

WRONG: If true, this statement would not most weaken the author's contention, as there was an orphanage-wide phenomena distinct from her favoritism.

C. Both Comber and Younger were female and sympathized more with the children in Orphanage A.

WRONG: If true, this statement would not most weaken the author's contention: sympathy may have come after the study and does not necessarily translate to the emotional state of the children.

D. It was later determined that all of the headmistress's rebukes were completely justified.

WRONG: If true, this statement would not most weaken the author's contention. Though this would contradict some of the passage information, it would not necessarily (if at all) weaken the relationship between emotional state and growth rate.

168. According to the study results, during the first six months, the children with the greatest weight gain would have been:

A. the females in Orphanage B.

WRONG: Female favorites would have higher weight gain than other females in either orphanage.

B. the females in Orphanage A.

WRONG: Female favorites would have higher weight gain than other females in either orphanage.

C. the female "favorites" in Orphanage B.

CORRECT: We know from passage information that "girls" had greater growth rates than boys in many situations. During the first six months, there was no dietary supplementation. Further, the "favorites" of the headmistress seemed to display higher growth rates than their peers.

D. the female "favorites" in Orphanage A.

WRONG: There were no "favorites in Orphanage A during the first six months.

169. If the passage information is correct, which of the following statements would be best supported by the fact that fifteen years later, many of the orphans were still below average in both height and weight?

    A. Those children had been with too little food for too long.
        CORRECT: This inference would be supported by the passage information: The human body "can make up the loss (of nutrition) later if the famine does not last too long and is not too severe" (lines 9-10).

    B. These orphans must be the children in Orphanage B whom the headmistress had most severely rebuked.
        WRONG: This inference is not justified by information in the passage. Although this population would be most at risk for low growth rates, they too had the ability to "make up the loss" in the fifteen years following the study.

    C. Those children had received supplementary food and a healthy diet too late.
        WRONG: The human body "can make up the loss (of nutrition) later *if* the famine does not last too long and is not too severe" (lines 9-10). The author does not specify an age beyond which this phenomenon is not true.

    D. The new headmistress had also been a stern disciplinarian.
        WRONG: This inference is not justified by the passage. What new headmistress?

170. What is the most serious apparent *weakness* of the research described?

    A. There was no way to determine how much of the "unlimited" food the children were eating.
        WRONG: This is not the most serious apparent weakness of the research. Although it may have been one of the weaker aspects of the study, it is not the most serious weakness.

    B. There was no way to gauge the degree of the headmistress's rebukes.
        WRONG: This is not the most serious apparent weakness of the research. It is true, yet it is too specific, and can be encompassed in Answer D.

    C. The scientists were predisposed to "find" what they had been looking for.
        WRONG: The scientists did not actually find what they expected.

    D. There were too many variables involved in the experiments.
        CORRECT: This is the most serious apparent weakness of the research. This answer encompasses the most possible answer choices.

171. Some recent studies have concluded that in the absence of sufficient food, males of all ages are likely to give up a portion of their food to females and children. How would these studies affect the passage's assertion that girls seem to resist malnutrition better than boys?

    A. It would support the assertion.
        WRONG: This is not how the studies would affect the passage's reasoning.

    B. It would support the assertion if it could be shown that the girls refused the food.
        WRONG: This is not how the studies would affect the passage's reasoning. If the supposition were true, it would be necessary to show that the girls had refused food if it had been offered to them. However, this *still* would not cause the supposition (which is an obvious attack on the passage's reasoning) to support the passage's reasoning.

    C. It would refute the assertion if this behavior occurred in the Guam, Hiroshima, and WWII studies, as well as the passage study.
        CORRECT: Only if this effect was occurring in the studies that describe female restorative advantage, would it refute the findings of these studies. See lines 20-28.

    D. It would refute the reasoning.
        WRONG: Notice in the question stem that "some" studies have concluded that males are "likely" to give up their food. This is not a well proven effect that could be considered universal. There is no indication that this effect occurred in the present study or those studies that describe female growth advantage.

172. The author claims, "by using experimental and control groups (and partly by accident) Dr. Comber made observations that establish a clear connection between emotional states and growth" (lines 34-36). The support offered for this conclusion is:

    A. strong: there was a clear correlation between the amount the children ate and their growth rate.
        WRONG: This answer does not address the emotional states relation to growth. In addition, there is no evidence that the children actually ate anything at all! They were offered the food, but whether they ate it, or how much, is open to speculation.

    B. strong: under difficult circumstances, an important discovery was made, albeit inadvertently.
        WRONG: The question is asking whether or not there is sufficient support for the correlation that was noted between emotional state and growth to be validated. This answer does not address the question and is ambiguous.

    C. weak: the results do not appear accidental.
        WRONG: The author states that the correlation

was stumbled upon inadvertently. Futhermore, how the correlation came to be discovered has nothing to do with whether or not it is valid.

D. weak: the control group was not in the same situation as the experimental group.

CORRECT: Orphanage A was the experimental group, while Orphanage B was the intended control group. In any such experimental setup, only one variable should be manipulated—in this case, the amount of food. With the introduction of the headmistress as a compounding factor, the two groups were no longer comparable. Since the experimental design was not solid, the results noted cannot be strongly supported.

Examination 04: Biological Sciences

Passage V (Questions 173-179)

173. A is correct. Portions of M. Geromanium's double stranded DNA are shown in the passage. Each primer will bind to a complementary sequence on one side of the double strand depicted. The 5´-GTGTCCTC-3´ primer binds 5´-C CATAAAACC...GAGGACACT-3´ strand of DNA, while 5´-CATAAAACC-3´ binds the 3´-GGTATTTTGG...CTCCTGTGA-5´ strand. The fact that the primers do not anneal to the entire sequence is insignificant, as the sequence is 687 bp long.

Note: Locating the complementary sequences is easier if one focuses on more readily identifiable details, such as four adenines in a row.

174. D is correct. The two primers are not complementary to any of the bacterial DNA sequences provided. Again, a quick scan of the bacterial genomes for an obvious sequence that is complementary to the primers [such as an AGGA sequence for primer a), or a TTTT sequence for primer b)] will yield the answer.

175. C is correct. Previously used polymerases were denatured in the DNA denaturation step of each cycle as a result of the high temperatures. Taq, which comes from bacteria found in geysers and hot springs, is not denatured in such conditions. The use of Taq has made PCR more efficient in that scientists no longer have to add enzyme during every PCR cycle.

176. B is correct. DNA is negatively charged and thus migrates towards the positive end. The smallest strands will travel the farthest along the gel. The identity of the 'known' samples in the control lane may be extrapolated from the DNA lengths provided in the passage. The DNA which travels the farthest is *M. roberium*, the smallest of the three. This band is not found in the experimental lane, indicating that *M. roberium* was not present in the patient sample.

177. A is correct. DNA Polymerase is the only enzyme needed for successful PCR. The double stranded DNA separates with heat, and primers bind DNA via hydrogen bonds.

178. D is correct. Only the original template contains radioactive adenine. This is relatively insignificant relative to the 33,554,434 copies that are produced in 25 cycles. However, since radioactive cytosine bases are used, all the copies will contain radioactive C and will thus test positive.

179. C is correct. If *Mycoplasma* were found in the joints of healthy patients, its presence in the joints of TMJ patients could be considered coincidental rather than causal. All of the other answer choices support a causal relationship.

Passage VI (Questions 180-186)

180. B is correct. The lac enzyme genes will undergo transcription if either lactose inhibits the repressor from binding the operator, or if cAMP activates CAP. In the presence of glucose, cAMP will remain at low levels, and the promoter is unlikely to be activated making RNA transcription of the genes downstream equally as unlikely.

181. D is correct. IPTG is an allosteric regulator of the repressor protein. It does not bind DNA

182. C is correct. A mutation in the operator site, would most likely interfere with repressor binding. Without a bound repressor, transcription of all lac genes will increase equally.

183. D is correct. The two mutations are phenotypically silent, or recessive, as repressor can be produced from the second DNA strand, and β-galactosidase from the first.

184. C is correct. Transformation describes bacterial incorporation of genetic material from surroundings into its own genome.

185. B is correct. The passage delineates how lactose binds the repressor in order to facilitate gene transcription. CAP activation and initiation complex formation enhancement are achieved by cAMP and CAP binding the A site, respectively.

186. B is correct. Glucose levels determine cAMP levels, which in turn modulate the positive control mechanism.

Independent Questions (Questions 187-188)

187. B is correct. PCR requires the use of two distinct primers ($2^0=1$). During the PCR cycle, the DNA would denature and only one strand would be able to bind a primer and elongate. The remaining DNA strand, however, would be unable to replicate and thus the only double stranded DNA at the end of the run would be the original.

188. A is correct. Because DNA replication is semiconservative, none of the daughter cells will look like the original one-stranded mutant. After the first round, one daughter will have normal sequence and the second daughter will have the wrong base on both strands. With faithful replication afterwards, all of the daughter cells will look like the first generation daughter cells.

EXPLANATIONS 05

Answers to Questions 189-235

ANSWERS TO EXAMINATION 5

PHYSICAL SCIENCES	VERBAL REASONING	BIOLOGICAL SCIENCES
189. C	205. A	220. C
190. D	206. C	221. C
191. B	207. C	222. C
192. D	208. B	223. D
193. B	209. B	224. A
194. A	210. C	225. D
195. D	211. D	226. B
196. C	212. B	227. A
197. B	213. A	228. C
198. D	214. D	229. D
199. A	215. B	230. C
200. B	216. B	231. D
201. B	217. C	232. D
202. D	218. D	233. A
203. B	219. A	234. B
204. C		235. B

Passage I (Questions 189-195)

189. C is correct. The molar mass for fluorine gas, F_2 is about 38. The molar mass for Ne is about 20, so the square root of 38/20 is about the same as the square root of 2, which is 1.4.

190. D is correct. From Graham's law, the lower the molar mass of a gas, the greater its average speed. Since the two gases are at the same temperature, their average kinetic energies will be the same.

191. B is correct. According to the passage, the process required repetition because the separation factor was so small. From the equation in the passage, a small separation factor results when there is little difference between the molar masses of the two gases.

192. D is correct. Choice D is the only option where the two gases have significantly different molar masses. Separation via successive effusion depends on the difference in the molar masses of the two gases.

193. B is correct. According to the passage uranium-238 is the most common isotope. All uranium isotopes contain 92 protons. Subtracting the number of protons from the atomic mass yields the number of neutrons: 238 – 92 = 146.

194. A is correct. From Dalton's law, the mole fraction of a gas is directly proportional to its share of the total pressure. The partial pressure due to helium, 152 mmHg, is exactly one-fifth of 760 mmHg.

Passage II (Questions 195-200)

195. D is correct. The work is equal to the gravitational potential energy gained by the barbell. Do not forget that there are two 60 kg plates on the barbell.

GPE = mgh = (120)(10)(2.5) J = 3000 J = 3 kJ.

196. C is correct. For an object in free fall, the speed at the moment it hits the ground is given by the formula:

$$v = \sqrt{2gh} = \sqrt{(2)(10)(2.5)} = \sqrt{50} = 7 \text{ m/s}$$

197. B is correct. The diagram below shows the torques on the bar.

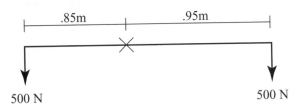

Figure 1 Torque diagram

Torque = (0.95)(500) – (0.85)(500) = (0.95 – 0.85)(500) = (0.10)(500) = 50 Nm

198. D is correct. Power = (Energy)/(time). So Power = (2 kJ)/(0.2 sec) = 10 kW.

199. A is correct. The strongman does no work in holding the barbell motionless over his head. If work is equal to zero, then power must also be zero.

200. B is correct. Calculate the torques by placing the axis at the 50 kg weight. Remember that the strongman pushes up on the bar with a force equal to the total weight on the bar, 900 N.

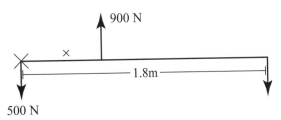

Figure 1 Torque diagram

(1.8)(400) = (x)(900)

x = (1.8)(4)/(9) = (0.2)(4) = 0.8 m = 80 cm

Independent Questions (Questions 201-204)

201. B is correct. Trials 1 and 2 demonstrate that the reaction rate doubles when [B] doubles, thus the reaction is first order with respect to B. In Trials 2 and 3, as both [A] and [B] are doubled, the reaction rate quadruples. One can expect the reaction rate to have doubled as a function of the concentration of B, thus doubling the concentration of A must be responsible for the rest of the increase in reaction rate. One can conclude that the reaction is also first order with respect to both A.

202. D is correct. When the bow is stretched, it behaves like a spring, creating elastic potential energy. The elastic potential energy is converted into kinetic energy as the arrow is released from the bow. As the arrow climbs higher and slows down, kinetic energy is converted into gravitational potential energy.

203. B is correct. The equilibrium expression is found by dividing the concentrations of the products by the concentrations of the reactants. The reaction coefficients are placed as exponents in the equilibrium expression. Solids and pure liquids are not included in the equilibrium expression; this is why water isn't included.

204. C is correct. Since the rocket is moving at a constant speed, there is no acceleration of the rocket, so the next force on it must be zero. The power of the rocket is used to overcome gravity and air resistance, both of which decrease as the rocket rises.

Examination 05: Verbal Reasoning

Passage III (Questions 205-212)

205. Which of the following statements is most clearly a thesis presented by the author?

A. We may be the ancestors of aliens.
CORRECT: This assertion is most clearly a thesis presented by the author. This is an even more attractive choice since it contains the qualifier, "may".

B. The SETI program will eventually discover alien life.
WRONG: This assertion is not most clearly a thesis presented by the author. Based upon the author's admiration for the scientists, it is reasonable to assume that the author believes in alien life. However, none of this confidence is projected toward the SETI program. He criticizes SETI's efforts as unpromising: "almost three-quarters of the heavens have been scanned with no discernible patterns discovered" (lines 8-9). In addition he comments on the impracticality of searching for radio signals.

C. Aliens intentionally spawned humankind.
WRONG: This assertion is not most clearly a thesis presented by the author. It is too strong. It is much easier to argue that Answer A is correct than this answer. Though the author apparently believes in aliens, and that they "shipped some microorganisms to Earth" (line 27), it is a far different matter to say that they intentionally spawned *humankind.* Perhaps they meant to spawn frogs...

D. Notable scientists believe in alien ancestors.
WRONG: This assertion is not most clearly a thesis presented by the author. What does "notable" mean? This answer is too simplistic and strong. More importantly, this is not a main idea of the passage.

206. Which of the following scientific advances would most seriously *challenge* the hypothesis involving aliens?

A. Association of efforts to detect alien life with

man's genetic structure.
WRONG: This answer is nonsensical. Does it mean that because of man's genetic structure he instinctively searches out his alien forbearers? How is an 'association of efforts' a scientific advance?

B. Proof of ancient alien landing sites in the southwest desert.
WRONG: This scientific advance would support the author's hypothesis.

C. The discovery of large molybdenum deposits in the earth.
CORRECT: This scientific advance would most seriously challenge the author's hypothesis. The *scarcity* of molybdenum is one of the two tenets of the scientists' arguments. "organisms [evolving spontaneously on earth] would not have placed such reliance on a rare element—unless they were descended from life forms that arose on a planet where molybdenum is more common" (lines 43-46).

D. Confirmation of TV-type transmissions emitting from another star system.
WRONG: This scientific advance would not most seriously challenge the hypothesis. So the author provides that these TV-type transmissions are "not likely" to be detected by SETI. This *might* challenge the information relating to SETI, but it has little effect on the hypothesis involving aliens.

207. According to the passage information, what would happen if life had evolved spontaneously here on earth without outside intervention of any kind?

I. The idea of the existence of alien life forms could be dismissed.
WRONG: This is not what would have happened, given the supposition in the question. The only thing that could be "dismissed" would be the idea that aliens were our ancestors. For instance, they might still have "seeded" this planet, albeit unsuccessfully. They might have seeded other planets. It has little bearing on the existence of aliens as a whole.

II. Organisms would not be dependent on a rare element.
CORRECT: This is what would have happened, given the supposition in the question. "In their [Crick and Orgel's] view, organisms [evolving independently on this planet] would not have placed such reliance on a rare element—unless they were descended from life forms that arose on a planet where molybdenum is more common" (lines 43-46).

III. There would be different molecules controlling the inheritance of at least some organisms.
CORRECT: This is what would have happened, given the supposition in the question. "Crick and

Orgel believe that if life originated on Earth, it would have arisen in many places and at many different times, and this would have resulted in a diversity of genetic codes" (lines 50-53).

A. I only

B. II only

C. II and III only
   CORRECT: See above answer explanations.

D. I, II, and III

208. If the hypothesis of the passage is correct, one should find that relatively weak TV-type transmissions:

A. cannot possibly reach our planet from nearby star systems.
   WRONG: "However, these signals are relatively weak and SETI *is not likely* to detect the equivalent of Earth type TV transmitters, even on the nearest stars" (lines 14-17). Although unlikely, the author does not say this is impossible.

B. travel at about the same speed as light.
   CORRECT: In lines 11-14, the author states:"As an example, early TV shows like I Love Lucy and Ed Sullivan *left the earth about 40 years ago, and have traveled 40 light years,* reaching several thousand nearby stars" If these signals have traveled the same distance (light years) in the same amount of time (years) as light, their speed must be the same as light (one light year/year)

C. might be the first signal that an alien planet receives from the earth.
   WRONG: "However, these signals are relatively weak and SETI *is not likely* to detect the equivalent of Earth type TV transmitters, even on the nearest stars" (lines 14-17). If we are not likely to detect them, then presumably, neither are the aliens.

D. are what SETI has been programmed to detect.
   WRONG: "However, these signals are relatively weak and SETI *is not likely* to detect the equivalent of Earth type TV transmitters, even on the nearest stars" (lines 14-17).

209. The author most likely believes which of the following statements:

A. SETI will eventually detect alien transmissions.
   WRONG: This supposition is not most clearly believed by the author. Based upon the author's advocacy of Crick and Ogel's theory, it is reasonable to assume that the author believes in alien life. However, none of this confidence is expressed toward the SETI program. He admits, "almost three-quarters of the heavens have been scanned with no discernible patterns discovered" (lines 8-9).

B. The evolution of our species is a foregone conclu-

sion.
   CORRECT: This supposition is most clearly believed by the author. The author refers to "the inexorable process of evolution …" (lines 29-30).

C. Crick and Orgel were geniuses.
   WRONG: This supposition is not most clearly believed by the author. Admiration for the two scientists, or support of their theory, cannot be equated with a belief that they were geniuses.

D. The "seeding" of earth was probably accidental.
   WRONG: In the passage the author states, "billions of years ago a sophisticated civilization on a planet circling some nearby star *shipped some microorganisms to Earth*" (lines 25-27). The aliens seem to play an active role in the process, which should convey the author's belief in intentioned seeding.

210. The word *perplexing* (line 30):

A. detracts somewhat from the author's main argument.
   WRONG: The word is central to the author's thesis introduction.

B. conveys that Crick and Orgel are the first to respond
   WRONG: This is a nonsensical answer. Perplexing is not used to convey the time course of the scientists' theory.

C. conveys that certain aspects of earthly life have not been satisfactorily explained.
   CORRECT: Crick and Orgel's hypothesis was born out of their effort to explain these aspects of earthly life. From paragraphs three and four we can glean that the author feels that these aspects (molybdenum dependency and the ubiquity of DNA) have not been satisfactorily explained by any other theories up until now.

D. suggest that further study needs to be undertaken.
   WRONG: This is an attractive answer because it presents a conventional response to something 'perplexing'. However, futher study did not resolve these two aspects, theoretical explanation did.

211. On the basis of the passage, it is reasonable to conclude that:

A. the aliens were probably "seeding" more than just one planet at a time.
   WRONG: This is not a reasonable conclusion. There is no support for this conclusion in the passage.

B. the aliens did not "seed" earth intentionally.
   WRONG: This is not a reasonable conclusion. The scientists "speculated that billions of years ago a sophisticated civilization on a planet circling some nearby star *shipped some microorganisms to*

Earth" (lines 25-27).

C. eventually SETI may yield the reasons why aliens chose earth for seeding.

WRONG: This is not a reasonable conclusion. The author does not argue that SETI will eventually yield any information, much less information as specific as this conclusion. This is not supported in the passage.

D. the aliens might not have known a great deal about earth.

CORRECT: This is a reasonable conclusion. "… organisms [evolving spontaneously here on earth] would not have placed such reliance on a rare element—unless they were descended from life forms that arose on a planet where molybdenum is more common" (lines 43-46). It is not unreasonable to conclude that the aliens *might* also not have chosen a planet where a critical element was so scarce if they had known more about earth.

212. Which of the following choices would the author of the passage be most likely to describe as *barren*?

A. a lifeless desert

WRONG: The author would not be most likely to describe this choice as *barren*. Though a desert may bear vegetation, this answer lacks the assurance that exists in Answer B.

B. a lifeless but fertile garden plot

CORRECT: The author would be most likely to describe this choice as *barren*. "These seeds, they suggest, took hold on the *then-barren* planet, and proceeded to set the inexorable process of evolution in motion" (lines 28-30). "The fear that foreign living matter could proliferate in a *barren* world has led scientists to routinely sterilize spacecraft sent from the earth to the moon and other planets to prevent contamination of alien soil" (lines 55-59).

C. a sterile woman without children

WRONG: The author would not be most likely to describe this choice as *barren*.

D. a massive rocky planet

WRONG: The author would not be most likely to describe this choice as *barren*.

Passage IV (Questions 213-219)

213. If the author's primary criterion for judging the '*realness*' of time were applied to human feelings, which of the following feelings would be the LEAST real?

A. Love

CORRECT: Considering the supposition in the question, this feeling would be the least real. "To ask whether time is real is to ask whether the changes—biological, astronomical, or atomic—by which we measure time, and which we measure by it, are real" (lines 23-26). Love is the only emotion offered as an answer and the most difficult, if not impossible to quantify in any way.

B. Hunger

WRONG: Considering the supposition in the question, this feeling would not be the least real. The effects of hunger and the physical responses to hunger can be analyzed and quantified. An emotion such as love would be less real.

C. Pain

WRONG: Considering the supposition in the question, this feeling would not be the least real. The effects of pain and the physical responses to pain can be analyzed and quantified. An emotion such as love would be less real.

D. Cold

WRONG: Considering the supposition in the question, this feeling would not be the least real. The effects of cold and the physical responses to cold can be analyzed and quantified. An emotion such as love would be less real.

214. On the basis of the passage, one may assume that as humans discover newer and more effective scientific methods:

A. what was once irreversible will become reversible.

WRONG: This may not be assumed on the basis of the passage.

B. what was once impossible will become possible.

WRONG: This may not be assumed on the basis of the passage.

C. what was once trivial will become important.

WRONG: This may not be assumed on the basis of the passage. "trivial, meaning that it is not worth answering" (lines 22-23).

D. what was once meaningless will become meaningful.

CORRECT: This may be assumed on the basis of the passage. "For the scientist, the question [of whether time is real or not] is meaningless, in the sense that it cannot be answered by scientific methods …" (lines 20-22). If more can be assessed with scientific method, more will be meaningful, to the scientist at least.

215. Which of the following statements would the author most likely *disagree* with:

I. A scientist must make certain assumptions in order to do his job.
WRONG: The author would agree: "And the scientist, … is compelled to *assume* that they—and therefore time—are real." (lines 26-29).

II. We cannot rely on common sense.
CORRECT "Common sense born of experience, however, teaches us that a backward-moving time is as fantastical as an unmoving time" (lines 66-68). Here the author suggests that common sense is important, and certainly reliable.

III. Philosophy is important to scientific discovery.
WRONG: The author provides examples of how scientists must disregard philosophy in order to continue their study.

A. I only

B. II only
CORRECT: See above answer explanations.

C. III only

D. II and II only

216. The author believes a philosopher may come to a conclusion that:

A. it is possible to go back in time.
WRONG: This is not the conclusion that the author believes a philosopher would come to. There is no basis for this answer.

B. defies common sense.
CORRECT: This is the conclusion that the author believes a philosopher would come to. Lines 32-43 provide a powerful glimpse of the authors beliefs regarding philosophers.

C. centers on only one of the fundamental questions.
WRONG: The author does not suggest a limited scope to philosophic conclusions..

D. cannot be taken literally.
WRONG: Although this may be true, it is not as good an answer choice as B as choice B is more directly supported by the passage.

217. According to the author, which of the following statements must NOT be true?

A. Time has no beginning or end.
WRONG: There is not information in the passage to support or refute the truth of this statement.

B. Time must be infinite.
WRONG: There is not information in the passage to support or refute the truth of this statement

C. Time can be moving and unmoving.
CORRECT: The author clearly states that time is not only moving, but is unidirectional. He suggests that the consideration of time not moving is one of

the dreamers, poets, writers, and perhaps the philosophers.

D. Time is real.
WRONG: It is fairly clear that the author does believe that time is real.

218. The assertion that time is paradoxical is NOT clearly consistent with:

A. the ironies of philosophical conclusions.
WRONG: This information is actually consistent with the assertion.

B. our yearnings for a return to a former period of our lives.
WRONG: This information does not have any clear relation to the assertion and thus can be neither consistent nor inconsistent.

C. time being rather easy to define.
WRONG: This information does not have any clear relation to the assertion and thus can be neither consistent nor inconsistent.

D. our abilities to use common sense born of experience.
CORRECT: This information is not clearly consistent with the assertion. "Time, … which is as straightforward as an alarm clock yet as paradoxical as relativity …" (lines 1-4). "Common sense born of experience, however, teaches us that a backward-moving time is as fantastical as an unmoving time" (lines 66-68). Common sense born of experience will not lead us to the theory of relativity.

219. On the basis of the passage, it is reasonable to conclude that:

A. alchemists must have believed that time was reversible.
CORRECT: This is a reasonable conclusion based on the passage. "For such a magical elixir of youth, the alchemists toiled long years over their alembics …" (lines 63-65).

B. many philosophers believe that time is an illusion.
WRONG: This is not a reasonable conclusion based on the passage. How many is "many"? Two are mentioned and there is nothing in the passage that would lead us to believe that their beliefs are indicative of all or "many" other philosophers.

C. time has no beginning and no end.
WRONG: This is not a reasonable conclusion based on the passage. The question regarding whether time has a beginning or end is not answered in the passage.

D. time is not intuitively obvious.
WRONG: This is not a reasonable conclusion

based on the passage. There is no basis for this answer.

Passage V (Questions 220-235)

220. **C is correct.** As per the passage, a heterologous vaccine is made up of a closely related organism of lesser virulence (in this case: the cowpox and/or vaccinia viruses), which displays antigens found on the virulent organism (in this case: the variola virus). The cowpox or vaccinia replicated in milkmaids, inducing an immune response which cross-reacted with variola antigens.

221. **C is correct.** A good vaccine elicits the appropriate immune response for the particular pathogen, provides long term protection (ideally life-long), does not cause clinical disease, and is inexpensive.

222. **C is correct.** A review of central dogma:

The conversion of DNA → DNA is **replication**.

The conversion of DNA → RNA is **transcription**.

The conversion of RNA → protein is **translation**.

According to the question stem, *expression* involves the transcription of DNA into RNA, a process that requires **RNA polymerase**. The rest of the enzymes listed are only involved in DNA replication. **RNA primase** synthesizes short stretches of RNA primer upon which the DNA polymerase binds: DNA polymerase cannot initiate DNA replication without a primer. (A primer is NOT needed for transcription). **DNA ligase** seals the lagging strand gaps between Okazaki fragments and is not involved in RNA synthesis.

223. **D is correct.** As per the passage, vaccination induces a "primed" state in the mother, which she passes on to her unborn baby. Thus, a 3 month old baby is expected to be primed to all diseases the mother is primed for. The baby's immune system is identical to the mother's at this age.

224. **A is correct.** A is correct. According to the passage, live recombinant vaccines are viruses with a recombinant gene coding for an immunogenic protein from a virulent virus. The recombinant virus must use the hosts' cellular machinery to transcribe and translate the viral proteins and sometimes replicate the viral genome. Protein synthesis not destined the cytoplasm of the host cell occurs on ribosomes docked on the rough endoplasmic reticulum. Viral genetic material will utilize the ribosomes on the rough endoplasmic reticulum. Lysosomes are digestive organelles which play a role in the digestion of molecules obtained from the extracellular environment. Peroxisomes are detoxifying organelles which synthesize hydrogen peroxide. The nucleus is not necessary for live recombinant vaccines to work because prokaryotic cells can replicate and transcribe genetic material without a nucleus.

225. **D is correct.** The passage introduces the concept of "primed" immune systems in vaccinated subjects. However, this information is not pertinent in answering the question. Only one of the organs listed is NOT involved in the immune response. The **adrenal gland** is part of the endocrine system, synthesizing aldosterone, epinephrine, norepinephrine etc. The correct answer choice is D.

The **bone marrow** gives rise to all cells of the immune system, including B-cells, T-cells, macrophages, etc. The **spleen** is a giant filter of the cardiovascular system. It is full of mature B and T-cells ready to respond to infection. **Lymph nodes** line the lymphatic system in search of invaders. A swollen lymph node indicates a host infected state because it implies active division of immune system cells housed in the node.

226. **B is correct.** As per the passage, killed (inactivated) vaccines are not as infectious and are therefore relatively safe. However, they are usually of lower immunogenicity (produces a poor immune response) and multiple doses may be needed to induce immunity. In addition, they are usually expensive to prepare.

Passage VI (Questions 227-235)

227. **A is correct.** In all cases, RG7 resulted in a reduction in protein levels, which was more pronounced than any effect on ATP levels. As bacteria lack membrane-bound organelles, including lysosomes and Golgi bodies, choices B and D are incorrect. If the Krebs cycle was the major site of RG7 action, a greater change in ATP levels would be expected.

228. **C is correct.** Bacteria do not have nuclei, nucleoli, or histones. They can contain circular DNA however, and require enzymes which specifically cleave circular DNA, in order to replicate and transcribe the genome.

229. **D is correct.** Neither human cells, nor the cells of any animal, have cell walls.

230. **C is correct.** Bacteria reproduce very rapidly (some divide every 30 minutes) and have high mutation rates due to high inaccuracy within their DNA duplication process.

231. **D is correct.** Patients often experience symptomatic relief as the bacterial load is reduced in the first few days of antibiotic treatment. However, significant amounts of bacteria remain at this time, which have now been exposed to antibiotic. If antibiotics are discontinued at this point, surviving bacteria have the opportunity to develop resistance. The passage states that bacteria which were previously susceptible to antibiotics, have now once again become serious health concerns. In other words, there are not new bacterial species, but rather the same bacteria with antibiotic resistance, such as Staphylococcus Aureus. Penicillin is still a first line treatment for many infections.

232. **D is correct.** Peroxisomes are not involved in protein synthesis. Bacteria have ribosomes, and although they lack nuclei, the question stem asks for an organelle involved in *posttranslational* processing. The nucleus is only involved in posttranscriptional processing of mRNA. The Golgi is responsible for protein modification in eukaryotic cells.

233. **A is correct.** Bacteria generally undergo binary fission, although some may engage in budding or even a type of sexual reproduction called conjugation. Bacteria cannot undergo mitosis as they do not have chromosomes.

Independent Questions (Questions 234-235)

234. **B is correct.** The acquired immune system is composed of humoral and cell mediated responses. The humoral response is accomplished by B-cells which mature in the bone marrow. If properly stimulated, B-cells are activated into plasma cells, which secrete antibodies.

Cell mediated immunity is carried out by T-cells, which mature in the thymus. T-helper cells are the gatekeepers of the immune response and regulate the activity of other T and B-cells. Macrophages are non-specific immune cells released by the bone marrow. They do not produce antibodies.

235. **B is correct.** In the absence of oxygen, facultative anaerobes switch from aerobic metabolism to fermentation.

338

EXPLANATIONS 06

Answers to Questions 236–282

ANSWERS TO EXAMINATION 6

PHYSICAL SCIENCES	VERBAL REASONING	BIOLOGICAL SCIENCES
236. C	252. C	267. B
237. D	253. A	268. B
238. B	254. B	269. B
239. A	255. D	270. C
240. D	256. D	271. C
241. B	257. C	272. B
242. A	258. D	273. C
243. A	259. B	274. D
244. C	260. D	275. A
245. A	261. D	276. B
246. B	262. A	277. C
247. D	263. B	278. C
248. B	264. C	279. D
249. D	265. D	280. B
250. C	266. B	281. C
251. A		282. D

Passage I (Questions 236-282)

236. C is correct. Gravitational potential energy is given by the formula:

$$GPE = mgh = (10)(10)(20) = 2000 \text{ J}.$$

The work accomplished is against a conservative force, resulting in an increases in PE. Note that the height is path-independent.

237. D is correct. The distance equals the total length of sections A – D in the diagram, or 30 m. The magnitude of the displacement equals the difference between the starting and ending positions, 20 m.

238. B is correct. The force due to friction is equal to the product of the coefficient and the normal force. Since the surface is flat, the normal force has the same magnitude as the weight.

$$F = \mu mg$$

$$20 = \mu(10)(10)$$

$$\mu = (20)/(100) = 0.2$$

239. A is correct. Power is work per unit time. Since the frictional force always acts directly against any motion, you can get the work done by multiplying the frictional force by the total distance.

$$P = Fd/t = (20)(30)/(40) = (600)/(40) = 15 \text{ W}$$

240. D is correct. In sections A and C, the object is moving parallel to the resisting force, so no work is performed. In sections B and D, however, the object is moving against the resisting force, so work must be done.

241. B is correct. Velocity is displacement divided by time. Even though the force acts over the entire distance of 30 m traveled in Example 2, the displacement is still only 20 m.

$$v = d/t = (20)/(50) = 0.4 \text{ m/s}$$

242. A is correct. When work is done against friction (nonconservative force), it is converted into the internal energy of the sliding objects, or heat. The passage states that nonconservative work is not converted into potential energy.

Passage II (Questions 243-248)

243. A is correct. The partial pressures are proportional to the number of moles of gas. Two moles of NO are required for every mole of Br_2. Since there are equal molar amounts of the two gases, NO will be depleted first.

244. C is correct. Because they are directly proportional, partial pressure ratios are the same as molar ratios. The partial pressure of NOBr increases from 0 to 0.30 atm. It only takes 1 mole of Br_2 to create 2 moles of NOBr, so Br_2 will lose half as much pressure as NOBr gains, so Br_2 lost $(0.30)/(2) = 0.15$ atm. 0.50 atm – 0.15 atm = 0.35 atm.

245. A is correct. Because 3 moles of the reactants form 2 moles of product, as long as the reaction moves in the forward direction, the pressure will decrease. As there is no product in the container at the start of the reaction, the reaction must proceed in the forward direction to reach equilibrium.

246. B is correct. One can gather from the chart that the pressure of nitrosyl bromide is increasing with the increase in initial bromine pressure. For every NOBr formed, an NO is depleted, thus the increase in the NOBr pressure coincides with the decrease in NO pressure.

247. D is correct. The equilibrium constant is equal to the partial pressures of the products divided by the reactants, with the coefficients of the balanced equation placed as exponents.

248. B is correct. The value of K_p is the same as stated in the passage; the change in initial pressures has no effect on the equilibrium constant.

Independent Questions (Questions 249-251)

249. D is correct. The diagram below shows the torques on the beam. Keep in mind that the weight of the beam acts at its center.

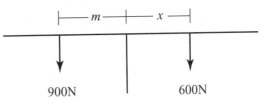

At the man's farthest position, the opposing torques have equivalent magnitude.

$$(900)(1) = (600)x$$

$$x = (900)/(600) = 1.5 \text{ m}$$

250. C is correct. The rate law equation for the situation described is as follows. The rate constant, k, can be calculated as follows:

$$\text{Rate} = k[A][B]$$

$$2.0 \times 10^{-3} = k(0.2)(0.2)$$

$$k = (2.0 \times 10^{-3})/(4.0 \times 10^{-2}) = 0.5 \times 10^{-1} = 5.0 \times 10^{-2}$$

251. A is correct. For an ideal gas, pressure and temperature are directly proportional, so when temperature increases at constant volume, pressure will increase too. The change in temperature will have no effect on the mass of the gas.

Examination 06: Verbal Reasoning

Passage III (Questions 252-258)

252. On the basis of the passage, it is reasonable to conclude that:

A. the signatories of the Declaration of Independence intended that all men are of equal intelligence.
WRONG: This is not a reasonable conclusion: 'created equally' does not translate to 'of equal intelligence'. This answer lacks any support within the passage.

B. those who espoused Jensenism were racists.
WRONG: This is not a reasonable conclusion on the basis of the passage. Although many may consider Jensen rascist at some level, the author clearly states that the psychological theory was "not [an] exponents of racism" (line 4).

C. even prior to 1973, attempts at compensatory education had been going on for some time.
CORRECT: This is a reasonable conclusion. "[In 1973, Jensen} did not retreat from the controversial position he had set forth in earlier years, that *compensatory education had failed"* (lines 16-18).

D. intelligence is largely hereditary.
WRONG: This is one of Jensen's conclusions, not that of the passage. The author presents several other factors affecting intelligence, such as the subjectivity of IQ test, nutrition, and parental literacy.

253. An important comparison is made in the passage between:

A. environment and heredity.
CORRECT: 'Nature vs. Nurture' is an important comparison in the passage. It lies at the crux of the arguments between the Jensenists (Nature) and those who believe that I.Q. and intelligence are the result of many factors (nurture).

B. genetic diversity and human equality.
WRONG: This is not an important comparison in the passage.

C. biased testing and future performance.
WRONG: This is not an important comparison in the passage.

D. educability and group differences.
WRONG: This is not an important comparison in

the passage. This is the name of Jensen's book.

254. That results of the researchers, whom had succeeded in helping to raise the I.Q. of deprived preschool children (lines 47-60), are most in accord with the view that:

A. one-on-one time with a "toy demonstrator" can raise a child's I.Q.
WRONG: The information is not most in accord with this view. The toy demonstrators were encouraging *parents* to play with their children. The children were not one-on-one with a toy demonstrator.

B. parents play a critical role in a child's I.Q. development.
CORRECT: The information is most in accord with this view. "Levenstein's project used trained "toy demonstrators" to visit toddlers at home and to encourage inarticulate or illiterate parents to play and talk with their children, stimulating them to use words and make observations" (lines 59-63). In this way, Levenstein claimed that she was able to raise children's I.Q.s.

C. intelligence and I.Q. are one in the same.
WRONG: This information is not most in accord with this view, in fact it is unrelated. The question does not deal with the validity of IQ tests.

D. the I.Q. tests were biased toward white middle-class culture.
WRONG: Although this may be one of the critiques of Jensen's theory, this is unrelated to the researchers results. The question does not deal with the validity of IQ tests.

255. Years later, in *The Bell Curve*, Herrnstein writes, "The difference in measured IQ between African Americans and Whites has remained at about 15 IQ points for decades". Passage information suggests that:

A. the Jensenists attributed this difference to inadequate stimulation of children.
WRONG: This is not suggested by passage information. Herrnstein believed "that intelligence depended mainly on heredity, varied among the races, and created inherent inequalities that could not be overcome" (lines 6-9). Hernstein, along with the Jensenists, most likely attribute the differential to genetic makeup.

B. without marked changes in I.Q. testing methodology, the Jensenists felt that this would not improve.
WRONG: This is not suggested by passage information. The Jensenists believed "that intelligence depended mainly on heredity, varied among the races, and created inherent inequalities that could not be overcome" (lines 6-9). They did not call into

question the effectiveness of IQ testing in truly measuring intelligence.

C. Jensenism's critics argued that these results had been falsified.
WRONG: This is not suggested by passage information.

D. the opponents of Jensenism found that this difference can be overcome.
CORRECT: This is suggested by passage information. Lines 47-59.

256. Which of the following statements most strongly *challenges* one of the assertions made in the passage?

A. There is no definitive proof that an I.Q. test will accurately measure intelligence.
WRONG: This statement is actually suggested by the passage.

B. High status within U.S. society consists of those who have wealth, power, and fame.
WRONG: This statement does not most strongly challenge one of the assertions made in the passage. It is unrelated.

C. It is genetics that can determine how a person will react to their environment.
WRONG: This statement *does* challenge a passage assertion, however, it *equally supports* another passage assertion. Thus is does *not "most strongly challenge* one of the assertions made in the passage" and is thus not the best answer.

D. A racist is one who believes that race is the primary determinant of human traits and capacities.
CORRECT: This statement most strongly challenges one of the assertions made in the passage. In the first paragraph the author writes that Jensen and Herrnstein were "not … exponents of racism" (line 4). Yet the statement in this answer seems to aptly describe them.

257. Assume that the Jensenists *agreed* with geneticist Dobzhansky that "high status requires not just intelligence but 'energy, self-discipline … persistence and other personal qualities'" (lines 73-75). How would Herrnstein interpret this information in the context of his theories on social stratification?

A. Without these qualities, any attempts to raise I.Q. would probably be unsuccessful.
WRONG: This is not the relevance of the new information to Herrnstein's theories. Herrnstein did not believe that I.Q. could be changed. The assumption does not modify this aspect of Herrnstein's viewpoint.

B. Environmental influences would still remain rela-

tively more important.
WRONG: Herrnstein did not believe that environmental influences were important to begin with. It is unlikely that he would renege a central tenet of his theory.

C. A person with a high I.Q. will also have these personal qualities.
CORRECT: This is the relevance of the new information to Herrnstein's theories. "[Herrnstein's] reasoning: 1) People with high I.Q.s, or high intelligence … had already risen to the top of U.S. society, and those with the low I.Q.s and low intelligence had remained at the bottom" (lines 28-32). Thus a person at the top of society would already have the personal qualities described in the assumption.

D. Given a high I.Q., these qualities are unnecessary to an individual born into high society.
WRONG: This answer would not be an incorporation of new information into Herrnstein's theory— it is simply refuting Dobzhansky's assertion.

258. The author's attitude toward the findings and conclusions of the Jensenists is most accurately described as:

A. favorable.
WRONG: This is not the most accurate description of the author's attitude.

B. neutral.
WRONG: This is not the most accurate description of the author's attitude.

C. mistrusting.
WRONG: This is not the most accurate description of the author's attitude.

D. disapproving.
CORRECT: This is the most accurate description of the author's attitude. Though the author , somewhat unconvincingly, offers that the Jensenists are not exponents of racism (line 4), the passage is not completely objective. For instance, the author calls Herrnstein's conclusions "disturbing" (line 25).

Passage II (Questions 259-266)

259. The word *astronomical* (line 36) is used in the sense of: ("This arrangement confronted them with *astronomical* problems that have plagued calendar makers for thousand of years.")

A. enormous.
WRONG: The word is not used in this sense. "Astronomical" can mean enormous, and the prob-

lems *may* have been enormous, but the problems were with the movement of the celestial/astronomical bodies. This is made clear by the next line: "The main problem stems from the fact that the *astronomical* cycles from which the day, the year, and the months are derived do not fit neatly together" (lines 41-43).

B. planetary.

CORRECT: This is the best answer choice as the author follows with a discussion of the problems being rooted in planetary factors. "The main problem stems from the fact that the *astronomical* cycles from which the day, the year, and the months are derived do not fit neatly together" (lines 41-43).

C. excessive.

WRONG: The word is not used in this sense.

D. heavenly.

WRONG: The word is not used in this sense. Though "heavenly" *may* mean "celestial" or "astronomical", it is somewhat nonsensical to have a heavenly problem.

260. According to the passage, the Sumerian's calendars were manufactured by:

A. priests.

WRONG: The passage states that priestly scribes manufactured the Sumerian's calendars.

B. the king.

WRONG: The passage states that priestly scribes manufactured the Sumerian's calendars.

C. each city-state administrator.

WRONG: The passage states that priestly scribes manufactured the Sumerian's calendars.

D. priestly scribes.

CORRECT: This is who manufactured the Sumerian's calendars. "The Sumerians had the specialists for calendar making: priestly scribes …" (lines 6-7).

261. Later in the passage, the author asserts, "For many centuries these calendar corrections were a matter of cut-and-try" (lines 56-57). This assertion most likely means that:

A. by the time of the Babylonians, the Sumerian's ability to make accurate calendar corrections had been lost.

WRONG: This is not the most likely meaning of the assertion. Based upon passage information, almost everything we know about the Sumerian's ability was based upon the Babylonian's ability. The relative accuracy of the calendars seems to be the same.

B. the Sumerians were no better at correcting the

calendar than the Babylonians.

WRONG: Though this answer may be a true statement, this is not the most likely meaning of the assertion.

C. during the reign of King Hammurabi, calendar corrections became even more capricious.
    WRONG: This is not the most likely meaning of the assertion. There is no information that would lead one to believe that they were any more or less capricious. Further, it is specified in the passage that it was the gods who were capricious, not the changes.

D. there were several methods whereby a deficient calendar year might be corrected.
    CORRECT: This is the most likely meaning of the assertion.

262. According to the passage, the Babylonians most likely continued the Sumerian practice of correcting their calendars by periodically inserting an extra:

A. month.
    CORRECT: The Babylonians most likely continued this Sumerian practice. Passage information tells us that the author's entire basis for what the Sumerian's did is based upon what the Babylonians did later. For instance, "We do know, however, that [the Sumerian's] Babylonian successors … [added] an occasional extra 30-day month to make up for lost days. Similarly, they kept the year in step with the sun by throwing in an extra month every three years or so" (lines 53-59), and "the [Babylonian] King ordered the insertion of an extra month whenever he happened to notice [a deficiency in the year]" (lines 63-64)

B. week.
    WRONG: The Babylonians did not most likely continue this Sumerian practice.

C. 29 days.
    WRONG: The Babylonians did not most likely continue this Sumerian practice.

D. few weeks.
    WRONG: The Babylonians did not most likely continue this Sumerian practice. Of course, this *could* be that a "few weeks" equals a month, but this is an extrapolation that is not warranted. Answer A is the best answer.

263. According to the information in the passage, the problems with the lunar calendar always stemmed from:

I. the calendar year being too short.
    WRONG: This is not what the problems of the lunar calendar stemmed from. See lines 41-51.

II. the calendar year not being long enough.
    CORRECT: This is what the problems of the

lunar calendar stemmed from. See lines 41-51.

III. the whims of the king.
    WRONG: This is not what the problems of the lunar calendar stemmed from. See lines 41-51.

A. I only

B. II only
    CORRECT: "We do know, however, that [the Sumerian's] Babylonian successors … [added] an occasional extra 30-day month to make up for lost days. Similarly, they kept the year in step with the sun by throwing in an extra month every three years or so" (lines 53-59), and "the [Babylonian] King ordered the insertion of an extra month whenever he happened to notice [a deficiency in the year]" (lines 63-64).

C. III only

D. II and III only

264. The author implies that the primary significance of the Sumerians was their:

A. ability to create the first truly accurate calendar.
    WRONG: This is not what the author's implies is the Sumerian's primary significance. Nowhere in the passage is there an allusion to a "truly accurate" calendar.

B. reliance upon the lunar cycles.
    WRONG: This is not what the author's implies is the Sumerian's primary significance.

C. faculty for writing and recording.
    CORRECT: This is what the author's implies is the Sumerian's primary significance. "The earliest clear examples of a society in which some people not only learned to keep records, but made it their business to do so …" (lines 1-3). And, "… that singularly gifted people who evolved the first literate, urban culture" (lines 5-6).

D. administrative and agricultural skills.
    WRONG: This is not what the author's implies is the Sumerian's primary significance. Perhaps, administrative, but not necessarily agricultural.

265. The author claims, "The earliest clear examples of a society in which some people not only learned to keep records, but made it their business to do so, occurred about 5,000 years ago on the banks of the Tigris and Euphrates Rivers, among the Sumerians" (lines 1-5). Thus, King Hammurabi's letter "written some 1,700 years before Christ" (line 58) would have been created:

A. 3300 years afterward.
    WRONG: This is not when Hammurabi's letter would have been created.

B. 6700 years ago.

WRONG: This is not when Hammurabi's letter would have been created.

C. 300 years after that.
WRONG: This is not when Hammurabi's letter would have been created.

D. 1300 years later.
CORRECT: This is when Hammurabi's letter would have been created. 5,000 years ago means 3,000 years before Christ. If the letter was written 1700 years before Christ, that would mean 1300 years after (or later than) the author's claims the occurrence of the example.

266. On the basis of the passage, it is reasonable to conclude that:

A. the written documentation on the Babylonians exceeds that of the Sumerians.
WRONG: This is not a reasonable conclusion. Apparently the Sumerians left quite a bit of documentation, their calendars among the most important. Further, there is no indication of the quantity of materials left behind by the Babylonians.

B. the Sumerians left behind voluminous written records of their culture.
CORRECT: This is a reasonable conclusion. This answer could have been arrived at using process of elimination with the other answers.

C. the Sumerians are not studied by scholars to the same extent as the Babylonians.
WRONG: This is not a reasonable conclusion.

D. the Babylonian kingdom consisted of small city-states.
WRONG: There is no support for this answer in the passage.

Examination 06: Biological Sciences

Passage V (Questions 267-272)

267. **B is correct.** This is a common MCAT question. As stated in the passage, *S. pyogenes* is a group A streptococcus. Cocci bacteria are round and can present as chains, pairs or clusters. Bacilli bacteria are rod-shaped while spirochetes are spiral in form. Staphylococus form clusters, while streptococcus form chains.

268. **B is correct.** According to the passage, the *S. pyogenes* exotoxin is able to digest surrounding tissue. Based in this information, it is safe to assume that the exotoxin is structurally similar to enzymes found in lysosomes, digestive cellular organelles which breakdown ingested macromolecules. The golgi apparatus is the cellular distribution center that also carries out post-translational protein modification. The smooth endoplasmic reticulum is not associated with ribosomes, but is involved in steroid synthesis and cellular detoxification.

269. **B is correct.** Based on Table 1, if the infection started 24 hrs ago, the infecting bacterium must be in the stationary phase of their growth curve. 5 hrs of lag + 10 hrs of log + 15 hrs of stationary = 30 hours, and the infection started 24 hours ago, therefore the bacteria are still in stationary phase. According to Figure 1, while penicillin has a higher killing efficacy during hours 10-20 (or the log phase of growth), clindamycin has higher killing efficacy during the stationary phase (hours 15-30). Since this patient is in the stationary phase of bacterial growth, clindamycin is the preferred antibiotic based on the Eagle effect.

270. **C is correct.** Many antibiotics exploit the differences between eukaryotic and prokaryotic cells in order to maintain selectivity. Prokaryotic cells (bacteria) have cell walls; penicillin can bind to and inactivate enzymes responsible for cross-linking peptidoglycan strands of bacterial cells walls. Effective penicillin treatment can result in bacterial cell lysis. Animal cells lack a cell wall and therefore are immune to penicillin's effects. The question stem states that penicillin is effective against other Gram positive bacteria, therefore answer choice B is incorrect.

271. **C is correct.** According to the passage, *S. pyogenes* consumes skin (the integumentary system) and also causes respiratory illnesses such as strep. throat and pneumonia.

272. **B is correct.** Figure 1 demonstrates that penicillin has the greatest bacterial killing efficacy during hours 5-15, which corresponds to the log phase of its growth curve (when correlated with Table 1.) The log part of the bacterial growth curve shown is labeled B.

Passage VI (Questions 273-280)

273. **C is correct.** Drugs which target ergosterol specifically attack fungal cells as mammalian cell membranes are formed from different sterols (cholesterol derivatives). According to the passage, "fungi are simple eukaryotes more similar to complex mammals than prokaryotes..." As a eukaryote, fungi possess an 80S ribosome, prokaryotes possess a 70S ribosome. Antifungal drugs that target the ribosome would likely target the host ribosomes also, and would not be an effective treatment. Mycorrhizae are structures formed between an infecting fungi and plant roots. Mammals do not possess mycorrhizae and they will not be present in a fungal infection of an animal. Mammals do not possess a chitin cell wall, making it a logical target for antifungal drugs. However, according to the passage, chitin is "a linear homopolymer containing β-(1 → 4)-linked N-acetylglucosamine

residues." As a homopolymer, only N-acetylglucosamine is present in chitin, not glucose.

274. **D is correct.** The passage states "Chitin fibers can be polyanionic, and interact with counterions to provide rigidity and stability to cells." Polyanionic implies the presence of multiple negative charges. A counterion for one or more negative charges would be a cation, or positively charged ion. Sodium is the only cation listed.

275. **A is correct.** The passage notes that "Hyphae form the structural units of the fungal body, known as a mycelium, which has a large surface-to-volume ratio adapted for nutrient absorption." This implies that fungi must obtain nutrients from the environment, making them heterotrophic. The formation of mycorrhizae with plant roots is an example of mutualism. Disease-causing fungi are parasites. Fungi are not autotrophs; they cannot make their own food (as they do not contain photosynthetic chlorophyll that plants do).

276. **B is correct.** A lichen is a mutualistic association of a photosynthetic organism (algae or cyanobacteria) and a fungus (usually a type of basidiomycete or ascomycete). Choices A and D describe saprophytic fungi (degrading dead material). Choice C can be classified as parasitic or predatory.

277. **C is correct.** The passage states "Attached fungal hyphae increase the effective surface area of the root" and "Hyphae form the structural units of the fungal body, known as a mycelium, which has a large surface-to-volume ratio adapted for nutrient absorption." These statements imply that the fungal hyphae enhance nutrient absorption, allowing plants to resist drought. Although it is possible that mycorrhizae may protect against some root parasites, the passage makes no mention of this. Answer choice B is incorrect, as the chitin cell wall provides rigidity and stability to cells of the fungus, not the plant root. Answer choice D is incorrect as fungi do not produce glycogen.

278. **C is correct.** The passage states "Multicellular fungi have cells that rapidly grow into filamentous structures called hyphae, which may be of different mating types." This implies that hyphae are the necessary structures for fungal reproduction. Answer choices B and D are eliminated. The exchange of chromosomes by conjugation is a prokaryotic phenomenon.

279. **D is correct.** The ability to switch between aerobic and anaerobic respiration makes yeast facultative anaerobes. The question stem implies that ethanol production is an adaptive mechanism. Obligate aerobes and anaerobes have a strict requirement for the presence or absence of oxygen, respectively. Answer choice C is incorrect, as fungi are not protista.

280. **B is correct.** Choices A and C are incorrect, as they represent the haploid and diploid states, respectively. Answer choice D is incorrect; XY refers to the presence of both female and male sex chromosomes.

Independent Questions (281-282)

281. **C is correct.** By definition, Gram (+) organisms stain blue. The reason is that Gram (+) have thicker cell walls than Gram (–) bacteria. Their thicker walls enable them to retain the blue color of crystal violet, one of the dyes used in Gram staining. Gram (–) bacteria, on the other hand, have walls that are too thin to retain this blue stain. They remain reddish pink, which is the default stain used in the Gram stain process.

282. **D is correct.** Anaerobic bacteria require an oxygen free environment in order to survive. This is opposite of aerobic bacteria, which require oxygen in order to survive (because they lack the equipment for anaerobic fermentation). Crevices of teeth and gums, nail beds, and alveoli are all exposed to oxygen.

348

EXPLANATIONS 07

Answers to Questions 283-329

ANSWERS TO EXAMINATION 7

PHYSICAL SCIENCES	VERBAL REASONING	BIOLOGICAL SCIENCES
283. C	299. B	314. A
284. D	300. A	315. D
285. B	301. C	316. B
286. A	302. B	317. C
287. D	303. D	318. C
288. D	304. C	319. A
289. B	305. A	320. A
290. C	306. B	321. C
291. A	307. C	322. D
292. A	308. D	323. C
293. B	309. D	324. B
294. D	310. C	325. B
295. B	311. A	326. B
296. B	312. B	327. C
297. A	313. D	328. D
298. D		329. B

Passage I (Questions 283-289)

283. C is correct. Work is equal to the product of force and distance. In this case, the distance is the circumference of the circle traveled by the handle. Additionally, centimeters must be converted to meters.

$$W = Fd = (120)(2)(3.14)(0.2) = 150 \text{ J}$$

284. D is correct. Efficiency is equal to AMA/IMA.

$$\text{Efficiency} = \text{AMA/IMA} = \left(\frac{480}{60}\right)/\left(\frac{20}{2}\right) = \frac{8}{10} = 80\%$$

285. B is correct. For the net to be held in static equilibrium, the net torques must be zero.

$$F_1 d_1 = F_2 d_2$$
$$(800)(0.02) = F(0.08)$$
$$F = 200 \text{ N}$$

286. A is correct. The ideal mechanical advantage is the ratio of the input distance to the output distance. An increase in handle length and decrease in spindle radius will increase the ratio, and thus ideal mechanical advantage. Changing the forces will change the actual mechanical advantage, not the ideal mechanical advantage.

287. D is correct. Tension is the type of force exerted by a rope on objects attached to either end.

288. D is correct. If less input force is required to achieve the same output force, then the actual mechanical advantage has increased. If the AMA is increased, then the efficiency is increased. The IMA depends only on the length of the handle and the radius of the spindle.

289. B is correct. If the machine is less than 100% efficient, then the input force must do more work than the output force to overcome friction.

Passage II (Questions 290-295)

290. C is correct. The final temperature is higher than the initial temperature in all three cases, indicating that energy was transferred to the water in the calorimeter. When a reaction releases energy into its surroundings, it is exothermic.

291. A is correct. The heat absorbed by the solution is given by the expresstion $Q = mc\Delta T$. The heat absorbed by the calorimeter and thermometer is given by $Q = C\Delta T$. The heat released by the reaction may be found by adding these two expressions. It is helpful to remember that 100 ml of the solution has an approximate mass of 100 g.

$$Q = mc\Delta T + C\Delta T = [(100)(4.18)(1) + (15)(1)] \text{ J}$$

292. A is correct. Percent error is calculated using the formula below.

$$\% \text{ error} = \left(\frac{\text{observed} - \text{actual}}{\text{actual}}\right)(100)$$
$$= \left(\frac{(-4.3) - (-5.0)}{(-5.0)}\right)(100)$$
$$= (-0.14)(100) = -14\%$$

293. B is correct. The temperature in trial 3 is increased, so the reaction is exothermic and ΔH is negative. The reaction is spontaneous, so ΔG is also negative.

294. D is correct. For this experiment to work perfectly, the water in the cup must absorb all of the energy released by the reaction so all of the energy released will be measured in the temperature change of the water. If some of the energy is lost to the surroundings, then the temperature change, and subsequently the magnitude of the enthalpy change, will be less than ideal.

295. B is correct. In a double displacement reaction, both the anions and cations of the reactants trade 'partners'.

Independent Questions (Questions 296-298)

296. B is correct. In order for trapeze artists to land, their momentum must be brought down to zero. Change in momentum is called impulse and it is given by the product of force and time. The more time that a collision takes, the less force is needed to change the momentum. Choices C and D are incorrect because the overall value of the impulse is not changed by the net. The net acts to spread the collision out over more time, thus decreasing the force.

297. A is correct. Use conservation of momentum. Remember, an alpha particle is the same as a helium nucleus, so it has a mass number of 4. If the isotope with a mass of 210 emitted a particle with a mass of $m_2 = 4$, then the remaining nuclide has a mass of $m_1 = 206$.

$$v_1 = \frac{m_2}{m_1} v_2$$
$$v_1 = v_2$$

298. D is correct. At low temperatures, enthalpy dominates, so in order for the reaction to be spontaneous at low temperatures, ΔH must be negative. At high temperatures, entropy dominates, so in order for the reaction to be nonspontaneous at high temperatures, ΔS must also be negative.

Passage III (Questions 299-306)

299. Suppose behavioral geneticists discover that many people who fall into deep credit card debt have a genetically predisposed condition, which compels them to purchase items that are on sale, or being auctioned, irrespective of their need for these items. The author of the passage would be most likely to respond to this information by:

A. suggesting that a strictly defined 'fair market value' could still be negotiated by such persons.

WRONG: The author does not delve into negotiations in her discussion. She presents the caveat, "neither [buyer nor seller] being under any compulsion to buy or sell" to excuse herself from exploring the topic. It is unlikely that anyone would respond as such, given that the question stem directly suggests such persons are genetically predisposed to *not* be able to negotiate.

B. proposing that this situation would fall under the nature of intrinsic value.

CORRECT: This is the author's likely response, as one's buying propensity (whether it is the result of genetic makeup or any other factor) is an individual characteristic and thereby subjective. According to the passage, "Social and emotional factors often affect an object's worth and in some cases to a very great degree. ... The highly subjective nature of the [intrinsic value] ..." (lines 4-10).

C. asserting that such factors are of little relevance to a discussion of value.

WRONG: The author would not be most likely to respond to this information in this manner. She describes two categories of value: intrinsic and monetary. One's purchasing attitudes have a great deal to do with intrinsic value.

D. explaining that most people probably feel some compulsion to buy to some degree or another.

WRONG: This statement does not reconcile the information in the question stem with the authors opinion, s presented in the passage.

300. According to the passage, when shopping for antiques, one should consider that:

I. the price is always negotiable.

CORRECT: This is a consideration. "Basic to the understanding of the monetary value of antiques is the fact that stated figures are *purely arbitrary*, and there is no such thing as a fixed price" (lines 1-3).

II. the price will usually be consistent with its value.

WRONG: This is not true. "... there is no such thing as a fixed price" (line 3). For example, inflation may cause a difference between price and value.

III. the price will usually be indicated in U.S. dollars.

WRONG: This may or may not be true. There is no support for this answer in the passage.

A. I only

CORRECT: See above answer explanations.

B. III only

C. II and III only

D. I, II, and III

301. Suppose the author had inserted the following sentence at line 6: "This may be particularly true when an object has been passed down through a family for generations and is considered an heirloom by the current owner". This example would best support the author's discussion of:

A. neither the seller or the buyer being under any pressure to sell.

WRONG: The author does not discuss, per say, unpressured business environments. She only describes these as the setting of her analysis. In addition, the question stem suggests a pressure present *not* to sell.

B. why some people might not be as willing to sell certain objects.

WRONG: Although this may be an effect of sentimental attachment to an object, the author never discusses factors involved in determining one's *willingness* to sell an object.

C. the difficulty of quantifying an object's intrinsic value.

CORRECT: Inserting the above statement would function to support the author's assertion of the subjective nature of intrinsic value. The insertion provides an example of how sentimental attachment may increase and object's intrinsic value. The author alludes to this concept in his admission that "intrinsic value" is "highly subjective in nature".

D. the factors which will further determine the value of an object.

WRONG: "...value is further determined by the factors: demand, rarity, and condition " The insertion is not relevant to any of these factors.

302. The ideas in the passage seem to derive primarily from:

A. evidence on the behavior of sellers and buyers.

WRONG: This is not where the ideas seem to derive primarily from. This answer does not include the information from *Webster's, Roget's,* or the U.S. Treasury.

B.   knowledge of ongoing antique transactions.
CORRECT: This is where the ideas seem to derive primarily from. "In other words – based on the store owner's experience and very close acquaintance with the antique market and the highly regarded authorities in the antique field …" (lines 49-52).

C.   speculation based on accepted theory.
WRONG: This is not where the ideas seem to derive primarily from. What is the accepted theory?

D.   facts observable in antique transactions.
WRONG: This is not where the ideas seem to derive primarily from. This is a possible answer that pales next to the correct answer. This answer does not include the information from *Webster's, Roget's,* or the U.S. Treasury.

03. At an estate sale, a relatively worthless item has been manipulated to look like a rare antique because the seller is desperate to recoup monetary losses in other areas. This situation best points out the author's emphasis that:

A.   all antiques should be certified as genuine.
WRONG: Although this may be a helpful practice, the author makes no mention of the topic.

B.   situations where the seller is in desperate need of money should be avoided.
WRONG: The author does not discuss transaction situations which should be avoided. Furthermore, a buyer would be at and advantage in such a scenario.

C.   it is difficult to assign monetary value to an object.
WRONG: Although this may be true, the situation in the question stem does not best emphasize this point of the author's.

D.   a buyer be fully informed about the pertinent facts.
CORRECT: This emphasis is best pointed out by the question stem. Here a buyer not "having reasonable knowledge of the relevant facts" (lines 31-32) would be up against a hard bargain.

304. The author would most likely *agree* with which of the following statements?

A.   It is unlikely that neither buyer nor seller would be compelled to act.
WRONG: There is no support in the passage indicating the author believes this, although the reader may (and should).

B.   A buyer should always begin negotiating well below the price she is willing to pay.
WRONG: The author would not necessarily agree with this statement.

C.   The thesaurus definition of "value" is too ambiguous to be useful.
CORRECT: The author presents this idea in the second paragraph..

D.   One can usually count on the accuracy of an antique's marked price.
WRONG: The author would not necessarily agree with this statement.

305. What is the most serious apparent *weakness* of the Department of the U.S. Treasury's concept of "fair market value" as described?

A.   The concept is based upon an unlikely set of assumptions.
CORRECT: This is the most serious weakness. Consider, "neither [buyer nor seller] being under *any* compulsion to buy or sell and *both* having reasonable knowledge of the relevant facts" (lines 30-32). If neither were under any compulsion (i.e. pressure, impulse, desire, etc.) to buy or sell then why would that transaction ever take place? This is a very artificial set of circumstances.

B.   "Legalistic sounding" does not mean that it would be legally binding.
WRONG: This is not the most serious weakness.

C.   As outlined, the concept is less rigorous than the Webster's definition.
WRONG: The Webster definition is unrelated.

D.   A "fair market" does not really exist.
WRONG: This is an extreme version of Answer A.

306. Elsewhere, the author of the passage states, "An item is only worth what someone is willing to pay for it". This statement most directly supports the passage assertion that:

A.   There is no such thing as a fixed price.
WRONG: This assertion is not most directly supported by the above statement.

B.   The ultimate factor determining value is demand.
CORRECT: This is a passage assertion, and it is directly supported by the statement. In other words, if a person will not pay what you are asking, the item is not worth what you are asking.

C.   An item's actual price may fluctuate dramatically from day to day.
WRONG: This is not really a passage assertion.

D.   The price of an object should be determined before it is put up for sale.
WRONG: This is not really a passage assertion.

307. The author's comparison of wood-firing and other types of firing indicates that:

A. wood firing is the method which the author uses.
WRONG: There is no support for this in the passage.

B. without wood firing, electric firing would not be possible.
WRONG: This is not a true statement.

C. the author has great respect for wood firing.
CORRECT: This is indicated by the author's comparison.

D. the results of wood firing are more predictable.
WRONG: This is not indicated by the author's comparison. The passage makes clear that wood firing is very unpredictable.

308. The author cites Garth Clark's description of the "generosity of the kiln" (line 18, and lines 42-44) to make the point that:

A. electric kilns provide a much more forgiving method of firing.
WRONG: Though this point may be true, it is not the point the author sought to make with Clark's quote.

B. without different methods, most ceramics would look very similar.
WRONG: This is not the point to be made by the author's citation.

C. wood kilns are relatively easy to learn to use.
WRONG: The author delineates the difficulty in using wood kilns as compared to electric kilns.

D. the firing of a wood kiln can be unpredictably destructive.
CORRECT: The author points out that Clark's statement does not apply to wood fire kilns. In lines 37-47, he discusses the dangers of "violent heat", etcetera.

309. The author is primarily concerned with demonstrating that wood firing:

A. has come a long way, in the last 20 years, towards acceptance in the ceramics community.
WRONG: The statement is not true. The 20 year mark is based on "raku and salt glazing", and has nothing to do with how far wood firing has come.

B. is a capricious practice requiring patience, knowledge, and strong determination.
WRONG: Although the author may believe this, it is not his main idea.

C. is tremendously unpredictable.
WRONG: The author is not primarily concerned with demonstrating this. It is clear that the author is providing this information. But it is tangential to the primary concern. The unpredictability of wood firing is something the author finds pleasing. This is one of the "good reasons" (Answer D) that wood firing is flourishing.

D. is flourishing for good reason, despite being consistently disregarded by ceramic critics.
CORRECT: This is the author's main idea in the passage.

310. The author's characterization of wood firing and how the practitioners of this craft have been perceived suggests that the retort/comment about "electric kilns and their *heated* but *unfired* wares" (line 68) was meant to:

A. explain why a clay sculpture might break more easily in a wood kiln.
WRONG: This is not the suggested meaning of the retort/comment. The comment does little to explain this.

B. make clear the differences between electric and wood kiln firing.
WRONG: This is not the suggested meaning of the retort/comment. This answer is quite similar to Answer A, and just as incorrect.

C. convey scorn for the more controlled conditions of electric kilns.
CORRECT: This is the suggested meaning of the retort/comment. The author is clearly scornful of the controlled, more predictable, and safer (to the ceramics) conditions of electrical firing. "It is humbling to note that [the shards of pots that have broken under the conditions of wood firing] could well fill a gallery from floor to ceiling as a **perverse** endorsement of electric kilns and their *heated* but *unfired* wares" (lines 69-72). Notice the "perverse" endorsement. The author likes the vagaries and variables of fire.

D. communicate the pride one feels after the successful firing of a wood kiln.
WRONG: This is not the suggested meaning of the retort/comment.

311. The contention that "chance favors only the prepared mind" (line 59) can most justifiably be interpreted as support for the idea that:

A. without suitable understanding, fortune is against you.
CORRECT: In other words, if you have an unprepared mind, chance will not favor you. One can draw from traditional logic theory: **If A, then B** can be translated equivalently to **If not B, then not A.**

354

B. if you prepare yourself well, the odds will always be in your favor.
WRONG: This idea cannot be justifiably supported by the contention. This answer reads, Chance *always* favors the prepared mind.

C. without some degree of luck, you have only your intellect.
WRONG: This idea is unrelated and nonsensical.

D. 'accidents' can actually assist you if you are ready for them.
WRONG: This idea cannot be justifiably supported by the contention. This answer leaves open the possibility that chance (i.e. accidents) can also favor the *unprepared* mind, or favors you if you are not ready for the accident.

312. Given the claims made in the passage, the idea that, "Despite the lack of critical savvy by contemporary ceramic historians, the movement has proceeded on level terrain, with neither a verbal headwind nor a boost from comprehending and appreciative writers who might have advanced the climate of acceptance for this type of work by the public at large" (lines 24-29), suggests:

A. The critics should realize that wood firing is fast gaining in popularity and support, rather than hinder it.
WRONG: This is not suggested by the idea, given the claims in the passage. First, this inaccurately implies that critics are hindering the rise in popularity instead of passively ignoring wood firing. Second, this implies an acceleration of popularity that is not implied in the passage nor the "level terrain" of the idea.

B. The popularity of wood firing has been steadily advancing despite its lack of critical acclaim.
CORRECT: This is not only a appropriate paraphrasing of the above excerpt, but the main idea of the passage.

C. Facing dismissive ignorance in the media, wood firing has nevertheless managed to gain in popularity among ceramicists.
WRONG: This is not suggested by the idea, given the claims in the passage. "Dismissive ignorance" connotes not being passively ignored, but being actively disregarded. The author does not discuss whether the lack of critical acclaim is intentional or not in the excerpt provided.

D. Wood firing has been exploding in popularity among ceramicists with virtually no help from critics.
WRONG: This is not suggested by the idea, given the claims in the passage. "Exploding in popularity" is not an accurate depiction of "proceeded on level terrain".

313. In organizing a group of ceramicists to try wood firing for the first time, the author would most likely advise them to approach wood firing with:

A. love, because fire can have such a beautiful effects on all of their wares.
WRONG: This is not the most likely advice the author would give. But the fire frequently/usually does not have beautiful effects. Thus "all" of their wares is an inaccurate statement.

B. an open-mind, because they might not initially like what little comes out of the kiln.
WRONG: This answer is true, but incomplete, and thus not the best answer. The author calls for three qualities, as presented in Answer D.

C. caution, because most pieces will be destroyed and many will look substandard.
WRONG: This is not the most likely advice the author would give. This is also possible, but again, the idea is encompassed in Answer D's call for "patience".

D. patience, because it requires experience and an expanded perspective to obtain good results.
CORRECT: This is the most likely advice the author would give. Patience is required in order to accept the inevitable breakages and unpredictable results (lines 39-47). Experience is necessary to take full advantage of the variability, or "chance" (lines 60-64). An expanded perspective is required in order to appreciate different types of beauty, techniques, and results (lines 48-59).

Examination 07: Biological Sciences

Passage V (Questions 314-319)

314. A is correct. If Gene B's protein were responsible for protein trafficking (choice B) or activation (choice D), then percent protein activity would near 0 in the absence of Gene B; Table 1 indicates this is not the case. Choice C is not a form of posttranslational modification, which the passages states as the function of Gene B's protein. Glycosylation, on the other hand, is a frequently cited method of posttranslational modification.

315. D is correct. Mitochondria, like prokaryotes, contain circular DNA, ribosomes, and the ability for independent replication. Neither, however, have a nucleus.

316. B is correct. Group 1 shows an average decrease of 50% in protein activity, which is less than the 72% decrease seen in Group 2, indicating a greater effect of Gene C.

317. C is correct. In the absence of Genes B and C, percent protein activity is decreased more than in the absence of one gene. The presence of continued protein activity in the absence of either Gene B or C suggests that neither posttranslational modification is imperative for protein function. A cumulative effect would suggest higher levels of percent protein function in the absence of both genes. A synergistic effect is seen instead, where the cumulative effect of both Genes is greater than the sum of the two gene's effects separately.

318. **C is correct.** The ribosome is the only organelle in the list that does not have a membrane, and thus it is the only organelle that is found in both prokaryotes and eukaryotes.

319. **A is correct.** Centrioles are only found in animal cells.

Passage VI (Questions 320-327)

320. **A is correct.** Epinephrine, also known as adrenaline, is responsible for the woman's exaggerated stress response. Epinephrine is a neurotransmitter in the sympathetic nervous system, and thus choices C and D are incorrect. Preganglionic sympathetic neurons, however, utilize acetocholine.

321. **C is correct.** The question stem reveals botulinum toxin to be an inhibitor of presynaptic acetylcholine release. An overdose should therefore lead to an extreme inhibition of actions mediated by acetylcholine. Even if you don't know what accommodation is, from the chart in the passage you can infer that A, B, and D are all actions of acetylcholine and that only C pupil dilation opposes the actions of acetylcholine. (Accommodation occurs as the lens shape is adjusted to focus on near objects).

322. **D is correct.** The sympathetic and parasympathetic systems are divisions of the autonomic nervous system.

323. **C is correct.** Acetylcholine functions as an excitatory neurotransmitter at the neuromuscular junction.

324. **B is correct.** The passage states that muscarinic receptors are coupled to G proteins. These proteins operate via a second messenger system.

325. **B is correct.** Postganglionic neurons are part of the peripheral nervous system, and peripheral nerves are surrounded by Schwann cells.

326. **B is correct.** The passage states that norepinephrine is removed from the synaptic cleft by monoamine oxidase. Noradrenaline and noepinephrine are the same compound.

327. **C is correct.** In the presence of acetylcholinesterase inhibitors, acetylcholine will not be degraded. Table 1 reveals that acetylcholine acts to decrease heart rate. Therefore, without consideration of the potassium channel, choices A, B, and D are incorrect.

Independent Questions (Questions 328-329)

328. **D is correct.** Microtubules are employed in mitosis to pull chromosomes apart, for movement in flagella and cilia, and for exocytosis by transporting vesicles from the Golgi to the cell membrane. Microtubules are not essential for cellular respiration, however.

329. **B is correct.** The cell wall helps to prevent lysis of the cell, such as when there is high osmotic pressure. Situations fatal for animal cells, such as solution with hypotonic medium, are safe for plant cells as a result of cell walls. Cellular infrastructure is maintained with intracellular components such as microtubules. Cell walls are extracellular components, and contribute instead to plant infrastructure.

EXPLANATIONS 08

Answers to Questions 330-376

ANSWERS TO EXAMINATION 8

PHYSICAL SCIENCES	VERBAL REASONING	BIOLOGICAL SCIENCES
330. B	346. A	361. C
331. D	347. D	362. B
332. B	348. A	363. D
333. D	349. D	364. D
334. C	350. B	365. D
335. A	351. D	366. C
336. A	352. A	367. D
337. D	353. B	368. B
338. B	354. A	369. C
339. D	355. C	370. D
340. A	356. D	371. D
341. D	357. D	372. B
342. B	358. D	373. D
343. D	359. A	374. C
344. D	360. C	375. C
345. D		376. B

Passage I (Questions 330-336)

330. B is correct. The atomic mass given for neon on the periodic table is 20.2. This is much closer to 20 than to 21 or 22, the mass numbers for the other two stable isotopes of neon.

331. D is correct. In beta decay, a neutron is converted to a proton and an electron, which is then emitted. So the mass number will remain the same (24), and the atomic number will increase by 2 (to 12), which is the atomic number for magnesium.

332. B is correct. After 1 half life, 50% of the original sample remains. After 2 half lives, 25% of the original sample remains. If 25% remains, then 75% is depleted. Two half lives of neon-19 total 35 seconds.

333. D is correct. In electron capture, an atom converts an electron and a proton into a neutron, lowering the atomic number by one. In positron emission, an atom converts a proton into a neutron and a positron (a positively charged electron), also lowering the atomic number by one. In beta decay, an atom converts a neutron into a proton and an electron, thus increasing the atomic number by one. So only electron capture and positron emission will result in the lowered atomic number that gives fluorine.

334. C is correct. Neon-20 contains 10 protons and 10 neutrons, so the ratio is 1 : 1.

335. A is correct. Neon-23 undergoes beta decay, which reduces the number of neutrons and increases the number of protons, so it must be undergoing decay because it has too many neutrons.

336. A is correct. Positron emission does not change the mass number, so Choices C and D are incorrect. If a positive charge is emitted, the original nucleus must have lost a proton. Sodium is the only choice with 11 protons.

Passage II (Questions 337-342)

337. D is correct. The answer can be derived from the formula in the passage, or alternatively, by using the law of conservation of mass.

338. B is correct. The standard entropy value for liquid water must be less than the value for water vapor (188.7), but greater than zero. Choice B is the only option that fits these parameters.

339. D is correct. The heat of reaction is found by subtracting the heats of formation of the reactants from the reactants. The standard heat of formation of oxygen gas is zero because it is an element in its normal state.

$$(2)(-393.5) + (-241.8) - (226.7) = -1307.7 \text{ kJ/mol}$$

You can round the numbers and still get pretty close to the right answer.

$$(2)(-400) + (-250) - (200) = -1250 \text{ kJ/mol}$$

340. A is correct. C_2H_2 is an alkyne, with the form C_nH_{2n-2}. Alkynes contain triple bonds between carbon atoms.

341. D is correct. Since the reaction is simply the formation of C2H4 from its constituent elements, the enthalpy change and free energy change for the reaction are synonymous with the values for the heat and free energy of formation, listed in Table I. The enthalpy change is positive, so the reaction is endothermic. The free energy change is also positive, so the reaction is non-spontaneous.

342. B is correct. Methane has an atomic mass of 16 grams, so 8 grams is 0.5 moles. From the balanced equation, 1 mole of oxygen gas is required to consume 0.5 moles of methane. At STP, 1 mole of gas occupies 22.4 liters.

Independent Questions (Questions 342-345)

343. D is correct. Using conservation of momentum:

$$m_1v_1 = m_2v_2$$
$$(0.02)(250) = (1.25)v$$
$$v = 4 \text{ m/s}$$

344. D is correct. A wrench operates like a lever. The larger the handle, the greater the torque on the screw and the more likely it is to turn.

345. D is correct. The enthalpy change is the change in energy from the energy level of the reactants to the energy level of the products.

Passage III (Questions 346-352)

346. If the public reacted to Einstein's theory of relativity to in a manner similar to the public response toward the Fox sisters phenomenon, most people would:

A. accept the theory readily and quickly revise their theories about natural laws.

CORRECT: Given the supposition in the question, most people would receive Einstein's theory in this manner. "The sisters attracted thousands of followers, among them the eminent physicist and chemist Sir William Crookes … [who] was convinced that they "were true, objective occurrences."" (lines 28-32). Since we know from the passage that these "occurrences" were considered to contravene natural laws, it is a logical conclusion that the 'thousands of followers' and Sir William Crookes chose to revise their theories about natural laws.

B. resist the theory initially but gradually modify their view of the universe.

WRONG: Given the supposition in the question, most people would not receive Einstein's theory in this manner. There is no evidence that Crookes or the "thousands of followers" resisted the theory initially.

C. claim to believe the theory but ignore its profound implications.

WRONG: Given the supposition in the question, most people would not receive Einstein's theory in this manner. This is a vague answer. What "profound implications" were ignored in the Fox sister event?

D. reject its version of reality as contrary to common sense.

WRONG: Although this was the public response to Einstein's theory, the answer does not reflect what happened with the Fox sisters.

347. On the basis of the passage, it is reasonable to conclude that:

A. Sir William Crookes was in collusion with the Fox sisters.

WRONG: It is more likely that he too was deceived.

B. without help, the Fox sisters could not have carried out their deception.

WRONG: This is not a reasonable conclusion on the basis of the passage.

C. the Fox sisters deception was not revealed until they were quite old.

WRONG: The sisters revealed their secret only 21 years later, making them 29 and 31 years old respectively.

D. Margaret and Kate deceived their mother.

CORRECT: This is a reasonable conclusion on the basis of the passage. Their "mother concluded that strange raps heard only in her youngsters' presence were spirit messages" (lines 26-28). The mother must have had significant faith in her conclusion to invite the scrutiny of scientists and the public. We must assume that the mother was deceived as the author reveals only the sisters' intended deception.

348. Regarding the history of extrasensory phenomena, the passage strongly implies that:

A. there has never been a legitimate occurrence of the phenomena.

CORRECT: This is strongly implied in the passage. For instance, "Indeed, the whole history of extrasensory phenomena is tainted with deception …" (lines 12-13).

B. only a very rigorous academic institution could prove or refute claims of the phenomena.

WRONG: This is not strongly implied in the passage. This idea might be derived from the author's reverent reference to Stanford, however, what makes a "very rigorous academic institution" is vague and subjective. Further, the author gives an example of how "eminent" scientists and physicists have been deceived or fooled themselves. This is not the best answer.

C. several cases have proven to be highly unusual in their claims.

WRONG: The very nature of ESP is unusual, however this is not the emphasis of the passage. Again, this answer is vague.

D. claims and occurrences of this nature will always be prevalent.

WRONG: The author makes no claim that ESP will always exist, much less be prevalent. There is no support for this answer.

349. The author would most likely *disagree* with which of the following statements?

A. William Crookes wrote that he had actually tested the Fox sisters.

WRONG: The author would agree with this statement.

B. Stanford Research Institute is located in Menlo Park.

WRONG: The author would agree with this statement.

C. Uri Geller was an Israeli with an unusual claim to fame.

WRONG: The author might or might not completely agree with this statement.

D. Henry Sidgwick apparently believed the claims of the young twins.

CORRECT: The author would not agree with this statement. They two young men were not "twins".

350. Assume that magicians were able to repeat Uri Geller's feats time after time with identical results to Geller's, and that these feats were performed in different laboratories. What is the relevance of this assumption to the author's views about the *sine qua non* of science?

Notice that there are two prongs to each of the answers, both of which must be satisfied.

A. It strengthens them by demonstrating that there are really only a few areas where ESP can be tested.
WRONG: In his despcription of the *sine qua non* of science, the author is describing how research results should be repeatable anywhere with similar experimental conditions. In other words, if a phenomenon truly exists, it should be demonstrable by anyone anywhere given an appropriate setting. Thus, this answer does not represent the authors views.

B. It is consistent with them in proving the feats are actually only illusions.
CORRECT: The *sine qua non* of science, "experiments that lead to identical results, time after time, when repeated by different scholars in different laboratories" (lines 70-72), is followed in the scenario depicted in the question stem. The magician's repeated results prove that Geller's feats were indeed illusion, and not psychic feats.

C. It weakens them by showing that ESP can still trick science and scientists.
WRONG: The author shows that ESP tricks science and this is precisely the reason why he invokes the sine qua non. The scenario in the question stem fulfills the authors description of the sine qua non, and thus, if the assumption did show that ESP can still trick science and scientists, the author's views would be strengthened..

D. It weakens them by supporting Geller's feats as provable psychic phenomena.
WRONG: First of all, the question stem scenario supports the author's views on the sine qua non of science. Secondly, Geller's feats would only be proven in this construct if he himself were performing and repeating these feats, and if no one else was able to duplicate his performance. The fact that, in the assumption, "magicians" are performing the feats is extremely relevant.

351. An important comparison is made in the passage between:

A. psychic studies and scientific studies of physics.
WRONG: This is not a comparison made in the passage.

B. science of the 19th and 20th century.
WRONG: This is not an important comparison made in the passage. There is no implication that science has evolved to be less gullible.

C. Stanford Research Institute and the Society for Psychical Research.
WRONG: This is not a comparison made in the passage.

D. deliberate trickery and wishful thinking.
CORRECT: This is an important comparison made in the passage. "Indeed, the whole history of extrasensory phenomena is tainted with deception—*either deliberate trickery or the wishful thinking* that makes honest experimenters see what is not there" (lines 12-15). These two factors are regarded as responsible for past scientific acceptance, or support of, ESP.

352. Suppose the immediate relatives and family members of those who have died are much more likely to "sense" the presence of the deceased during a psychic séance than others who are present. Does this discovery support the author's argument?

A. Yes; it supports the author's argument.
CORRECT: The discovery does support the author's argument in this way. "wishful thinking" (line 14) is presumably a component of the "immediate relatives and family members of those who have died".

B. ; it does not affect the author's argument.
WRONG: The discovery does support the author's argument regarding wishful thinking in the fifth paragraph.

C. No; it weakens the author's argument.
WRONG: The discovery does support the author's argument regarding wishful thinking in the fifth paragraph.

D. No; it disproves the author's argument.
WRONG: The discovery does support the author's argument regarding wishful thinking in the fifth paragraph.

Passage IV (Questions 353-360)

353. Suppose the author had inserted the following sentence at line 21: "Though the terrible and notorious massacre of the Cheyenne chief Black Kettle and his peaceful contingent on the banks of the Washita rightfully supports some of these accusations, it is anecdotal and not necessarily indicative of the man." This example would best illuminate the author's discussion of:

A. Custer's tactical Indian-fighting capabilities.
WRONG: This is not one of the topics the author discusses.

B. false assumptions about Custer.
CORRECT: The example, in accordance with the author's main purpose in the passage, tries to discredit Custer's notoriety, "questionable cowardice, certain ignorant pride, poor decision-making" as

false. Granted, it is not the strongest example the author could use, however, it attempts support the author's assertion that the " true nature of the man is more complex."

C. Custer's poor decision-making.
WRONG: The only mention of Custer's poor decision-making was in the author's description of his notorious [and, in the author's opinion, undeserved] reputation. The author does not discuss this aspect of Custer, per say. The clause,"it is anecdotal and not necessarily indicative of the man" refutes the assertion of Custer being a poor decision-maker.

D. why Custer was misunderstood.
WRONG: The example does not best illuminate this discussion. This answer is similar to Answer B, but it is not as clear. It is more specific to say that the author feels that the assumptions about Custer are false, rather than that he was misunderstood.

354. The assertion that Custer ignored his Crow scout's warnings about the size of the Indian force is NOT clearly consistent with the information about:

A. Custer's lacking awareness of the situation as he split his forces.
CORRECT: The Crow scout had made Custer cognizant of the situation.

B. the size of Indian encampments in future years.
WRONG: The assertion has little to do with the information in the question stem.

C. Custer's courage in battle.
WRONG: This assertion is also unrelated.

D. why Custer was so intent on destroying the Indians.
WRONG: There is no information in the passage which suggests that Custer was intent on destroying the Indians.

355. The author most likely believes that modern historians:

A. have an agenda.
WRONG: The passage discussion does not most clearly suggest this hypothesis. This is vague.

B. know little about what actually happened at the Little Bighorn.
WRONG: The passage discussion does not most clearly suggest this hypothesis. Given the information from Sitting Bull, this does not seem to be true.

C. treat the subject of Custer unfairly.
CORRECT: The passage discussion does most clearly suggest this hypothesis. With remarks like, "From the perspective of *historical revisionism …*"

(lines 14-15), and elsewhere, the author seems to be arguing strongly that Custer was a courageous and accomplished soldier.

D. focus solely on Custer's accomplishments.
WRONG: The passage discussion does not most clearly suggest this hypothesis. The author feels that Custer has been maligned by history.

356. Which of the following findings would most *compromise* the author's conclusions about George Armstrong Custer?

A. Custer believed that the Indians could never defeat him.
WRONG: This finding would not most compromise the author's conclusions about Custer. It seems possible that blinding hubris as a military commander might compromise the seeming conclusion by the author that Custer was a great military commander. However, one would need more information about the Indians for this finding to compromise that idea. Perhaps Custer was right. It is pointed out in the passage that the gathering of such a large force of Indians was an anomaly never to be repeated.

B. Jeb Stuart's forces had been surprised by Custer.
WRONG: This finding would not most compromise the author's conclusions about Custer. This refers to the passage information that Custer "once fought the legendary Confederate cavalryman, Jeb Stuart, to a standstill" (lines 28-29). However, if would have mattered little if Custer surprised him or not.

C. The moment 'captured' in the painting occurs just before Custer is killed.
WRONG: This finding would not most compromise the author's conclusions about Custer.

D. Custer was shot in the back attempting to run away from the battle.
CORRECT: This finding would most compromise the author's conclusions about Custer. The author believes that Custer is courageous: "lest it be believed that Custer's Civil War accomplishments were aberrations, it must be remembered that courage ran in the Custer's blood." If Custer were attempting to run away from the battle, this would call into question his courageousness.

357. Which of the following conclusions is best supported by the passage?

A. George Custer was a supreme military tactician.
WRONG: This is not a passage conclusion. Though he allegedly fought Stuart to a standstill, the author admits that Custer was "impetuous" and his tactics against the Indians were unimpressive.

B. George Custer's achievements were legendary.
WRONG: Not unless one equates legendary with notorious. The two are not synonymous.

C. George Custer simply did not have enough information about the size of the Sioux gathering.
WRONG: This is not a passage conclusion. "it was Custer's impetuous side that came to the fore and caused him to ignore his Crow scout's warnings regarding the size of the Indian force he was facing" (lines 36-39), though the author clouds this information at the beginning of the next paragraph by opining that Custer "unknowingly" arrayed his forces against the large gathering.

D. George Custer was not a coward.
CORRECT: The passage offers the most support for this conclusion. Indeed, this is a main idea.

358. The author probably mentions that there had never been before or ever would be again, such a large gathering of Indians (lines 39-40) in order to:

A. demonstrate the weakness of the information that Custer was getting from his scouts.
WRONG: This is not the probable reason for the author's mentioning the information in the question. Crow scout provided accurate information, and this is the only example of scout information in the passage.

B. provide an example of the types of gatherings the Indians arranged in later years.
WRONG: If there never "would be again" such a gathering, this answer choice cannot be true.

C. illustrate the persistence of the myths about Custer.
WRONG: The author's mention of the unexpected size of the Indian gathering serves to weaken the myths about Custer's ignorant pride.

D. support the idea that Custer was not a foolhardy commander.
CORRECT: The author is trying to justify Custer's irreverence of the Crow Scout's information. If the general relied on trends form his own experience, he could hardly be considered foolhardy.

359. According to the Passage, which of the following statements must be true?

A. Custer's forces could not have defeated the Sioux on that day.
CORRECT: Passage information indicates that this statement must be true. For one thing, the author refers to the Indians that day as an "*indomitable* force" (line 49).

B. Tom Custer also graduated from West Point.
WRONG: Passage information does not indicate that this statement must be true.

C. George Custer's Civil War victories were not aberrations.
WRONG: Passage information does not indicate that this statement must be true. There is no argument made to this effect.

D. Sitting Bull saw Custer being killed.
WRONG: Passage information does not indicate that this statement must be true.

360. According to the author, why did Custer repeatedly split his soldiers into smaller groups before attacking the Indian encampment?

A. To ensure that the Indians were completely surrounded
WRONG: This answer is possible, however, not as feasible as Answer C. The words *ensure* and *completely* make the answer speculative.

B. To enable them to capture Sitting Bull
WRONG: There is no support for this answer in the passage.

C. To reduce the chances that the Indians could escape from his soldiers
CORRECT: This is why Custer repeatedly split his forces.

D. To follow the advice of his scouts
WRONG: The scouts would have advised the opposite, given their knowledge of the size of the Indian contingent.

Examination 08: Biological Sciences

Passage V (Questions 361- 367)

361. **C is correct.** Fructose-6-phophate has 3 chiral centers so there are 8 (2^3) possible optical isomers.

362. **B is correct.** In the topmost carbon the priority groups are arranged in a clockwise order, however the lowest priority group extends out of the page, so the configuration is actually **S**. The second carbon's priority groups are arranged in counterclockwise order, however once again the lowest priority group extends out of the page, designating an **R** configuration. The third carbon also has its priority groups arranged in counterclockwise order with the lowest priority group extending out of the page, assigning its configuration as **R** as well.

At the top of the page are three Fischer projection structures each with CH$_2$OH, C=O, HO—C—H, and CH$_2$OPO$_3^{2-}$ groups, with numbered carbons and curved arrows.

363. D is correct. The Emden-Meyerhoff-Parnas scheme delineates the release of carbon dioxide. As this is the only gas produced, it must be responsible for the bread rising.

364. D is correct. Molecule 12, an aldehyde, is converted to an alcohol (Molecule 13).

365. D is correct. The spatial arrangement is tetrahedral as the central carbon is sp^3 hybridized with four substituent groups.

366. C is correct. Lactic acid has a hydroxyl group while pyruvic acid is a ketone. As lactic acid has a greater number of Hydrogens and the same number of Oxygen atoms, the oxygen:hydrogen ratio is lower.

367. D is correct. The passage states that each molecule of glucose produces 31 kcals. 62 kcals indicates 2 molecules of glucose underwent the reaction. The process yields 2 moles of ethanol for each mole of glucose. Thus 4 moles of ethanol are produced.

Passage VI (Questions 368-373)

368. B is correct. The chiral carbon is indicated by the grey area.

A structural diagram of thalidomide with the chiral carbon highlighted.

369. C is correct. The passage states that the drug racemizes at the pH of the body (pH = 7.35 – 7.45 on average).

370. D is correct. The enatiomer shown is in the "S" configuration. The lowest priority group extends back into the page, and the other groups are prioritized counterclockwise (shown below). The passages states that the S isomer is responsible for thalidomide's healing proper-

ties, which would include anti-inflammatory applications. The passage further states that at the pH of the human body, the S isomer will racemize. Thus human use of the S isomer may still result in serious birth defects.

A structural diagram of thalidomide with numbered atoms 1, 2, 3, 4 and a curved arrow.

371. D is correct. Replacing the topmost Nitrogen with an Oxygen atom results in an anhydride.

A structural diagram of an anhydride.

372. B is correct. All of the atoms adjacent to Nitrogen atoms are sp^2 hybridized Carbons.

373. D is correct. In structure D, a Hydrogen atom is added. As this involves more than electron shifting, structure D is not a resonance structure.

374. C is correct. Enantiomers are also known as stereoisomers. Geometric isomers are diasteriomers. Structural isomers have differing connectivity instead of differing absolute configuration.

Independent Questions (Questions 375-376)

375. C is correct. Aspirin lacks chiral carbons and is thus optically inactive.

376. B is correct. Aspirin contains the two functional groups shown on the structure below.

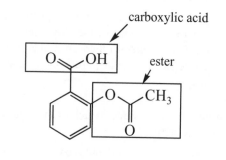

EXPLANATIONS 09

Answers to Questions 377-423

ANSWERS TO EXAMINATION 9

PHYSICAL SCIENCES	VERBAL REASONING	BIOLOGICAL SCIENCES
377. B	393. C	408. B
378. A	394. B	409. D
379. D	395. A	410. A
380. D	396. B	411. C
381. A	397. C	412. C
382. C	398. D	413. A
383. D	399. B	414. D
384. A	400. B	415. B
385. B	401. A	416. C
386. A	402. D	417. A
387. C	403. D	418. C
388. C	404. B	419. D
389. A	405. C	420. C
390. C	406. C	421. C
391. A	407. C	422. D
392. D		423. A

377. B is correct. The surface tension is given by the ratio of the force to the length over which it acts. The length of the ring is the circumference, $2\pi r$, but since surface tension acts on both sides of the wire, the circumference is doubled to $4\pi r$.

378. A is correct. From the table, pure water has a higher surface tension than soapy water, and cold water has a higher surface tension than hot water.

379. D is correct. As indicated by the equation in the passage, height is directly proportional to surface tension and inversely proportional to density. The surface tension of water is more than double that of ethyl alcohol, while the density of ethyl alcohol is only slightly less than water. Thus water's greater surface tension will have a much larger effect and the water will climb higher.

380. D is correct. The cohesive forces in mercury are stronger than the adhesive forces between mercury and the walls, so the meniscus will be inverted (apex above sides), and the level in the tube will be below the normal level.

381. A is correct. From the equation in the passage, height is inversely proportional to the radius of the tube. Thus, doubling the radius will halve the height.

382. C is correct. The intermolecular forces in fluid determine its surface tension. The stronger the forces, the more the fluid attempts to minimize surface area and the more it will push against objects that press on its surface.

Passage II (Questions 383-389)

383. D is correct. The solubility product is found by multiplying the concentrations of the products of the solvation and turning the coefficients into exponents.

384. A is correct. Each mole of lead nitrate produces one mole of lead ions, so the number of moles of Pb^{2+} ions is the same as the number of moles of lead nitrate.

$$\text{moles} = MV = (0.015)(0.010) = 1.5 \times 10^{-4}$$

385. B is correct. According to the passage, lead iodide solution is colorless and so its concentration cannot be measured with a spectrophotometer. The spectrophotometer is only useful after the iodide ions have been converted into diatomic iodide.

386. A is correct. The concentration of I_2 measured by the spectrophotometer is used to calculate the concentration of I^- ions. In order for this measure to be accurate, all of the I^- must be consumed in Reaction 2.

387. C is correct. According to the passage, the solvation of lead iodide is endothermic, so an increase in temperature would favor the formation of products at equilibrium. The lead iodide would become more soluble and the equilibrium constant would increase.

388. C is correct. Adding KI will increase the concentration of I^- ions in the solution. Because of the common ion effect, some of these additional I^- ions will combine with Pb^{2+} ions and precipitate out of the solution, thus decreasing the concentration of Pb^{2+}.

389. A is correct. Based on Reaction 1, there is 1 lead ion produced for every 2 iodide ions. Since all of the ions must come form the lead iodide sample, the concentration of lead ions must be half as large as the concentration of iodide ions.

Independent Questions (Questions 390-392)

390. C is correct. In an ideal flow system, volume flow is the same at all points. In such a system, fluid must move faster through narrower parts of the system and slower through the wider parts.

391. A is correct. $P = \rho g y$. As P and y are directly proportional to each other, the graph is linear and increasing.

392. D is correct. $MgCl_2$ dissociates into 3 charged particles, while each of the others dissociates into only two. The more charges in the solution, the better it will conduct electricity.

Passage III (Questions 393-399)

393. Which of the following conclusions can justifiably be drawn from the *Richmond Enquirer* excerpt (lines 1-10)?

    A. Only the men of Virginia believed that their state should secede.
        WRONG: This conclusion cannot be justifiably drawn from the article.

    B. By this time Virginia had seceded from the Union.
        WRONG: This conclusion cannot be justifiably drawn from the article.

    C. Virginia was probably not the first state to secede from the Union.
        CORRECT: This conclusion can be justifiably drawn from the article. In order to "unite our des-

tinies with our sister Southern States", there had to have been southern states that had already chosen this destiny.

D. One of the last states to secede from the Union was Virginia.
WRONG: This conclusion cannot be justifiably drawn from the article.

394. Each state is allotted Representatives according to state population along with two Senators per state. Given the information in the passage, if increasing "emphasis was now placed on maintaining parity in the Senate" (lines 17-18) the South could probably only have accomplished this by:

A. increasing each state's population.
WRONG: Given the information in the passage, this is not the only way that maintaining parity in the Senate could have been accomplished. Representatives were allotted by population, not Senators.

B. adding even more states to the Union.
CORRECT: Given the information in the passage, this is the only way that maintaining parity in the Senate could have been accomplished. The only way to increase Senatorial representation was by adding more states to the Union.

C. electing Jefferson Davis as their President.
WRONG: Given the information in the passage, this is not the only way that maintaining parity in the Senate could have been accomplished.

D. seceding from the Union.
WRONG: Given the information in the passage, this is not the only way that maintaining parity in the Senate could have been accomplished.

395. The author would argue that an understanding of the factors which led the South to form the Confederacy is important to the study of Civil War because it:

A. provides a basis for understanding the importance of a strong central government.
CORRECT: The lack of a strong central government was undoubtedly a major factor in the evolution of the civil war. This is also a main idea in the passage.

B. explains the reasoning behind Jefferson Davis's decision to form the Confederacy.
WRONG: Jefferson Davis did not make the decision to form the Confederacy.

C. indicates the strength of the feelings Southerners had about being forced into the Union.
WRONG: This answer does not address the relation between The forming of the Confederacy and the Civil War.

D. illustrates how little can be gained through violent resistance when other options are available.
WRONG: The author does not mention violent defensive strategy. If anything, the author would argue that the use of the Union's offensive force may have been unconstitutional. There is no support for this answer in the passage.

396. The author's discussion regarding the position of the southern states in the Union could most reasonably be extended to:

Note: "if a state or section of the country no longer felt itself represented by, or fairly treated by, the Federal Government, then it had the right to dissolve its association with that government. It could secede from the Union. No provision had been made for such an eventuality in the Constitution." The author discusses how the separation of the southern states was not provisioned for.

I. citizens of a country.
WRONG: There are provisions for citizens to separate from a country, or renounce their citizenship.

II. auto workers in a factory.
WRONG: Auto workers may form Unions at a factory, or even simply quit and leave that factory to find work elsewhere.

III. sailors at sea on a warship.
CORRECT: Sailors at sea, particularly on a warship, are certainly not free to simply no longer follow orders; such 'mutiny' would be similar to the way the Union viewed the secession of the southern States. There are no provisions for the sailors to dissolve their association with the ship.

A. I only

B. III only
CORRECT: See above answer explanations.

C. I and II only

D. I and III only

397. Which of the following objections, if valid, would most *weaken* the argument presented regarding the unconstitutionality of the Union's use of force?

Note: In order to answer this question correctly, one first must know and/or understand the argument. "The use of force to stop a state from seceding was, the argument went, unconstitutional, since the Union itself was a creature of the states. They had wholly created it." (lines 35-38).

A. No means other than force could be found that would hold the Union together.
WRONG: This objection would not most weaken the argument for the unconstitutionality of using force. Assuming that this is a valid objection, it still does not bear on the constitutionality or unconstitutionality of using force.

B. An amendment to the Constitution authorizing the use of force in cases of secession had not been passed.
WRONG: This objection would not most weaken the argument for the unconstitutionality of using force. This objection does not change the status quo as described in the passage.

C. The citizens of the states, not the states, had created the Union.
CORRECT: This objection would most weaken the argument for the unconstitutionality of using force. This objection responds directly to the supporting statement that the States "had wholly created" the Union (see note above).

D. Jefferson Davis gradually changed his views on slavery in the South.
WRONG: This objection would not most weaken the argument for the unconstitutionality of using force.

398. The author's characterization of Jefferson Davis suggests that his reference to Davis as Lincoln's "Southern counterpart" (lines 57-58) meant that:

A. Davis was, for a short time, the President of the Confederacy.
WRONG: This is not suggested by the author's characterization, as the passage does not present Lincoln in the role of a president. Lincoln was only characterized as a supporter of strong central unity.

B. slavery repulsed Davis in the same manner it had repulsed Lincoln.
WRONG: This is not suggested by the author's characterization. There is no information that slavery repulsed Lincoln. This answer relies on information outside of the scope of the passage, and would be speculative based on passage information.

C. Davis had tried desperately to overcome Lincoln's attempts at outlawing slavery.
WRONG: This is not suggested by the author's characterization. there is no information that Lincoln had attempted to outlaw slavery. This answer relies on information outside of the scope of the passage, and would be speculative based on passage information.

D. Davis in some ways mirrored Lincoln's role in the North.
CORRECT: The last paragraph describes how Davis mirrored Lincoln in his eventual support of strong central unity, and efforts to create this within the Confederacy.

399. Which of the following conclusions about the Constitution can be inferred from the passage?

A. The Constitution explicitly authorizes the use of force to prevent state's secession.
WRONG: This conclusion cannot be inferred from the passage. The exact opposite is expressly noted.

B. The use of force to prevent secession was arguably unconstitutional.
CORRECT: This conclusion can be inferred from the passage. "The use of force to stop a state from seceding was, the argument went, unconstitutional, since the Union itself was a creature of the states." (lines 35-37).

C. The authors of the Constitution did not foresee a state's wish to secede.
WRONG: This conclusion cannot be inferred from the passage. This is speculative. Perhaps they had foreseen it, yet did not find it wise to make provisions for such a situation. There is stronger support from the passage for Choice B.

D. A state had a Constitutional right to secede from the Union.
WRONG: This conclusion cannot be inferred from the passage. The exact opposite is expressly noted.

Passage IV (Questions 400-407)

400. According to information in the passage, a loss of nutritional value would be likely to occur when food is:

A. slowly cooked to remove moisture.
WRONG: This is not when a loss of nutritional value would be likely to occur. There is no support for this answer in the passage.

B. dried in the sun.
CORRECT: This is when a loss of nutritional value would be likely to occur. "A few vitamins, particularly, tend to be destroyed or depleted by the light of sun-drying" (lines 8-9). Later the author mentions the destruction of Vitamin C by sun-drying as well.

C. dehydrated by almost any means.
WRONG: This is not when a loss of nutritional value would be likely to occur. For instance, the more "modern" method of drying apparently prevents "some of this loss".

D. bottled or canned.
WRONG: This is not when a loss of nutritional value would be likely to occur. There is no support for this answer in the passage.

401. The author of the passage apparently associates the degree of development in nations, such as Turkey (lines 33-39), with:

A. industrialization.

CORRECT: This is what the author apparently associates with a nation's degree of development. Line 24 refers to "under-developed nations". In line 33 he then contrasts this paragraph with "industrialized nations".

B. their method of drying food.

WRONG: This is not what the author apparently associates with a nation's degree of development. Industrialization is not necessarily indicated by the advanced ability to dehydrate foods. Clearly, the author is not using "industrialized nations" in this sense.

C. the nutritional value of their food.

WRONG: This is not what the author apparently associates with a nation's degree of development. Clearly, the author is not using "industrialized nations" in this sense.

D. agriculture.

WRONG: This is not what the author apparently associates with a nation's degree of development.

402. The assertion that the "canning of food was developed little more than 200 years ago, by a man who set out to solve a specific problem in the spirit of modern science and technology" (lines 42-44) is NOT clearly consistent with the information about:

A. the methods of sun-drying in use at that time.

WRONG: The assertion is unrelated to this information.

B. what difficulties would need to be overcome in order to be successful.

WRONG: The assertion is unrelated to this information.

C. Appert's family legacy.

WRONG: The assertion is unrelated to this information.

D. what actually led Appert to begin his tests.

CORRECT: This assertion is not clearly consistent with this information. Later in the passage, at lines 57-59, the author asserts that Appert *"spurred by the prize offer, … embarked upon a series of tests that occupied him for more than a decade"*. This assertion and the one in the question (and earlier in the passage) are not consistent. The first is altruism, while the second is self-aggrandizement.

403. According to the passage, one drawback of dehydrating food that has been ameliorated by more modern techniques of dehydration is:

A. simplicity.

WRONG: This is not a drawback that has been ameliorated by more modern techniques of dehydration.

B. the need for sunlight.

WRONG: This is not a *drawback* that has been ameliorated by more modern techniques of dehydration. It is true that the need for sunlight has been eliminated in more modern techniques. However, this was not necessarily a *drawback*. To the author, the "disadvantages" of sun-drying were "far outweighed by dehydration's … *simplicity"* (lines 10-11). There is no indication that the author thought that "the need for sunlight" was a *drawback, according to the passage.*

C. rehydration.

WRONG: This is not a drawback that has been ameliorated by more modern techniques of dehydration. Presumably, even foods that were dehydrated using modern methods would have to be rehydrated.

D. loss of flavor.

CORRECT: This is a drawback that has been ameliorated by more modern techniques of dehydration. Sun-drying, "while preserving food, dehydration also affects its taste – usually adversely" (lines 4-5). "In [more modern] industrialized nations, some of this loss of nutritional quality and flavor is prevented by newer drying techniques" (lines 33-35).

404. Which of the following conclusions regarding the method of canning, for which Nicolas Appert was awarded a prize by the French government in 1809, can be inferred from the passage?

A. The 'stoppers' were probably made from natural cork.

WRONG: This is not a conclusion which can be inferred from the passage.

B. Cans were not actually used in the process.

CORRECT: This is a conclusion which can be inferred from the passage. The passage repeatedly refers to "bottles" and "filled bottles" not cans.

C. The technique would have worked at any altitude.

WRONG: This is not a conclusion which can be inferred from the passage. Further, at higher altitudes, the boiling water would have boiled at a much lower temperature, perhaps not neutralizing whatever it was that Appert thought was causing the food to spoil.

D. Appert invented the method too late to help his countrymen.

WRONG: This is not a conclusion which can be inferred from the passage. This is speculation based on information outside of the passage.

405. Based on passage information, the most effective situation for sun-drying food would be found during:

A. a hot sunny day in a desert.
WRONG: The heat provides no benefits based on passage information. Heat is used for a different process of food preservation: canning.

B. a hot sunny day high on a mountain.
WRONG: The heat provides no benefits based on passage information. Heat is used for a different process of food preservation: canning.

C. a cold sunny day high on a mountain.
CORRECT: This would be the most effective situation for sun-drying food. From the more effective "industrialized nations" method of dehydration we know that cold is helpful. Sun is required for sun-drying. Finally, if one realizes that the near-vacuum described in paragraph 33-40 is simply increasingly low air pressure, one will also realize that increasing altitude will also provide lower and lower air pressure.

D. a cold sunny day in a desert.
WRONG: The "desert" provides no benefit based on passage information.

406. Apparently, an attractive benefit of dehydration which has been lost through modern processes is:

A. usefulness.
WRONG: This is not an attractive benefit of dehydration which has been *lost* through modern processes. The food and methods would still be useful.

B. flavor.
WRONG: This is not an attractive benefit of dehydration which has been lost through modern processes. The modern processes have improved the loss of flavor resulting from sun-drying.

C. simplicity.
CORRECT: This is an attractive benefit of dehydration which has been lost through modern processes. "These disadvantages [of sun-drying] are far outweighed by dehydration's usefulness and *simplicity*" (lines 10-11). In the past only the sun was required. A vacuum-type "chamber" (line 36) is briefly described as required for the modern processes of dehydration. This places the process into the commercial arena and is certainly not as simple as it once was.

D. nutritional value.
WRONG: This is not an attractive benefit of dehydration which has been lost through modern processes. Apparently, the loss of nutrition has been improved upon.

407. Though both processes preserved foods, the sun-drying and canning methods of food preservation described in the passage differed in that one of them did not:

A. adversely affect flavor.
WRONG: This is not a difference which one of the processes failed to provide. We do not know if the canning method adversely affected flavor or not. Canning may still adversely affect flavor, but less so than sun-drying.

B. resist spoilage as well.
WRONG: This is not a difference which one of the processes failed to provide. There is no comparison made between the two methods of food preservation in this regard.

C. eliminate moisture.
CORRECT: This is a difference which one of the processes failed to provide. The canning method of preservation was not based on dehydration, and did not eliminate moisture at all.

D. require a vacuum.
WRONG: This is not a difference which one of the processes failed to provide. According to the passage, neither of the processes required a vacuum.

Examination 09: Biological Sciences

Passage V (Questions 408-414)

408. B is correct. If parathyroid glands do not develop, they cannot secrete PTH. The resulting PTH deficiency allows serum calcium levels to remain low. In the absence of PTH, calcium is not reabsorbed by the kidney or released by bone.

409. D is correct. Increased serum calcium exerts negative feedback inhibition on PTH secretion. Parathyroid glands are only sensitive to serum calcium levels, not bone density. PTH does not inhibit itself. Choice C is incorrect as hyperphosphatemia indirectly stimulates PTH secretion although this is beyond the scope of the passage. Furthermore, phosphate was not mentioned in the passage.

410. A is correct. PTH is a peptide hormone, and thus must utilize secondary messengers (knowing that the secondary messenger for PTH is cAMP is not necessary in this case). Only steroid hormones are able to act at the level of transcription. $1,25\text{-}(OH)_2D$ is not a gene product and thus cannot be transcribed. Further, the passage states that PTH catalyzes the conversion of vitamin D, not transcription. PTH does not affect Na^+ transport across the cell membrane.

411. C is correct. Hormones are released into the bloodstream, enabling them to exert effects on distant tissues. The activity of a neurotransmitter is confined to the synapse. There is no mention in the passage of vitamin D affecting a reaction rate, as an enzyme or coenzyme would.

412. C is correct. The persistence of low serum calcium in the presence of elevated PTH, points toward end-organ resistance to PTH. As PTH is a peptide hormone, G protein dysfunction is a reasonable hypothesis. Choice A is wrong because peptide hormones do not bind to nuclear receptors. There is no mention in the passage of osteoblasts or their autostimulation. In the case of nonfunctional osteoclastic cells, PTH and $1,25\text{-}(OH)_2D$ would still be able to elevate serum calcium levels through their respective actions on the kidney and intestine.

413. A is correct. Cortisol and aldosterone are steroid hormones. Epinephrine and norepinephrine are derived from tyrosine. Prolactin and oxytocin are peptide hormones. Adenine and guanine are purine bases found in DNA and RNA.

414. D is correct. When the action potential reaches the axon terminal, voltage-gated Ca^{++} channels open and Ca^{++} enters the cell. The Ca^{++} influx causes vesicles containing neurotransmitters to fuse to the presynaptic membrane, releasing their contents into the synapse. Thus, a decrease in calcium levels would decrease neurotransmitter release.

Passage VI (Questions 415-420)

415. B is correct. The passage states that imbalances of hormones, as would be seen in choices A and C, often result in fertility problems. As the egg must traverse the fallopian tube in order to be fertilized, inflammation the tubes may interfere with successful fertilization (as seen in Pelvic Inflammatory Disease). Multiple follicles, on the other hand, may lead to multiple conception, not infertility.

416. C is correct. As Group C is a placebo, the number of follicles harvested is unlikely to be a reflection of treatment conditions.

417. A is correct. The corpus luteum secretes estrogen, progesterone, and relaxin.

418. C is correct. Since providing an LH agonist induced follicular development in subject 2s, LH receptors are most likely functional. The cause for infertility then lies either in a lack of LH production or production of nonfunctional LH. A mutation in the LH gene could result in the latter.

419. D is correct. The passage states that the average female rat has a maximum of 10-12 mature follicles. Subject 2 in Group A has 15, the only subject with greater than 12 mature follicles. Thus, this rat best exemplifies therapeutic overstimulation. Note that in order to demonstrate a therapeutic phenomenon, the subject had to be in an experimental group.

420. C is correct. In human eggs, meiosis I produces a haploid cell and an inert polar body. After meiosis II (which only occurs when sperm cell has bound to the egg), a haploid cell and a polar body are produced. Then, the haploid egg and haploid sperm join to produce the diploid zygote.

Independent Questions (Questions 421-423)

421. C is correct. Spermatogenesis proceeds as follows: spermatogonia → spermatocytes → spermatids → spermatozoa.

422. D is correct. Microtubules form the flagellar tail which is essential for sperm movement into the fallopian tubes and eventually into the egg. Acrosomal enzymes digest the zona pellucida in order to facilitate sperm entry. Testosterone is essential for proper spermatogenesis. Sperm do not need mitochondria, however, as they rely on anaerobic metabolism alone

423. A is correct. Osteoclasts have white blood cells progenitors. Along with macrophages, osteoclasts are derived from monocytes. Both cell types engage in nonspecific phagocytosis and breakdown of their surrounding matrix. Chondrocytes are terminally differentiated, as are erythrocytes. Osteoprogenitor cells become osteoblasts, not osteoclasts.

EXPLANATIONS 10

Answers to Questions 424–470

ANSWERS TO EXAMINATION 10

PHYSICAL SCIENCES	VERBAL REASONING	BIOLOGICAL SCIENCES
424. A	440. D	455. B
425. D	441. B	456. D
426. D	442. A	457. B
427. C	443. B	458. D
428. D	444. C	459. D
429. B	445. D	460. A
430. B	446. B	461. B
431. A	447. A	462. D
432. B	448. B	463. B
433. D	449. B	464. A
434. C	450. A	465. A
435. A	451. D	466. D
436. B	452. D	467. D
437. C	453. C	468. B
438. A	454. B	469. A
439. B		470. C

Passage I (Questions 424-430)

424. A is correct. Since the specific gravity of the sensor is 0.8, 80% of the ball will be submerged. The volume of the submerged portion equals the volume of water displaced: $(0.8)(300) = 240 \text{ cm}^3$. One cubic centimeter of water has a mass of 1 gram, so the mass of water displaced is 240 g.

425. D is correct. The flow speed will be greater for spigot C as the water travels farther to reach it, gaining speed on its way down. Since the radii of the spigots are the same, the cross-sectional areas are the same, and volume flow $= Av$, So if the flow speed is greater through spigot C, then the volume flow must also be greater.

426. D is correct. The radius at point E is half that at point D, so the area at point E must be one-fourth the area at point D. Since volume flow $= Av$, if the area is one-fourth as large, then the speed must be four times as large.

427. C is correct. Using Torricelli's theorem:

$$v = \sqrt{2gh} = \sqrt{(2)(10)(10)} = \sqrt{200} = 14 \text{ m/s}$$

428. D is correct. Using the formula for gauge pressure:

$$P = \rho gh = (1000)(10)(15) = 1.5 \times 10^5 \text{ Pa}$$

429. B is correct. Mass is equal to the product of density and volume.

$$m = \rho V = \rho \pi r^2 h = (1000)(3.14)(16)(5) = 250,000 = 2.5 \times 10^5 \text{ kg}$$

430. B is correct. The water flowing out of spigot C passes through both points, while the water flowing out of spigot B will pass through point D but not point E, Thus, there is greater volume flow through point D than through point E.

Passage I (Questions 431-436)

431. A is correct. Each mole of silver chloride produces 1 mole of silver ions and 1 mole of chloride ions. One can use the solubility product:

$$K_{sp} = [Ag^+][Cl^-] = x^2$$

$$x = \sqrt{K_{sp}} = \sqrt{1.8 \times 10^{-10}} \ M$$

432. B is correct. According to the table, the solubility product, and thus the solubility, of the silver salts decreases as the halogens get larger. There is no clear trend in the lead halogen salts.

433. D is correct. The NaBr dissociates completely, so $[Br^-] = 0.2 \ M$. Using the K_{sp} expression:

$$K_{sp} = [Pb^{2+}][Br^-]^2$$

$$4.0 \times 10^{-5} = [Pb^{2+}](0.04)$$

$$[Pb^{2+}] = (4.0 \times 10^{-5})/(0.04) = 1.0 \times 10^{-3} \ M$$

434. C is correct. AgCl is the least soluble of the chloride salts in the solution, so as more chloride ions are added with the NaCl, the AgCl will precipitate out of the solution first. If the chemist continues to add the NaCl solution, the $PbCl_2$ will also precipitate.

435. A is correct. AgCl has a higher solubility product at higher temperatures, so the forward reaction is favored by increased temperature. The forward reaction then must be endothermic, and ΔH is positive. ΔS is positive because the transition from solid to aqueous particles increases randomness.

436. B is correct. AgF is soluble, so all of the sample will dissolve. The molar mass of AgF is 127 g/mol, so the sample contains 0.1 moles. By the definition of molarity:

$$\text{Molarity} = (\text{moles})/(\text{liters}) = (0.1)/(2) = 0.05 \ M$$

Independent Questions (Questions 337-339)

437. C is correct. Force is equal to the product of pressure and area.

$$F = PA = (\rho gh) \ A = (1000)(10)(3)(0.2) = 6000 \text{ N}$$

438. A is correct. Young's modulus is a constant equal to stress/strain. Doubling the radius of the wire increases the cross-sectional area by a factor of 4. This decreases the stress (F/A) by a factor of 4. If the stress is decreased by a factor of 4, then the fractional change in length will also be decreased by a factor of 4.

439. B is correct. The vapor pressure of the solution will lie in between the vapor pressures of the solute and solvent. Because the solvent is non-volatile, it will have the lower vapor pressure of the two, so the vapor pressure of the solution will be greater than that of the solvent.

Examination 10: Verbal Reasoning

Passage III (Questions 440-447)

440. Assume that only the 'felsic' compositional group of igneous rock is composed mostly of quartz. Based upon this new information:

A. the author has made an error.
WRONG: This is not correct based upon the new information/assumption.

B. White Sands is an abundant source of felsic rock and rock particles.

WRONG: This is not correct based upon the new information/assumption. White sand is almost pure gypsum. The passage would lead one to believe that gypsum is "another" form of sand.

C. most sand would have to come from some other type of igneous rock.

WRONG: This is not correct based upon the new information/assumption. From passage information we know that "most sand starts as tiny crystals of *quartz* which break off granite and other hard igneous rocks" (lines 44-46).

D. most sand would probably come from felsic rock.

CORRECT: This is correct based upon the new information/assumption. The passage states that "most sand starts as tiny crystals of *quartz* which break off granite and other hard igneous rocks" (lines 44-46). If 'felsic' is the only igneous rock composed mostly of quartz, then most sand would be felsic in origin.

441. Which of the following conclusions is best supported by the author's description of how sand particles change shape?

A. Heavier rocks in water would abrade more quickly than smaller windblown particles.

WRONG: There is insufficient information in the passage to support this conclusion. Furthermore, it is unclear whether this abrasion would be quantified via percentage of weight abraded, amount of weight abraded, or shaping, etcetera.

B. Most of the rounded sand grains in the world have been exposed to wind abrasion at one time or another.

CORRECT: This is the most reasonable conclusion that can be drawn from the author's description. There is a clear relationship presented between wind abrasion and round-shape in the last paragraph.

C. Weight seems to be more significant than size in determining particle shape.

WRONG: This is not the most reasonable conclusion as erosion, or shaping of particles in *water* seems to be influenced by weight *and* size (lines 55-61). Although wind has a faster effect, there is no indication that it more significant an influence on particle shape.

D. Most sand particles are spherical in shape.

WRONG: This is not the most reasonable conclusion that can be drawn from the author's description. For example, if the majority of sand particles have remained underwater, this statement is untrue. Further information would be required to support this conclusion.

442. Which of the following assertions is most clearly an idea presented by the author?

A. Windblown sand is capable of eroding metal.

CORRECT: This assertion is most clearly an idea presented by the author. "The abrasive, sandblast effect of the blown sand is greatest at ground level and insignificant above a height of 18 inches. ... telegraph poles are neatly amputated at their bases unless specially sheathed in metal, and even then they last only a few years" (lines 21-26).

B. Large areas of the desert are relatively uninhabited.

WRONG: Although this assertion may be true, it is not an idea presented by the author.

C. Most areas of a desert are actually polished and free of sand.

WRONG: Although the author mentions that "large areas of many deserts are left sand-free", there is no indication that the majority of the desert is without sand. The use of the word *most* makes this answer choice incorrect.

D. Gypsum is only found in dried-up lakebeds.

WRONG: This assertion is incorrect due to the qualifier 'only'. The passage does not place any limits on the location of gypsum.

443. The passage suggests that the heavier particles of wind-blown sand:

A. cannot usually be lifted above the ground.

WRONG: This is not suggested by the passage. "But sand, being heavier and coarser, rarely gets more than *a few feet* off the ground" (lines 14-15). Additionally, the passage mentions that sand particles may be blown across the desert in a blanket as high as chin-level.

B. produce the most significant erosion effects.

CORRECT: The height that particles can be lifted by the wind seems to be weight dependent, from dust which can be lifted thousand of feet into the air to sand which can be lifted a few feet off the ground (lines 13-15). "The abrasive, sandblast effect of the blown sand is greatest at ground level and *insignificant* above a height of 18 inches" (lines 21-23).

C. are sometimes compacted into a "gibber plain".

WRONG: This is not suggested by the passage.

D. are not eroded by water.

WRONG: This is not suggested by the passage.

444. During an interview on desert life, a zoologist remarks that the desert-dwelling *Stenocara* beetles' ability to collect water from wind-borne fogs is being emulated in certain devices which will be used to collect water for drinking and irrigation in the desert, to collect vapors in industrial condensers, and even to dispell fog at airports. This information would most *weaken* the passage assertion that:

A. wind essentially renders the desert devoid of any water.
WRONG: This is not a passage assertion. The passage only implicates the wind as a dehydrating factor, however, does not go as far as to say that deserts are devoid of water.

B. the desert offers nothing in the way of usable water.
WRONG: This is not a passage assertion.

C. desert winds dehydrate all living things.
CORRECT: This is a passage assertion and it is weakened by the fact that beetles', living creatures, are not dehydrated by the desert winds.

D. deserts are devoid of any sizeable vegetation.
WRONG: The passage indirectly acknowledges the presence of desert vegetation in line 4: " [Desert wind] Impeded not at all by vegetation".

445. The contention that, "As an agent of erosion the wind is secondary..." (line 1), can most justifiably be interpreted as support for the idea that:

A. the crucial cause of erosion is movement.
WRONG: This idea cannot be most justifiably supported by the contention. Furthermore, there is no indication as to what is moving.

B. the principal agent of erosion is water.
WRONG: This idea cannot be most justifiably supported by the contention. Answer choices B and C are synonymous, and therefore most likely incorrect.

C. the chief means of erosion is wind. Answer choices B and C are synonymous, and therefore most likely incorrect.
WRONG: This idea cannot be most justifiably supported by the contention.

D. the key player in erosion is sand.
CORRECT: This idea can be most justifiably supported by the contention. It is clear from the passage that it is the movement of the sand particles as a result of the wind that is the key to erosion.

446. According to the passage, one may conclude that in the desert, above a height of 18 inches.

A. wind-blown sand is essentially non-existent.
WRONG: This conclusion is not supported by the passage. "[S]and, being heavier and coarser, *rarely* gets more than a few feet off the ground" (lines 14-15). Additionally, the heavier particles can be blown in a blanket up to chin-level.

B. there is significantly less erosion.
CORRECT: "The abrasive, sandblast effect of the blown sand is greatest at ground level and insignificant above a height of 18 inches" (lines 21-23).

C. it may be easier to breathe in a duststorm.
WRONG: This conclusion is not supported by the passage. In fact the passage states that dust can rise and permeate the air for thousands of feet.

D. the air is much cooler.
WRONG: This finding is not supported by the hypothesis of the passage.

Passage IV (Questions 447-)

447. According to information in the passage, rolling would be less likely to occur when a seagoing liner:

I. is driving into the oncoming waves.
CORRECT: This is when rolling would be less likely. Rolling is caused by "...wave trains [that] keep hitting the side of the ship just as it is starting its roll, and under this constant nudging [rolling] soon builds to a dangerous degree" (lines 23-26). Therefore, if the ship could be maneuvered so that the waves were hitting the bow or some other area this would conceivably diminish rolling.

II. is beset by rough and irregular waves.
WRONG: This is when rolling would be *more* likely to occur.

III. has a longer hull.
WRONG: This is not when rolling would be less likely. A longer hull has to do with diminishing pitching.

A. I only
CORRECT: See above answer explanations.

B. II only

C. III only

D. I and III only

448. According to the passage, the ship's rolling period is considered a result of all of the following factors EXCEPT:

A. the shape of the ship's hull.
WRONG: This is considered a factor in the ship's rolling period, not an exception. "A ship's rolling period is determined by the *shape of its hull*, its beam, and the distribution of weight" (lines 14-15).

B. the length of the ship.
CORRECT: This is an exception, and not considered a factor in the ship's rolling period.

C. the distribution of the ship's weight.
WRONG: This is considered a factor in the ship's rolling period, not an exception. "A ship's rolling period is determined by the shape of its hull, its beam, and the *distribution of weight*" (lines 14-15).

D. the beam of the ship.
WRONG: This is considered a factor in the ship's rolling period, not an exception. "A ship's rolling period is determined by the shape of its hull, its *beam*, and the distribution of weight" (lines 14-15).

449. The ideas in the passage seem to derive primarily from:

A. facts observable in a ship's log.
WRONG: This is not where the ideas in the passage seem to derive primarily from. Presumably a ship's log would allow for conclusions for that particular ship. The information in the passage concerns all ships.

B. evidence on the behavior of ships and waves.
CORRECT: The ideas in the passage are presented as a science—a set of conclusions based on evidence.

C. speculation based on an accepted theory.
WRONG: The passage ideas are not presented as speculative, and there is no mention of a source of accepted theory.

D. knowledge of ongoing hydrology studies.
WRONG: The ideas in the passage cannot be attributed primarily to hydrology; there are also numerous ideas on shipbuilding and seamanship.

450. The ideas discussed in this passage would likely be of most use to:

A. a ship designer.
CORRECT: The ideas would most likely be of use to this person. Choices B, C, and D are all essentially sailors. A ship designer would be most concerned about the physics of the ships interaction with the water in order to design ships with minimal danger. Furthermore, the first line of the last paragraph suggests ship designers as the target audience for the science of ship-wave interaction.

B. a captain of a large liner.
WRONG: The "captain of a large liner" might have all of the antirolling and antipitch devices and not require knowledge on the physics of the ship's interaction with the water. Rather, one sailing a ship requires knowledge of what troubleshooting maneuvers must be made. Further, a "captain" would probably not need information on the six basic ship's movements. See the explanation for answer choice A.

C. a sailing hobbyist.

WRONG: The ideas would not most likely be of use to this person. Sailboats rarely require such extensive devices. See the explanation for answer choice A.

D. a competitive yachtsman.
WRONG: The ideas would not most likely be of use to this person. A "competitive yachtsman" would probably not need information on the six basic ship's movements. See the explanation for answer choice A.

451. In 1928, the clipper *Ellis Spethman* broke apart in heavy seas with a loss of all hands. Subsequent investigation revealed that her back had broken due to excessive pitching. Given the information in the passage, this result was probably due to:

A. not immediately changing her speed and course.
WRONG: This is not the probable reason for the results. It is *roll*, not pitch, that can be counteracted by immediately changing course and speed. "When … a ship [rolls badly] a much more drastic change of course or rate of speed must be made to break the motion" (lines 29-31).

B. the ship heading straight into the oncoming waves.
WRONG: This is not the probable reason for the results. There is no mention of a pejorative effect of a ship sailing into oncoming waves.

C. poor design.
WRONG: This is not the probable reason for the results. This is a plausible answer, but its vagueness renders it not the best answer when compared to the specificity of Answer D.

D. the clipper encountering waves that were longer than her hull.
CORRECT: This is the probable reason for the results. "… waves shorter than the ship will not make it pitch, even though they are in synchronism with its natural pitching period" (lines 46-47), it is the waves that are as long or longer than the hull that cause pitching.

452. Assume that all vessels are now required to have antirolling devices when they are built. This assumption necessitates which of the following conclusions?

Note: In order to answer this question correctly you must remember that, according to the passage, there exist ships without antirolling devices. "To counteract [roll] most modern vessels are equipped with antirolling devices of one kind of another" (lines 32-33).

A. It was most likely determined that roll was more serious than pitch.
WRONG: This conclusion is not necessitated by the assumption. There is no information that an an-

tipitch device exists. What if antipitch devices had been mandated also, but this information had not been given to us?

B. The requirement apparently does not apply to all vessels.
WRONG: This conclusion is not necessitated by the assumption. The assumption clearly states that the requirement is for "all" vessels.

C. Vessels without the devices were probably determined to have long enough hulls.
WRONG: This conclusion is not necessitated by the assumption. Longer hulls has to do with pitch, not roll.

D. Those vessels without the devices had been built before the requirement.
CORRECT: This conclusion is necessitated by the assumption. From the passage we know that, "To counteract [roll] *most* modern vessels are equipped with antirolling devices of one kind of another" (lines 32-33). Therefore, there exists at least one or more ship(s) that do not have the devices.

453. The passage presents an important relationship between:

A. airplanes and ships.
WRONG: This is not an important comparison made in the passage. The reference to an aircraft's aileron (lines 36-37) is for comparison of the antirolling device to an aircraft component, not the ships themselves.

B. pendulums and swings.
WRONG: This is not a comparison made in the passage.

C. wave regularity and minor speed changes.
CORRECT: This is an important relationship presented in the passage. "When the waves are fairly regular, a minor change of course or speed usually ends synchronous rolling" (lines 17-19).

D. hull length and rolling period.
WRONG: This is not an important comparison made in the passage. Hull length has to do with pitch, not roll.

454. According to the passage, pitching is, in part, a function of a ship's:

A. weight distribution.
WRONG: Weight distribution is related to roll, not pitch.

B. speed.
CORRECT: A ship designer "knows that the longer he can make his ship the *faster she can go before pitching becomes violent*" (lines 51-52).

C. date of manufacture.
WRONG: This is not what pitching has some relationship to.

D. beam.
WRONG: This is not what pitching has some relationship to. This has a relationship to roll.

Examination 10: Biological Sciences

Passage V (Questions 455-461)

455. B is correct. Hydroboration gives anti-Markovnikov orientation which would place the hydroxyl group at the less substituted carbon, C3, on allyl chloride.

456. D is correct. Hydrogen bonding in water stabilizes the carbocation that is generated in the S_N1 pathway. It is evident that the transition state is stabilized by the drop in the activation energy.

457. B is correct. In carbon tetrachloride the preferred mechanism is S_N2, so the product should have inversion of stereochemistry. A quick answer would be to look at figure 1 and replace Cl with Br in the S_N2 product.

458. D is correct. Isoprenyl chloride has an extra electron donating group (methyl) to help stabilize the positive charge. Furthermore, isoprenyl may form a tertiary cation while the other three have primary or secondary. This stabilization is also evident by the lower activation energy for the S_N1 mechanism for the molecule.

459. D is correct. The mechanism is S_N2 pathway. Although S_N2 reaction rates are dependent on two substrates, S_N2 occurs in one step.

460. A is correct. The mechanism is S_N1 pathway. All the rest of the answers are true of a S_N2 pathway.

461. B is correct. The conversion of an alkene to an alkane is a reduction and hydrogenation is the only reducing reagent listed.

Passage II (Questions 462-467)

462. D is correct. Atoms need to be moved in order to convert isopulegone to pulegone so none of the other answers are possible.

463. B is correct. The presence of an acid implies that a protonation step is occurring. Protonation effectively removes nucleophilic electrons, so protonation will not make a nucleophile stronger. Acids do not oxidize carbonyls nor do they cleave double bonds under most conditions.

464. A is correct. See the structure below. The group priorities are arranged clockwise and the lowest priority is going back making the absolute configuration R.

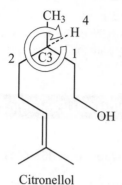

Citronellol

465. A is correct. The product has a higher substituted double bond so it is more stable than the reactant. Sodium hydroxide cannot oxidize and the ring closure is catalyzed by acid.

466. D is correct. When a primary alcohol is oxidized, it can be converted to an aldehyde or a carboxylic acid. To stop at the aldehyde the weaker oxidant is needed.

467. D is correct. Hot sulfuric acid is the condition for dehydration. Only D is a product of dehydration.

468. B is correct. Ethanol is a much smaller alcohol and would have a much lower boiling point making it the first compound to come across.

Independent Questions (Questions 468-470)

469. A is correct. The longest possible Carbon backbone forms butene. The chloro group takes precedence over the double bond.

470. C is correct. Hydrogenation of an alkene involves the addition of two bonds. Forming new bonds releases energy, which is exothermic.

EXPLANATIONS 11

Answers to Questions 471–517

ANSWERS TO EXAMINATION 11

PHYSICAL SCIENCES	VERBAL REASONING	BIOLOGICAL SCIENCES
471. B	487. D	502. A
472. C	488. A	503. A
473. C	489. C	504. C
474. C	490. C	505. D
475. A	491. D	506. C
476. D	492. C	507. A
477. C	493. B	508. B
478. B	494. B	509. C
479. C	495. D	510. C
480. B	496. A	511. B
481. B	497. D	512. A
482. A	498. A	513. D
483. C	499. B	514. A
484. D	500. A	515. C
485. C	501. A	516. B
486. C		517. B

Passage I (Questions 471-479)

471. **B is correct.** There must be total destructive interference for there to be no signal at the receiver. In order for this to occur, the waves must arrive at the receiver exactly one-half wavelength out of phase. Choices A and D differ from the length of tube A by multiples of the wavelength, so they will be in phase. Choice B differs by 1.5 wavelengths, so when the waves arrive at the receiver, they will be one-half wavelength out of phase.

472. **C is correct.** Use $v = d/t$ to find the speed of the sound.

$$v = d/t = (7.0)/(0.02) = 350 \text{ m/s}$$

According to Table 1, this speed is in between the speed of sound in air at 298 K and 373 K, so the temperature must be in between 298 K and 373 K. 305 K is the only answer choice that fits these parameters.

473. **C is correct.** Frequency remains constant for a wave, regardless of the medium. According to the wave equation, $v = \lambda f$, if frequency is the same for different speeds, then the wavelength must be different.

474. **C is correct.** The dB level of a whisper is 30, which means that it's intensity is 1000 times as great as the threshold of hearing: $(10^{-12})(10^3) = 10^{-9} \text{ W/m}^2$

475. **A is correct.** The speed of sound increases with increasing resistance to compression and decreasing density. As water is more dense than air, the greater speed of sound in water must be attributed to water's greater resistance to compression.

476. **D is correct.** Using the wave equation, $v = \lambda f$:

$$\lambda = v/f = (346)/(174) = 2$$

477. **C is correct.** The specific gravity reveals that seawater is more dense than fresh water. If the speed of sound is greater in seawater, it must be more resistant to compression.

478. **B is correct.** The molar masses of helium (4 g/mol) and argon (40 g/mol) differ by a factor of 10. According to the equation in the passage, their sound speeds will differ by a factor of $\sqrt{10}$, or about 3. Argon has a larger molar mass, thus its speed of sound will be slower. The answer can be approximated by dividing the speed of sound in helium, from Table 1, by 3.

972/3 = 325, which is pretty close to 307.

The answer may also be approximated using the equation in the passage.

Passage II (Questions 479-483)

479. **C is correct.** $MgSO_4$ dissociates into particles with +2 charges, while NaCl dissociates into particles with +1 charges. The greater charges exert more pull on each other in solution and are more likely to pair up.

480. **B is correct.** Use the formula. 9.5 grams of $MgCl_2$ is equal to 9.5/95 = 0.1 moles. (0.1 moles)/(1 kg) = 0.1 m.

$$T = kmi = (1.86)(0.1)(2.7) = 0.5° \text{ C}.$$

If the boiling point elevation is 0.5° C, the boiling point is 100.5° C.

481. **B is correct.** The solution with the highest freezing point will have the least freezing point depression. All other things being equal, that will be the solution with the smallest Van't Hoff factor.

482. **A is correct.** The more ion pairs formed, the smaller the Van't Hoff factor. We would expect that increased concentration would lead to more interaction among ion pairs and a lower Van't Hoff factor.

483. **C is correct.** The Van't Hoff factor is always smaller than the expected dissociation, so the boiling point elevation and freezing point depression will be smaller than expected. So the boiling point will be lower and the freezing point will be higher.

Independent Questions (Questions 484-486)

484. **D is correct.** The specific heat of copper is three times as large as that of gold, so the same heat will increase the temperature of three times the mass of gold by the same amount.

485. **C is correct.** A colligative property depends only on the number of particles present in a solution, not on their identities. pH is a measure of the number of H+ ions in a solution, so the identity of the particle is important in this case.

486. **C is correct.** Osmotic pressure causes water to move toward more concentrated solutions. If there is salt water in the stomach and intestines, water is drawn out of the body and into the intestines and from there it is lost.

Examination 11: Verbal Reasoning

Passage III (Questions 487-492)

487. Evidence shows that until 1889 about 20,000 rail employees were killed or injured each year, a third of them while stepping between cars to connect the primitive link and pin couplers. This fact tends to support the hypothesis concerning railway safety because:

A. Westinghouse had not yet come up with a solution to this problem.
WRONG: This is not why the fact tends to support the hypothesis concerning railway safety. Westinghouse came up with automatic brakes, not the automatic couplers that presumably enabled cars to be coupled without stepping between them.

B. automatic brakes were invented before automatic couplers.
WRONG: This is not why the fact tends to support the hypothesis concerning railway safety. This reasoning is not clearly related to the fact or the hypothesis.

C. it is clear that the powerful people who ran the railroads cared only about money.
WRONG: This is not why the fact tends to support the hypothesis concerning railway safety. This reasoning is not clearly related to the fact or the hypothesis.

D. up until this time automatic couplers were not in use.
CORRECT: This is the reason the question stem supports the hypothesis concerning railway safety. According to the question stem, "stepping between cars to connect the primitive link and pin couplers" accounted for a third of the injuries. The automatic couplers presumably enabled cars to be coupled without stepping between them. The date and the reference to automatic couplers lend credence to the hypothesis.

488. It is possible to determine if the railroads actually were able to increase their scheduling after instituting the improvements of Westinghouse and Janney by closely examining their yearly accident reports and taxes. Such information would support the author's mention of increased revenue by:

A. demonstrating that due to the improvements the railroads made more money.
CORRECT: This is why the information in the question would be relevant. Instituting the automatic brakes and couplers "would mean that longer trains could be operated reliably and economically on much *tighter schedules*. In other words, more freight, more passengers and, after an initial investment for the brakes and couplers, *much more revenue*" (lines 48-53).

B. demonstrating that more money could be made by marketing safety to passengers.
WRONG: This is not why the information in the question would be relevant. This is speculation not supported by the passage.

C. proving that the automatic braking and coupling systems actually worked.
WRONG: This is not why the information in the question would be relevant. This answer is specious and does not address "scheduling" or "revenues".

D. proving that tighter scheduling made more money.
WRONG: This is not why the information in the question would be relevant. This answer is not as complete as Answer A. Apparently "longer trains" were equally important. Instituting the automatic brakes and couplers "would mean that *longer trains* could be operated reliably and economically on much *tighter schedules*. In other words, more freight, more passengers and, after an initial investment for the brakes and couplers, *much more revenue*" (lines 48-53).

489. According to the passage information, what would have been most likely to happen if the automatic air brakes had been used *without* the automatic couplers?

A. Without the slack between the automatic couplers, the cars would have been too stiffly joined.
WRONG: This would not have been most likely to happen if the automatic air brakes had been used *without* the automatic couplers. This answer is speculative.

B. Without a tight coupling, the cars brakes would only have worked on a few of the cars.
WRONG: This would not have been most likely to happen if the automatic air brakes had been used *without* the automatic couplers. This answer is speculative.

C. Without a reliable connection, the trains might have stopped in a jerky manner.
CORRECT: This would have been most likely to happen if the automatic air brakes had been used *without* the automatic couplers. Referring to the test of the safety devices on the long freight train in Burlington, "When the brakes were set, "the train came to a standstill *within 500 feet* and *with hardly a jar*"" (lines 33-34). We can use this description to imagine what the *usual* (i.e. an attempt without the automatic brakes and couplers) sight of an emergency attempt to halt a long freight looked like.

D. With only the air brakes, each car would be stopping on its own.
WRONG: This would not have been most likely to happen if the automatic air brakes had been used *without* the automatic couplers. This answer is speculative.

490. The author would most likely agree that the owners of the railroads had a vested interest in:

I. making the most money possible.

CORRECT: Information in the passage suggests that this was one of the interests of the owners of the railroads. "Far more important to the *profit-minded group*, however, it would mean that longer trains could be operated reliably and *economically on much tighter schedules*." In other words, much more revenue (lines 45-50).

II. silencing complaints.

CORRECT: The author presents this as one of the interests of the owners of the railroads. "Together the brake and coupler were difficult for calloused railroad conservatives to ignore, for it gave them the means of silencing the everlasting hue and cry about safety and slaughter on the rails" (lines 43-45).

III. avoiding litigation.

WRONG: Information in the passage does not suggest that this was one of the interests of the owners of the railroads.

A. I only

B. II only

C. I and II only

CORRECT: See above answer explanations.

D. I and III only

491. Which of the following statements most strongly *challenges* one of the assertions made in the passage?

A. Westinghouse's device might have been much less effective without Janney's invention.

WRONG: This statement does not challenge one of the assertions made in the passage. There is no assertion that Westinghouse's device was less effective with Janney's. The inverse may have been true.

B. Lorenzo Coffin did not actually invent anything.

WRONG: This statement does not challenge one of the assertions made in the passage. There is no assertion that Lorenzo Coffin invented anything.

C. The use of the automatic brakes and couplers did not result in the saving of many lives.

WRONG: This statement does not most strongly challenge one of the assertions made in the passage. There is certainly no *explicit* assertion that the automatic brakes and couplers resulted in the saving of many lives. Moreover, this *implied* assertion is certainly not as strong as the *explicit* assertion which is challenged by Answer D.

D. After the successful trial of 1887, almost all of the owners opted to institute the brakes and couplers.

CORRECT: This statement *most strongly* challenges one of the assertions made in the passage. "Nevertheless, there was a *formidable bloc of holdouts*—But they were flogged into line in 1893"

(lines 50-53). A "formidable bloc of holdouts" is strongly challenged by this stated answer that "almost all" of the owners opted to institute the brakes and couplers.

492. According to the passage, which of the following is most likely to be true about the relationship between the 1887 trial of the automatic safety devices, and the state of Iowa?

A. It was in this state that all of the trials for railroad safety equipment were performed.

WRONG: This is not most likely true about the relationship. This is speculative.

B. Burlington, Iowa, was where Janney planned to retire.

WRONG: This is not most likely true about the relationship. We don't know where Janney "planned" to retire, but we do know that he *actually* did retire in Virginia (lines 54-58).

C. Lorenzo Coffin was Commissioner of Railroads there.

CORRECT: This is most likely true about the relationship. "Lorenzo Coffin, Commissioner of Railroads for the State of Iowa" (lines 5-6).

D. This was the most visible place to perform the test with the long freight trains.

WRONG: This is not most likely true about the relationship. This is speculative.

493. At the age of 22, George Westinghouse saw a wreck in which two trains had crashed together on a smooth, straight, level stretch of track in broad daylight. "What was the matter? Wouldn't the brakes work?" demanded Westinghouse of an employee. "Sure," said the man, "but there wasn't time." The author would most likely use this anecdote to:

A. expand on the dangers of train travel prior to the safety devices.

WRONG: This is not the most probable use that the author would make of this description. This might be the best answer if Answer B were not available.

B. explain why Westinghouse invented air brakes.

CORRECT: This is the most probable use of the anecdote. This description would help the author explain the zealousness that the he tries to convey in his depictions of Westinghouse, Janney, and Coffin.

C. justify the costs of forcing railroad owners to institute the automatic brakes.

WRONG: The author is primarily concerned with conveying the importance of the contributions of these three men to railroad safety, not in justifying the use of any of the inventions discussed.

D. clarify why Westinghouse went from a railroad owner to an inventor.

WRONG: This is not the most probable use that the author would make with this description. There is nothing in the passage that would indicate that Westinghouse was ever a railroad owner.

Passage IV (Questions 494-501)

494. According to passage information, the "old woman in Shropshire" (lines 14-15) was most likely attempting to:

A. alleviate her patients heart problems.

WRONG: This is not what the "old woman in Shropshire" was most likely attempting. There is no passage information which indicates that dropsy was associated with heart problems in 1775.

B. ease swelling in her patients.

CORRECT: This is what the "old woman in Shropshire" was most likely attempting. Foxglove was known as "a folk remedy esteemed…for its ability to relieve the swelling of dropsy" (lines 11-13).

C. relieve her patients of excess fluid.

WRONG: Though this may, in fact, have been the effect of the foxglove remedy administered by the "old woman in Shropshire", this is not what she was most likely *attempting*. Foxglove was known as "a folk remedy esteemed, … for its ability to relieve the swelling of dropsy" (lines 11-13). It seems that the old woman was treating symptoms. She may, or may not, have realized that dropsy (excessive swelling) would be relieved by ridding her patients of excess fluid.

D. teach the more legitimate practitioners.

WRONG: This is not what the "old woman in Shropshire" was most likely attempting. The recipe "had long been kept a secret" (line 14) by the woman.

495. Which of the following statements is the most reasonable conclusion that can be drawn from the author's description of the foxglove?

A. This plant could be harvested at almost any time of the year in England.

WRONG: This is not the most reasonable conclusion that can be drawn from the author's description of foxglove. Depending upon the purpose for the harvest, this may or may not be true. However, Withering "learned to obtain leaves of uniform potency by gathering them at a particular stage of the plant's growth" (lines 29-31). This "particular stage" may or may not have been at "almost any time of the year".

B. This plant had been relatively unknown for its medicinal properties.

WRONG: This is not the most reasonable conclusion that can be drawn from the author's description of foxglove. "This drug was long an old wives' remedy; it was first prescribed by a physician for heart trouble nearly 200 years ago" (lines 2-4). And, with no specificity, the passage provide that the remedy "had *long been kept a secret* by an old woman in Shropshire" (lines 14-15).

C. In England the plant was only available in early summer.

WRONG: This is not the most reasonable conclusion that can be drawn from the author's description of foxglove. Regarding the English summer, there is only the information that the foxglove's "pretty purple flowers dot English gardens in early summer" (lines 23-24).

D. Digitalis was derived from the leaves of the plant.

CORRECT: This is the most reasonable conclusion that can be drawn from the author's description of foxglove. Withering "suspected that the active principle of the mixture was to be found in only one of the ingredients – the *leaves of the foxglove*" (lines 21-23). Withering "began to treat dropsical patients with a tea made with foxglove leaves. In many cases it did indeed relieve them…" (lines 25-27).

496. If the author of the passage was asked, "When is the most effective time to treat a patient with digitalis?" The author's most likely response would be:

A. prior to the heart becoming enlarged.

CORRECT: This would be the author's most likely response to the question. From lines 61-62 we know that Vulpian's theory was somewhat backwards regarding the use of digitalis. Vulpian "concluded, [incorrectly] that the time to use the drug was *after* the heart had become enlarged …".

B. when urine output drops below normal.

WRONG: This would not be the author's most likely response to the question. There is no support in the passage for this answer.

C. after verifying initial indications that the heart is becoming enlarged.

WRONG: This would not be the author's most likely response to the question. This may or may not be accurate from a modern medical perspective. However, from the perspective of the passage, this is purely speculative and not the best answer.

D. before swelling has advanced beyond the limbs.

WRONG: This would not be the author's most likely response to the question. This answer has no support.

497. Dropsy occurs when "fluid is drawn from the blood into the tissues when there is a higher osmotic pressure in the tissues than in the blood." From this information we can assert that digitalis most likely:

A. equalizes the osmotic pressure in the blood and tissues.
WRONG: This assertion is not most likely. This would lead to equilibrium at a time when a patient is suffering from dropsy (i.e. swelling). This is not the best answer.

B. decreases the osmotic pressure in the blood.
WRONG: This assertion is not most likely. This would lead to more fluid in the tissues.

C. increases the osmotic pressure in the tissues.
WRONG: This assertion is not most likely. This would lead to more fluid in the tissues.

D. decreases the osmotic pressure in the tissues.
CORRECT: This assertion is most likely. It may be that digitalis more accurately increases the osmotic pressure in the blood *thereby relatively* decreasing the osmotic pressure in the tissues. However, that answer choice is not available.

498. It is little known fact that the English physician was honored for his work in botany when his name was given to a common plant malady. His name is most likely used to describe:

A. the results of a plant going without water for too long.
CORRECT: This is the most likely description of the naming. An "Englishman named William *Withering*" (lines 10-11). "Withering" results when a plant has gone too long without water.

B. the petals of the foxglove.
WRONG: This is not the most likely description of the naming. An "Englishman named William *Withering*" (lines 10-11).

C. when a plant has some medicinal value.
WRONG: This is not the most likely description of the naming. An "Englishman named William *Withering*" (lines 10-11).

D. a plant that has grown too large.
WRONG: This is not the most likely description of the naming. An "Englishman named William *Withering*" (lines 10-11).

499. Assuming all of Dr. Withering's discoveries were novel, then prior to Withering which of the following properties of digitalis was unknown:

A. that the drug worked primarily on the kidneys.
WRONG: It is clearly *not* accurate that the drug worked primarily on the kidneys. Therefore this answer cannot be a choice. "By 1855, at least one basic fact had become clear: digitalis, ... did not act directly on the kidneys" (lines 52-54).

B. how to obtain an unvaryingly potent form of the drug.
CORRECT: Based upon the assumption this was not known prior to Withering. Withering "learned to obtain leaves of uniform potency by gathering them at a particular stage of the plant's growth" (lines 29-31).

C. in what form the drug should be given.
WRONG: Nowhere does it say that Withering discovered the best form which the drug should be given. It is not asserted that Withering was the first to give the drug in a drinkable for such as tea.

D. why the drug also caused increased urine output.
WRONG: It is not clear that it was ever understood why the drug increased urine output. This was not presented as one of Withering's findings.

500. According to the passage, "Vulpian was confusing cause and effect" (lines 63-64). Which of the following distinctions is implied in the passage between "cause and effect", respectively?

I. enlarged and inadequate
CORRECT: "Vulpian was confusing cause and effect. In congestive failure, the heart is *not* inadequate because it is enlarged; it becomes *enlarged because it is inadequate*" (lines 63-65).

II. inadequate and enlarged
WRONG: This is not "respectively".

III. congestive failure and enlarged
WRONG: This may or may not be medically accurate according to today's standards. However, this is purely speculative based upon passage information.

A. I only
CORRECT: See above answer explanation.

B. II only

C. III only

D. I and III only

501. According to the information contained in the passage, an appropriate theory of pharmacological research for new medicines would state that discovering new medicines involves:

I. understanding the full spectrum of effects associated with that medicine.
CORRECT: This is an appropriate theory of pharmacological research for new medicines. "But neither [Withering] nor his successors for generations afterward had either the knowledge or the techniques to *determine the effects of the drug inside*

the body – and therefore the diseases for which it could best be used. Later promiscuously used as a "remedy" for all forms of edema, and sometimes for totally unrelated conditions, the foxglove's effects were so uncertain that many physicians stopped using it entirely" (lines 46-50). "The *halting progress* of digitalis from potion to modern prescription illustrates how inadequate knowledge of pharmacology can nullify the value of even an effective drug" (lines 6-9).

II. experiencing the effectiveness of a medicine through native research.
WRONG: This is not an appropriate theory of pharmacological research for new medicines. It is clear that the drug was being used in an ignorant fashion by the herbalists and natural healers. "The medicine, like many of the period, was a complicated concoction, with more than 20 different ingredients" (lines 16-18) only one of which was the active ingredient.

III. communicating the needs of the medical community to local herbalists and natural healers.
WRONG: This is not an appropriate theory of pharmacological research for new medicines. The remedy had been kept a secret from the regular practitioners (lines 14-15). There is no reason to suppose that communicating a need would change this situation.

A. I only
CORRECT: See above answer explanations.

B. II only

C. I and III only

D. II and III only

Examination 11: Biological Sciences

Passage V (Questions 502-510)

502. **A is correct.** The question stem states that heroin is an opioid, and thus an *agonist* of opioid receptors. The passage states that casein, like heroin, binds opioid receptors. The graph of the experiment's results shows that ingestion of casein decreases overall food intake (ie, increases one's satiety despite a smaller amount of food). Therefore, it can be inferred that heroin must also increase satiety and decrease overall food intake.

503. **A is correct.** Figure 1 shows that blockade of opioid receptors with an opioid antagonist reverses the satiety-increasing effects of a casein pre-load, causing the animals to consume more food. It can be inferred that use of an opioid antagonist alone would also cause increased consumption of food.

504. **C is correct.** According to the passage, satiety is dependent on several factors, including the volume of food ingested, the rate of gastric emptying, and the fat content of food consumed. All of these factors are part of the digestive system, which includes the activities of the mouth, esophagus, stomach, intestine, and accessory digestive organs such as the pancreas and gallbladder.

505. **D is correct.** The question states that morphine is a type of opioid. According to the passage, binding of opioid receptors in the small intestine causes decreased motility of the gastrointestinal tract. Decreased motility of the GI tract causes stasis of fecal material within the intestine, resulting in constipation. In fact, morphine-based painkillers are often administered with laxatives or stool softeners to avoid this common side effect.

506. **C is correct.** Casein is a peptide (stated in the passage), and therefore is first broken-down by the enzyme *pepsin*, which is secreted by *chief cells* of the stomach. Pepsin is an enzyme that helps digest protein and works best in an acidic environment. Parietal cells of the stomach secrete hydrochloric acid, which ensures that the stomach remains acidic. Goblet cells in the stomach secrete mucous, which helps protect the lining of the stomach from the acids that there. Once protein is broken down in the stomach, it continues its digestion in the small intestine, where bile and pancreatic enzyme release is stimulated.

507. **A is correct.** As stated in the question stem, CCK is released by the duodenum in response to food, which then stimulates the release of pancreatic enzymes and bile. In fact, CCK is the strongest stimulator of pancreatic enzyme and bile release. Pancreatic enzymes include such enzymes as trypsin (used to digest protein) and lipase (used to digest fats). Bile, which is released from the gallbladder, is also used to help digest and emulsify fats. It can therefore be assumed the foods high in fat *and* protein (such as a cheeseburger) would stimulate the strongest CCK response. Although an oil-based salad dressing is high in fat, it has little protein, which a cheeseburger has both high fat and protein content. Reduced-fat milk and fruit have less fat and protein than a cheeseburger.

508. **B is correct.** In general, increasing the number of study subjects (n) increases the validity of results. The larger the number of subjects, the less likely that biases are affecting the results seen. Using a control group that received a pre-load of saline would have also strengthened the validity of the study. All studies should use a control group against which the experimental groups are compared. Changing the dose of casein used or using an alternate opioid antagonist would not have impacted the study's validity.

509. **C is correct.** As exemplified by the results of the study in the passage, a pre-load of casein may result in premature termination of a meal. The passage states that casein

is a peptide found in dairy products. Therefore, it can be inferred from the passage that consumption of cheese before a meal may result in earlier satiety.

Passage VI (Quesitons 510-516)

510. **C is correct.** Spironolactone antagonizes aldosterone receptors, thereby decreasing the amount of sodium reuptake and potassium secretion. When potassium secretion is lowered, serum potassium levels rise. Choices A, B and D either lower or do not affect serum potassium.

511. **B is correct.** Sodium is driven through the Na^+/Cl^- cotransporter by a concentration gradient created by the Na^+/K^+ ATPase in membrane on the interstitial side of the cells. Although ATP is not directly used to bring sodium and chloride into the cell, the process is called *secondary* active transport because ATP is used to maintain the concentration gradient. Choice A is incorrect because primary active transport involves the use of ATP by the cotransporter itself (as in the case of Na^+/K^+ ATPase). Choice C is incorrect because passive diffusion involves the movement of molecules through leakage channels in the membrane. A transporter is not part of the process. Choice D is incorrect because pinocytosis involves invagination of the plasma membrane to form fluid-filled vesicles.

512. **A is correct.** Hemorrhage decreases intravascular volume and the body will respond by conserving as much salt (and thus water) as it can. By secreting angiotensin II, the body upregulates aldosterone and promotes salt retention. Choice B is incorrect because the body does not want to conserve salt when the blood pressure is high. Choices C and D are incorrect because although they do not directly affect angiotensin II levels, although they are both risk factors for high blood pressure.

513. **D is correct.** The $Na^+/K^+/2Cl^-$ cotransporter does not change the membrane potential because there is no net movement of charge across the membrane: 2 positive charges (sodium and potassium) and 2 negative charges (chloride) move through the transporter.

514. **A is correct.** ADH, made by hypothalamus and released by the posterior pituitary, increases the permeability of the collecting ducts to water. Thus in the presence of ADH, water reabsorption is increased. Choice B is incorrect because ACTH stimulates the adrenal cortex to release glucocorticoids. Although oxytocin is also released by the posterior pituitary, it stimulates uterine and mammary contraction. Choice D is incorrect because angiotensin I is converted to angiotensin II which then stimulates the release of aldosterone.

515. **C is correct.** The countercurrent multiplier in the medullary loop of Henle very effectively reduces the volume of filtrate in the nephron. In the descending loop, water is removed from the filtrate and in the ascending loop, salt is removed from the filtrate. Choices A, B and C are incorrect because they are all functions of the proximal tubule.

516. **B is correct.** The juxtaglomerular apparatus monitors filtrate pressure and therefore volume. It is located adjacent to the distal tubule and would sense the change in filtrate volume caused by furosemide.

Independent Question (Question 517)

517. **B is correct.** Aldosterone, like other mineralocorticoids, is made in the adrenal cortex.

EXPLANATIONS 12

Answers to Questions 518–564

ANSWERS TO EXAMINATION 12

PHYSICAL SCIENCES	VERBAL REASONING	BIOLOGICAL SCIENCES
518. C	534. C	549. C
519. D	535. B	550. B
520. B	536. A	551. D
521. D	537. C	552. A
522. D	538. D	553. B
523. A	539. B	554. B
524. A	540. A	555. C
525. D	541. C	556. D
526. C	542. B	557. A
527. D	543. B	558. D
528. A	544. D	559. C
529. C	545. B	560. D
530. B	546. C	561. A
531. B	547. B	562. A
532. B	548. D	563. B
533. A		564. B

Passage I (Questions 518-523)

518. C is correct. When x is equal to A, the expression for speed in the passage reduces to zero. You can get this one without the equation if you realize that for vibrating objects, the speed of the object has to be zero at maximum displacement because that's when the object has to stop and reverse direction.

519. D is correct. Frequency is equal to the reciprocal of period. $f = 1/T$.

520. B is correct. Simple harmonic motion is depicted by a sine or cosine wave. Since the motion began at the point of maximum displacement, we need a cosine wave. The sine wave in choice A is wrong because it starts at $x = 0$.

521. D is correct. The smaller the period of vibration, the more vibrations will occur in one minute. According to the equation in the passage, the smallest period will result from the largest spring constant and a smallest mass.

522. D is correct. From the period equation, a smaller mass makes for a shorter period, and thus greater frequency. Changing the maximum displacement has no effect on the frequency of motion.

523. A is correct. At the point of zero displacement, the block is at maximum speed and the spring is neither stretched nor squished, so there is no elastic potential energy. There is also no heat, as this is a frictionless system.

Passage II (Questions 524-530)

524. A is correct. The high specific heat of water tends to moderate the climate near the ocean, so the city on the landmass will be hotter in the summer and cooler in the winter.

525. D is correct. Freezing point depression is given by the expression $k_f m$. m can be found by adding the molalities of the various ions on the table to get about 1.1 m.

$$\Delta T = -k_f m = -(0.52)(1.1) = -0.60° \text{C}$$

526. C is correct. In distillation, seawater is boiled and the vapor which condenses will be fresh water. Salt particles are too small to be separated by filtration.

527. D is correct. The quantities in the table are given in g/kg and must be converted to mg/kg.

528. A is correct. The dissolved particles in ocean water create vapor pressure depression, so the vapor pressure will be lower for ocean water. Vapor pressure does not depend on exposed surface area.

529. C is correct. Molality measures moles per kilogram of solvent.

530. B is correct. Bonds are formed when water freezes, which is a process that releases energy. 180 g is equal to 10 moles of water so (10 moles)(6.01 kJ/mole) = 60 kJ

Independent Questions (Questions 531-533)

531. B is correct. When the frequencies of two waves differ by a small amount, a beat frequency equal to the difference can be heard. That means the frequency of the second wave must have been either 436 Hz or 444 Hz.

532. B is correct. Water is unusual in that it is more dense as a liquid than as a solid. So when the pressure is increased on ice at constant temperature, the ice will melt. All of the other phase changes require a decrease in pressure at a constant temperature.

533. A is correct. The harmonics for a pipe closed at one end are given by the formula below.

$$L = \frac{n\lambda_n}{4} \quad (n = 1, 3, 5...)$$

So the wavelengths are (12)/(1), (12)/(3), and (12)/(5).

Examination 12: Verbal Reasoning

Passage III (Questions 534-541)

534. The author of this passage is most likely a(n)

A. Anatomy lab instructor
WRONG: Though is the closest to the correct answer, it is not the best answer. A lab instructor's advice would most likely not include this degree of insight into the difficulties face by a first time dissector. Also, see C below.

B. Editor for a dissection manual
WRONG: There is no evidence to indicate this. Also, the statement "the lab manual is of questionable assistance" steers one away from this choice.

C. A medical student
CORRECT: This is most clearly indicated in line 45 where the author writes, "The fledgling dissector, such as I must invariably be categorized..." Furthermore, the author's insight into the difficulties faced by a novice dissector is more consistent with one that is going or has just gone through his or her initial dissection experience. Also, the subtle tenor of the passage indicating the author's difficulty and stress with dissection in general are consistent with this choice.

D. A board-certified physician
WRONG: This is not the best answer. Line 45 contraindicates this choice.

535. The author would be most likely to agree that dissection is

A. a tedious process
WRONG: Though this answer is correct as evidenced by the statement, "random, hesitant pokings to show for tedious moments thus passed," it is not the author's primary attitude toward dissection

B. an acquired art*
CORRECT: This is the best answer. The figurative language the author uses in the first gives the impression that the author views masterful dissection as an art. The fact that it can be acquired is most clearly expressed in the last sentence of the passage:

"However, as the days steady his hand and labor his markers, the student's scalpel too begins to swing, just a bit."

C. a fun pastime
WRONG: If anything, the author would seem to feel the opposite way because of difficulty, labor, and time involved in dissection.

D. loathsome experience
WRONG: Although, we do get the impression that dissection is laborious, there is no evidence to indicate strong hatred towards dissection as is implied by the word loathsome.

536. According to the passage above, to become an apt and dexterous dissector requires:

A. A strong knowledge base, experience, and patience*
CORRECT: The last paragraph states the most prominent difficulty in dissection is applying a yet fragile knowledge base practically on the cadaver. Overcoming this difficulty would then most likely lead one to becoming a good dissector as compared to any of the other choices. Also, the last line of the passage talks about experience steadying the student's hand and time making firm his or her knowledge base as preconditions for the novice to progress in his or her ability.

B. Patience and a passion for anatomy
WRONG: The author never indicates passion as a factor.

C. A strong knowledge base and steady, skillful hand
WRONG: This is true, but not the best answer. Although the author admires the skilled hand of a master dissector, we are not told that a steady hand is a requirement to become an apt dissector. As

such, the dexterity that the author admires is more a manifestation of long experience than a primary requirement for masterful dissection.

D. Ability to discern how deep to cut the cadaver and navigate around vasculature
WRONG: These are both difficulties that a beginning dissector faces, but they are not the most important ones.

537. Netter is most likely

A. a lab instructor
WRONG: A lab instructor would most likely not be lying on the gurney

B. an anatomy student
WRONG: An anatomy student would most likely not be lying on the gurney

C. an author of an anatomy atlas*
CORRECT: The next sentence talks about how an anatomy atlas with its two dimensional picture is not of much use in the lab. Mostly likely then, "Netter" is name of the editor of such an atlas but the term has been used to refer to atlas itself.

D. the name of the cadaver
WRONG: The following sentence would not fit well with the flow of the passage if this were the correct answer.

538. If the anatomy lab in discussion were to be remodeled to provide a more warm, relaxing ambiance, this would

A. make the dissection process less stressful and distasteful
WRONG: There is no support for this answer in the passage.

B. increase the efficiency with which dissection is done in the lab
WRONG: There is no support for this answer in the passage.

C. facilitate the application of anatomic knowledge in spatial decision making
WRONG: There is no support for this answer in the passage.

D. make little or no difference*
CORRECT: This is supported by the statement: "The cold, dead stare of the cadaver, the distinct, permeating stench of formaldehyde in the lab, the loud, steady buzzing of tube lights overhead- all of these are of little consequence." (lines 8-10).

539. If one were to generalize, most first time dissectors feel

A. bewildered because they do not have a strong foundational knowledge of anatomy

WRONG: This is true, but it is not the only reason why they feel bewildered.

B. frustrated by an inability to make appropriate and/or definitive decisions during the dissection process *

CORRECT: This is the best answer because the second and third paragraphs speak to the lack of surety that a first time dissector experiences, uncertainty that could reasonably result in a certain degree of frustration. Also, the author feels that the inability to make appropriate and/or definitive decisions is part of the fundamental difficulty involved in dissection (lines 43-49).

C. excited by the challenge and promise of dissecting a cadaver
WRONG: Nothing the author expresses indicates the emotion of excitement

D. angst because of the long hours required of anatomy lab
WRONG: Though, students may feel this way, this is not the main emotion that dissectors would probably feel.

540. Which of the following changes would result in the greatest benefit to new dissectors?

A. More lab instructors to dissect out and demonstrate important lab structures*
CORRECT: The author states that despite the difficulties associated with dissection, instructors present the important lab structures which results in learning for inexperienced dissectors (lines 51-52).

B. More colleagues per cadaver
WRONG: It does not seem that this is as important of a factor as the presence and aid of lab instructors.

C. Shorter laboratory sessions
WRONG: This is not indicated.

D. Better ancillary reading materials
WRONG: This is not indicated.

541. From the author's tone, it can be most directly inferred that the lab dissection manual is

A. Helpful but verbose
WRONG: The author feels rather that the lab manual is of questionable value.

B. Circumlocutory
WRONG: Though the quote reads as one that is loquacious, this would be the reader's personal impression. This is not directly implied by the author's tone.

C. Difficult to read and apply *

CORRECT: The next sentence, "A student is not left entirely to his own devices though," would seem to indicate that the manual is difficult to handle but that the student thankfully has some alternative.

D. Well written but too advanced for starting dissectors
WRONG: There is nothing to indicate this in the passage.

Passage IV (Questions 542-)

542. From the first paragraph we can infer that the author

I. is an enthusiast of literature from the Romantic genre

II. feels that society must actively participate in their existence

III. believes that life is unpredictable

A. I and II
WRONG: Even if you knew that the quote given in the first paragraph was from Moby Dick, there is nothing in the passage that indicates that the author favors this genre of literature. Furthermore, to know where the quote is from and what genre of literature it belongs to would be calling on totally irrelevant, outside information. This something that you would not be required to do on the verbal section as it is extraneous to the verbal reasoning skills tested on the MCAT.

B. II and III*
CORRECT: We know that author feels that society must actively participate in their existence from the statement, "It is of singular import for all those who traverse the capricious road of life, to understand the nature of that which they traverse." (lines 3-5). The author qualifies the road of life as being capricious indicating the he sees it as unpredictable.

C. I, II, and III
WRONG: Choice I is not correct. See explanation under A.

D. only II
WRONG: Choice III is also correct. See explanation under B.

543. According to the framework set up by the passage, an ascetic monk who has no worldly desire or wants would most like be characterized by

A. "Newtonian" metaphysics
WRONG: "Newtonian" metaphysics are used by the author to refer to the rules that govern general

human behavior. Such an individual is described as having no wants which obviates all the three rules of Newtonian metaphysics as all of them require some want or desire on which to operate (lines 10-15).

B. "Einsteinian" metaphyics
CORRECT: This is the best answer. An individual such as described in the question is clearly not normative and his behavior most appropriately would be categorized in the extremes of human behavior which is the realm of Einsteinian metaphysics (lines 20-22). Also such a person seems to hold spiritual values above material ones and this would further include him under the purview of Einsteinian physics. (lines 22-24).

C. Frankenstein logic
WRONG: Frankenstein logic, in its more abstract form, refers to an individual rationalizing his behavior because of his or her intense desire to acquire something (lines 55-56).

D. Such an individual does not fit into the framework of this passage
WRONG: This is not the correct answer because the correct answer is B.

544. What is the role of the "outside forces" of media and culture (line 43)?

A. They accelerate human wants according to Newtonian metaphysics
WRONG: Though this statement is true as evidenced by statement, "act in the same direction as this want- giving it impetus, accelerating it" (lines 44-45). However, C is also correct making the correct answer D.

B. The "outside forces" are metaphysical manifestations of the Frankenstein monster
WRONG: There is nothing the in the passage that supports this answer. In fact, the passage would suggest that society itself is the Frankenstein monster (line 51-52).

C. The "outside forces" reinforce man's desire to be wanted and in doing so form a basis on which he can rationalize otherwise unethical behaviors
WRONG: This answer is in and of itself correct. The author states that the "outside forces" accelerate man's desire to be wanted (lines 43-44). Later, the author states that this desire to be wanted drives all of human action and is so intense that it is used to justify even unethical actions (lines 52-56).

D. A and C are both correct
CORRECT: For explanation see A and C above.

545. "If an individual likes chocolate, seeing a chocolate ice cream cone will be more motivating than a vanilla ice

cream cone." This statement illustrates which of the author's Newtonian metaphysical principles?

A. The first Newtonian metaphysical principle
WRONG: This principle states that one's wants are in a steady state until something occurs to alter that homeostasis (lines 10-14). This does not apply to the statement given in this question.

B. The second Newtonian metaphysical principle
CORRECT: This principle states that the change in one's desire is directly proportional to the magnitude of force acting on it (lines 20-21). If one likes chocolate, we can assume that the magnitude of its effect is greater than vanilla. Thus a chocolate stimulus will elicit a greater change in desire that than a similar stimulus that is not chocolate.

C. The third Newtonian metaphysical principle
WRONG: The third principle is concerned with the predicted consequences of an action and how those consequence drive action (lines 23-25). This does not directly apply to the statement given in the question.

D. It doe not illustrate any of the Newtonian metaphysical principles of the author
WRONG: B is the correct answer.

546. Which of the following most directly challenges the author's views?

A. Victor Frankenstein was not a genius
WRONG: This does not challenge the author's views because he does not necessarily hold this view. Even the statement, "Victor Frankenstein a genius" is predicated by and "if" (Line 57)

B. The Frankenstein monster is a symbol of society's readiness to overlook the morality of means in their eagerness to acquire a certain end.
WRONG: This does not challenge the authors view. In fact, it supports the author's view (lines 52-54).

C. The underlying motivator of people's action is not to gain the favor of others, but rather to ultimately avoid incurring physical harm
CORRECT: This goes directly against one of the major points made by the author in this passage: "This desire [gaining the favor of others] now underlies all society's actions" (lines 46-47).

D. Newtonian physical and metaphysical laws are not absolute
WRONG: The author would agree with this because he states that the Newtonian metaphysical laws do not hold up when addressing the extremes of behavior just as his physical laws do not hold up at velocities close to the speed of light (lines 29-31).

547. What world does the author refer to when he states that he would rather "live in an Einsteinian world of Frankenstein physics ruled by Newtonian logic?" (lines 62-64).

  I.   The present world as defined by postmodernist theory

  II.   A world in which spiritual goals are primary and metaphysics are subordinate to this goal

  III. A world in people action are guided by logical and constrained by the parameters of normative human behavior

A. I and III
WRONG: Choice I is not correct. In the second to last sentence the author indicates that the present world is adequately defined by David Russell's characterization if one agrees to the premises laid out in the beginning of the last paragraph (lines 60-61). Also, there is nothing about postmodernism in the passage.

B. II and III
CORRECT: This is the correct answer. This is a potentially time-consuming question. This question is probably the most difficult question of the section, and in general, the final sentence is a very loaded philosophical commentary. The Eisteinian world refers to one in which spiritual values are prized over material ones. Frankenstein physics refers to a situation in which the way man operates on a metaphysical and psychological level is subordinate to the attainment of the spiritual goals of the Einsteinian world. Newtonian logic refers to man acting overwhelmingly on the basis of reason and logic so as to keep his wants and desire from distracting him from the attainment of spiritual values.

C. I, II, and III
WRONG: This is not correct because Choice I is not correct. See A for explanation.

D. None of the above
WRONG: This is not correct because B is the correct answer.

548. The author's purpose in writing this passage is best characterized by which of the following

A. to offer a conceptual framework to help the reader understand human nature
WRONG: Though this is something that the author sees as important, this is not the main reason. as is made clear by the sentence, "What is greater, such an understanding does not simply elucidate what is, but more importantly will guide one to what should be. This is the intent." (lines 5-7).

B. to equate physical laws to their corresponding metaphysical realities
WRONG: This is not the main reason for writing the passage. This just sets up a conceptual framework so that subsequent ideas may be better understood.

C. to define the rules of logic
WRONG: This is the most unlikely of the given choices to be correct. The passage is not a discussion on the topic of logic.

D. to convince the reader of the author's worldview
CORRECT: This is most clearly stated in the sentence, What is greater, such an understanding does not simply elucidate what is, but more importantly will guide one to what should be. This is the intent." (lines 5-7). Much of the passage, is then just background so that the reader can understand what the author's ideas and what he thinks "should be" (line 7). His worldview is best characterized by the last sentence of the passage (lines 62-64).

Examination 12: Biological Sciences

Passage V (Questions 549-555)

549. **C is correct.** Benzoyl chloride is an acid chloride.

550. **B is correct.** The lone pair of electrons on the nitrogen categorizes compound 3 as a Lewis base. A solution of a basic compound will have a pH greater than 7.

551. **D is correct.** The extra oxygen of the sulfonamide anion provides more resonance structures. Thus there is greater delocalization of the negative charge than the benzamide anion.

552. **A is correct.** Compound 4 in Reaction 2 would yield a benzamide product with a methylated Nitrogen.

553. **B is correct.** According to the passage, only a secondary amine will produce a white solid before acidification. Only Compound 2 is a secondary amine.

554. **B is correct.** The solid is benzesulfonamide, which is in column 1 of Table I. The Hinsberg test results indicate a primary amine. The primary amine with a melting point closest to the observed value is compound 3. Note: Crude melting points are lower than purified.

555. **C is correct.** The reaction of hydroxide with an acid chloride produces a carboxylic acid.

Passage VI (Questions 509-515)

556. D is correct. See below for the first step of the mechanism. Tetrahedral shape requires sp^3 hybridization. Furthermore, the intermediate is most likely charged if the transition state is charged.

557. A is correct. The nitro group is the only electron-withdrawing group in the answers. Electron withdrawing would stabilize the negative charge in the ring.

558. D is correct. The passage states that the reaction is quenched with acid. HCl is the only acid on the list.

559. C is correct. The fastest reaction step would have the smallest ΔG of activation, and thus the lowest energy barrier to progression. Formation of the acid salt is shown to be the fastest in the reaction coordinate diagram.

560. D is correct. The benzoate anion has the resonance structures that stabilize the negative charge.

561. A is correct. Carboxylic acid is a much higher oxidation state than benzyl group, and would require an oxidizing agent.

562. A is correct. According to the passage, sodium hydroxide catalyzes the hydrolysis of methyl benzoate, the reverse reaction.

Independent Questions (Questions 563-564)

563. B is correct. NH_3 will form an amide and amides are less reactive than esters. Cl^- and CH_3COOH form an acid chloride and anhydride which a more reactive. CH_2OH would form an ester.

564. B is correct. The enantiomer, D-lactic acid, will rotate light by an equal amount in the opposite direction.

398

EXPLANATIONS 13

Answers to Questions 565–611

ANSWERS TO EXAMINATION 13

Physical Sciences	Verbal Reasoning	Biological Sciences
565. B	581. B	596. A
566. A	582. C	597. C
567. B	583. B	598. D
568. C	584. C	599. B
569. D	585. C	600. A
570. D	586. B	601. D
571. A	587. A	602. B
572. D	588. C	603. D
573. D	589. D	604. D
574. C	590. B	605. B
575. B	591. B	606. D
576. B	592. D	607. A
577. C	593. C	608. C
578. B	594. B	609. B
579. D	595. A	610. C
580. B		611. C

Passage I (Questions 565-571)

565. B is correct. According to the temperature equation, a raise in temperature necessitates that $R > R_o$. According to the length-area equation, increasing the length will increase resistance and increasing the area will decrease resistance.

566. A is correct. Copper has the lowest resistivity and resistance per unit length. Since it offers the least resistance it will consume the least power.

567. B is correct. Keep in mind that the temperature change is negative.

$$R = R_o[1 + (T - T_o)]$$

$$R = (0.31)(1 + (5.0 \times 10^{-3})(-20))$$

$$R = (0.31)(1 - 0.1) = (0.31)(0.9) = 0.28 \ \Omega$$

568. C is correct. Iron has the greatest value for the temperature coefficient of resistivity, α. Thus, it will undergo the greatest change in resistance for a given change in temperature.

569. D is correct. $P = i^2/R$. The current, i, is given in the question as 10 A. From Table 1 we see the resistance of copper is 0.05 Ω/m. We multiply this by 1000 m to get 50 Ω. So we have $P = 10^2 \times 50 = 5000$ W

570. D is correct. The new wire has twice the radius, so four times the cross-sectional area. From the equation in the passage, R = $\rho L/A$, the resistance is decreased by a factor of 4. From $V = iR$, the current increases by a factor of 4.

571. A is correct. 0.96 mm is three times as large as 0.32 mm, the radius for the figures on the table. If the radius is increased by a factor of 3, the area will be increased by a factor of 3^2, or 9. If the area is increased by a factor of 9, then the resistance will be decreased by a factor of 9. (0.9)/9 = 0.01 Ω/m

---

Passage I (Questions 572-576)

572. D is correct. The base reaction for fluorine ion is shown below.

$$F^-(aq) + H_2O(l) \rightarrow HF(aq) + OH^-(aq)$$

The equilibrium constant is found by dividing the concentrations of products by those of reactants. Pure liquids such as H_2O are not included.

573. D is correct. HS^- is amphoteric, which indicates that it may behave as either an acid or a base. To tell whether the solution will be acidic or basic, you need to compare K_a and K_b for HS^-. If K_a is greater, the solution will be acidic and if K_b is greater, the solution will be basic. To find K_a for HS^-, one must employ the K_b for its conjugate S^{2-}.

$$K_a = K_w/K_b = (1 \times 10^{-14})/(7.7 \times 10^{-2}) = \text{about } 1 \times 10^{-12}$$

From the table, K_b for HS^- is 1.8×10^{-7}

As K_b is much larger than K_a and the solution will be basic.

574. C is correct. K^+ is the conjugate of a strong base, so will thus not react in aqueous solution. ClO^- is the conjugate of a weak acid, so it will react to form the acid, producing hydroxide ions as shown below:

$$ClO^-(aq) + H_2O(l) \rightleftharpoons HClO(aq) + OH^-(aq)$$

575. B is correct. The strongest acid will have the lowest pH and the weakest conjugate base. Of the choices listed, HF has the weakest conjugate, F^-. You can tell that F^- is the weakest base as it has the smallest value for K_b.

576. B is correct. For a buffer solution with equal concentrations of an acid and its conjugate base, the pH will be equal to the pK_a. The K_a of $HC_2H_3O_2$ may be calculating using the formula:

$$K_a = K_w/K_b = (1 \times 10^{-14})/(5.6 \times 10^{-10})$$

The pK_a is then found by taking the negative logarithm.

Independent Questions (Questions 577-580)

577. C is correct. For magnetic force, $F = qvB\sin$. The particles have equal and opposite charges, so if they are traveling in the same direction at the same speed, they will experience the same magnitude of force, but in opposite directions.

578. B is correct. pH is equal to $-\log[H^+]$. Because HNO_3 is a strong acid, it dissociates completely, so $[H^+] = 0.015 = 1.5 \times 10^{-2}$. $-\log(1.5 \times 10^{-2})$ is between 1 and 2; choice B is the only option.

579. D is correct. An important property of a buffered solution is that the pH will remain constant when water is added.

580. B is correct. H_2SO_4 is a strong acid and will dissociate completely in solution into H^+ and HSO_4^-, so there will only be a negligible amount of H_2SO_4 in the beaker. HSO_4^- is a weak acid, so it will dissociate to a lesser extent, producing more H^+ ions, so the number of H^+ ions will be slightly greater than the number of HSO_4^- ions, and both of these will be much greater than the number of H_2SO_4 molecules.

Passage I (Questions 581-595)

581. The main purpose of the passage is

A. To institute economic reform in the face of globalization
WRONG: There is no discussion about economic reform and globalization in the passage.

B. To convince the reader to abandon materialism
CORRECT: This is the most plausible of the given choices. The body of the passage mainly consists of various arguments against materialism designed to convince the reader. The final portion of the passage seeks a solution to what the author views as the problem of materialism.

C. To show the inherent flaws in materialism
WRONG: One might have a hard time deciding between this choice and B. However, one must be aware that the question is asking what is main purpose of the passage. The author expounds on the inherent flaws of materialism in order to show that materialism should be abandoned; his purpose in showing the flaws is not simply expository. His intent to persuade the reader can be gleaned from these strong statements and language against materialism, his proposal to abandon materialism (line 49), and his presentation of the benefits of abandoning materialism in the last few sentences of the passage.

D. All of the above
WRONG: This is not the correct answer because A and C are not correct.

582. What factors does the author believe argue against materialism?

A. Politics, psychology, and economics, and morality
WRONG: There is no mention of a political argument against materialism.

B. Psychology, logic, and economics
WRONG: Psychology was never mentioned per say as a factor. Even though some of the arguments would make it seem that there are psychological drawbacks to materialism, psychology was never stated explicitly as a factor. This is not the best answer.

C. Experience, logic, morality, and economics
CORRECT: This is the best answer. Experience, logic, and economics were mentioned at the beginning of the paragraphs, so most likely you would not have missed them. Morality, unlike the other factors, was not mentioned at the beginning of a

paragraph and might have been missed. It is stated as a factor that argues against materialism in line 3.

D. Logic, experience, and economics
WRONG: Though all of these are factors, the moral factor is missing in this choice.

583. What alternative does the author offer to materialism?

A. To accept materialism without reservation so as to break the vicious cycle created by Keynesian and classical economists
WRONG: The author never states that materialism should be accepted. One might get confused with the vicious cycle part that was lifted from lines 45-46, but notice that this has nothing to do the first part of the answer and is there just to throw you off.

B. To leave attachment to material but retain material possessions
CORRECT: This is the best answer. It is clearly found in line 60.

C. To renounce all material objects
WRONG: This answer is only partly correct. Answer B is a better answer.

D. To modify materialism to generate a new construct that is new and distinct yet still related to the original ideation of materialism
WRONG: The author talks about modifying the idea of materialism in the fifth paragraph but he does so in an entirely different context. Modifying the concept of materialism is never offered as a solution.

584. Which of the following most naturally and powerfully strengthens a gap in the argument presented in paragraph 2, "Logic speaks against materialism…" (lines 8-18)?

A. Human desire, like the scope of his determinations of the marginal amount, is infinite.
WRONG: his statement would be out of place in this paragraph. Also, it does not relate to the main idea of the paragraph which is society's inability to define the marginal amount.

B. It is impossible to acquire something that you cannot be defined by society.
WRONG: This is the argument that is already being made. This does not add anything to the already present argument.

C. The magnitude of the marginal amount cannot even be determined individually, as a person's psychological perception of what is satisfying is in constant flux.
CORRECT: This bridges a gap in the argument. Just because society cannot agree on a designation of the marginal quantity does not mean that any

given individual cannot settle on his own determination. For the individual then, the marginal quantity could very well be defined, and the author's argument (see B above) would hence fail. This answer addresses this gap in the author's argument.

D. The argument is well formed and there is no gap in the argument
WRONG: This is not true. See C above.

585. Which of the following is the biggest shortcoming of the argument presented in paragraph 5, "Materialism cannot be corrected..." (lines 42-51),

A. Not expounding on the internal flaws in materialism.
WRONG: This was done in the previous paragraphs.

B. Not addressing the ramifications of gross conceptual modification of materialism as an idea
WRONG: The ramifications were discussed. The author states that if there is a gross modification, then the object of debate would be an entity entirely different from materialism, and thus, beyond the scope of the present debate which is centered on materialism.

C. The structural fallacies proposed by the author were not defined and the possibility of such fallacies not arising was not addressed.
CORRECT: This is the best of the given choices. The author does not elaborate on what the structural fallacies are, and he quite apparently does not discuss what would happen if a slight modification occurred and gave rise to a modified concept of materialism that did not have any structural fallacies (read new inherent flaws). All this while he acknowledges, by implication, that the possibility of such a concept emerging is not impossible (line 53)

D. The argument is sound and has absolutely no shortcomings.
WRONG: This is not the correct answer. See C above.

586. If the government were to institute a new federal program to equally distribute societal resources, the author would most likely respond with

A. Exuberance as it resolves the socioeconomic disparities that the author is primarily occupied with.
WRONG: This is a decent answer choice. However, it is not the best answer as even though the author feels that perpetuation of economic disparities is not moral (lines 2-3), the government's action does not speak directly to the main idea of the passage which is to convince the individual against materialism.

B. Reserved approbation because such a program would not address or resolve the individual attachment to material wealth and acquisition
CORRECT: We can assume that the author would be moderately pleased with this action, since he is not a proponent of economic disparities (lines 1-3). However, as the answer states, the government's action would not resolve the issue of materialism itself and this is the central idea of the passage.

C. Sadness at the materialistic backlash from the bourgeoning class that would inevitably ensue
WRONG: This is answer reaches too far beyond the information provided in the passage.

D. Fear because such a move would diminish the validity of the theory of diminishing marginal utility
WRONG: Such a move does not apparently have anything to do with this theory. They are unrelated. Even if the two were to be related it is unlikely that the author would experience fear in response to the governmental action threatening the theory of diminishing marginal utility.

587. All of the following are examples of an internal flaw of materialism EXCEPT

A. It helps the rich get richer and this is to the severe disadvantage of the impoverished
CORRECT: This is an external consequence of materialism. It is not an example of the implications inherent in the concept of materialism itself. Also, this answer is the one that is most unlike the other answers.

B. Less pleasure is derived with the acquisition of successive material goods, moving one away from the aim of materialism which is to find pleasure in material goods
WRONG: This is an internal flaw because it shows how adopting materialism is self-defeating and leads one away from what materialism purports to offer.

C. Materialism tends to lead one to place greater emphasis on the acquisition of means rather than ends
WRONG: This is an internal flaw because materialism here leads one away from what it seeks to offer (i.e. pleasure/satisfaction). It is self-defeating. This is not a physical consequence of materialism as is A. Rather, it a phenomenon that is by its nature tied to materialism. According to the passage, materialism drives the individual to lose sight of this goal and focus on the means (houses, cars, money) that carry one to this goal rather than the end (pleasure/satisfaction) (lines 28-31).

D. Materialism's nature and goals are difficult constructs to define, making the aims of materialism impossible to acquire

WRONG: This is an internal flaw because, according to the passage, the benefits or goals of materialism cannot be acquired since they cannot be defined. This is something internal to the theoretical construct of materialism itself, not a physical or external consequence of materialism.

Passasge IV (Questions 588-595)

588. Which of the following can be directly ascertained from the passage

   I.   Variability in the amount of *Sabaq* recited depends on teachers' preferences.

   II.   The amount of *Sabaq-e-Para* recited daily depends on the teacher requirements

   III.   Teachers assign varying amounts of *Amukhta* to their students

  A. I and III
     WRONG: Choice I is not correct because the passage indicates that the amount of *Sabaq* a student does depends on the students ability which is not the same as the teacher's preference (lines 4-5).

  B. II only
     WRONG: Choice III is also correct.

  C. II and III
     CORRECT: Both *Sabaq* and *Sabaq-e-Para* are dependent on the teacher's requirements (lines 36-37, lines 39-40).

  D. I, II, and III
     WRONG: Choice I is not correct

589. According to the passage, which of the following is a similarity between *Sabaq-e-Para* and *Amukhta*

  A. Both require a lot of time to memorize and recite
     WRONG: The time required to memorize and recite was never explicitly discussed in the passage.

  B. Both must be completed daily by the beginning memorizer
     WRONG:*Amukhta* is not assigned to a beginning memorizer. It is only after the student finishes his first *Juz* that *Amukhta* is assigned (line 53-55). Also, we know that a beginning student only has two lessons, *Sabaq* and *Sabaq-e-Para*.

  C. Both can potentially require reciting more than one *Juz* depending on the teacher
     WRONG: *Sabaq-e-Para* can never be more than one *Juz* because by definition it is the recitation of previous *Asbaaq* within the current *Juz* that the student is memorizing (lines 45-49).

  D. None of the above
     CORRECT: Since all of the other choices are incorrect, this is the correct answer.

590. "Spot"-tested in line 62 most likely refers to which of the following

  A. Asking the student to recite everything that they have memorized so far
     WRONG: The word "spot" would seem to imply something limited rather than comprehensive such as would be involved in reciting everything one had memorized.

  B. Prompting the student from random points and asking them to recite what comes afterward
     CORRECT: This is the best choice. It includes the concept of limited testing implied by the word "spot" yet would also seem to fulfill the requirements of a formal examination, i.e. test the student's level of mastery in memorization.

  C. Asking the student to recite verses from different *Juz* while looking into the Quran
     WRONG: Reading straight out of the Quran would not fulfill the purpose of testing the student's memorization which would in turn obviate the purpose of formally testing a student who is memorizing the Quran.

  D. Request the student to clean any soilage, discoloration, or spots in their Quran to test their reverence and love for the Quran
     WRONG: Testing a student's reverence is out of context here and has nothing to do with testing the student's memorization which would seem to really be the purpose of formally testing a student who is memorizing the Quran

591. From the passage, one can infer that which of the following characteristics are most integral to the process of memorizing the Quran

  A. Patience and perseverance
     WRONG: This was never mentioned in the passage. One might be tempted to pick this as the whole process of *Tahfeezul Quran* might seem to the reader to require a lot of patience and perseverance. However, this was neither stated nor implied in the text as an integral component of memorizing.

  B. Repetition and revision
     CORRECT: All three of the lessons involve repetition and/or revision making these two entities integral to the process of memorizing the Quran.

  C. A teacher who has high standards for *Amukhta* and *Sabaq-e-Para*
     WRONG: Though the author only mentions that there are different standards for *Sabaq-e-Para* and

Amukhta. He never states that more rigorous standards are integral to memorize the Quran.

D. Ample time
WRONG: This was never mentioned in the passage.

592. Which of the following statements is INCORRECT:

A. *Sabaq-e-Para* may consists of six to nine *Asbaaq* daily
WRONG: This statement is correct (lines 45-48)

B. Final revision of the Quran consists of revising one to ten *Ajzaa* daily
WRONG: This statement is correct (lines 64-66)

C. *Amukhta* consists of one-fourth to two *Ajzaa* daily
WRONG: This statement is correct (lines 57-59)

D. *Sabaq* can never be longer than *Sabaq-e-Para*
CORRECT: This statement is not correct. For example, take a person who just recently started a *Juz* and is about to recite his second *Sabaq*. Further suppose that his or her first *Sabaq* was shorter than his or her second *Sabaq*. In this case, the *Sabaq-e-Para* (the first *Sabaq* of the *Juz*) will be shorter than his *Sabaq* (which is the second *Sabaq* of the *Juz*). This question requires strong control of the concepts laid out in the passage which are likely to be foreign to the reader. The best strategy with such a question is process of elimination. One can know for sure that the other three choices are incorrect leaving this as the only correct answer.

593. Consider a student who has is on his forty-fifth unit of the fifty units that comprise his current *Sabaq*. He usually repeats about eighteen units previous to the unit he is currently memorizing. Based on the information given in the passage, when he finishes the fiftieth unit, which of the following is most likely true about the first thirty-two units of his current *Sabaq*?

A. He will recite twenty seven of the units with the next day's *Sabaq* and the remaining five with today's *Sabaq*
WRONG: This choice is overly complicated and uses twenty-seven (45 minus 18) just to throw the reader off. Nothing in the passage indicates that a student splits his *Sabaq* to be recited over two days.

B. He will revise them with today's *Sabaq-e-Para* after reciting the last eighteen units as *Sabaq*
WRONG: *abaq-e-Para* includes the previous *Asbaaq* of the *Juz* and not the current *Sabaq* of the student (lines 41-43)

C. He will join them to the last eighteen units and see if he can recite them all without looking
CORRECT: This is the process that is discussed in lines 23-27.

D. He will save them to recite them when his *Amukhta* cycles around to include this portion
WRONG: Nothing would indicate this in the passage. *Amukhta* is separate from *Sabaq*.

594. According to the passage, if a teacher only assigns seven *Asbaaq* as *Sabaq-e-Para*, and the student is on the fourteenth *Sabaq* of the *Juz*, then what first becomes of the first seven *Asbaaq* of that *Juz*?

A. They are recited in *Amukhta*
WRONG: Though these passages might eventually be recited in *Amukhta*, this occurs secondary to their recital when one finishes the *Juz*. The question asks what <u>first</u> becomes of the seven *Asbaaq* in question.

B. They are recited once the student finishes the *Juz*
CORRECT: This is the correct answer. Please refer to lines 51-52.

C. They are never recited again because the *Sabaq-e-Para* shifts forward with each *Sabaq*
WRONG: This is not correct. Please refer to lines 49-51. Also, the seven *Asbaaq* would, in fact, be recited again in *Amukhta* as the student proceeds in his memorization.

D. The student must rememorize these as *Sabaq*
WRONG: This was not indicated in the passage.

595. The main theme of the passage would seem to be

A. To show the reader what is required to memorize the Quran
CORRECT: The whole passage is centered on showing one how to memorize the Quran. It outlines the different steps involved and also touches on some issues dealing with evaluation. The tone is more or less expository which is befitting given this theme.

B. To show the reader that memorizing the Quran is a difficult and arduous process
WRONG: Difficulty was not addressed in the passage neither directly nor indirectly. This would be an assumption on the part of the reader.

C. To motivate the reader to memorize the Quran
WRONG: The tone of the passage is more explanatory than persuasive. There are few emotional or loaded words in the passage. Most statements made are matter-of-fact and merely informational in nature.

D. To show the difference between *Sabaq, Sabaq-e-Para,* and *Amukhta*
WRONG: Though, the passage does show the difference between *Sabaq, Sabaq-e-Para,* and *Amukhta*, this is not the primary objective of the passage. The primary objective is to define what

these lessons are so that an individual can understand what is involved and required in memorizing the Quran. Also, the passage includes other things such as testing that do would not fit if the main objective was only to show the difference between *Sabaq*, *Sabaq-e-Para*, and *Amukhta*.

Examination 13: Biological Sciences

Passage V (Questions 596-603)

596. A is correct. Contractility is dependent on cross-bridge formation. Once stretched beyond a certain point, actin and myosin are pulled past each other, and the cross-bridges cannot form. Choices B and C are incorrect because the length of the muscle fiber does not affect the troponin C to calcium ratio or the sympathetic stimulation of the heart. Choice D is incorrect because it is contraction (and not stretch) that causes a decrease in blood flow to the cardiac muscle.

597. C is correct. Increased contractility of the heart muscle causes an increase in stroke volume. Thus, sympathetic stimulation increases stroke volume. Choice A is incorrect because parasympathetic stimulation directly lowers the heart rate and indirectly decreases cardiac contractility. Choice B is incorrect because a decrease in end-diastolic volume lowers stroke volume. Choice D is incorrect because a decrease in the coronary blood flow compromises oxygen delivery to the heart and thus decreases its ability to contract.

598. D is correct. The sarcomere falls between the Z lines. A bands correspond to the full length of the thick filaments, while the H zone corresponds to the region of the think filament which does not overlap with the thin filaments. The I band corresponds to the region of the thin filament that does not overlap with the thick filaments.

599. B is correct. Sympathetic stimulation occurs in a fight-or-flight situation that would require and increase of heart rate. Parasympathetic stimulation occurs in a rest-and-digest environment that would not require a fast heart rate. Therefore, sympathetic stimulation increases heart rate and parasympathetic stimulation decreases heart rate.

600. A is correct. A decrease in intravascular volume results in a decrease in the amount of venous blood returned to the heart. Therefore, the amount of blood in the heart at the end of diastole falls and the cardiac muscle does not stretch as much.

601. D is correct. According to the passage, sympathetic stimulation results in increased calcium concentrations in the myocyte cytoplasm. In muscle cells, the rapid increase in calcium concentration is acheived via calcium release from the sarcoplasmic reticulum. T-tubules are tunnels in the sarcolemma, also known as the myocyte plasma membrane, through which the action potential travels.

602. B is correct. The arterioles are responsible for peripheral vascular resistance. As they contain significant amounts of smooth muscle in the vessel wall, arterioles are a major site for blood pressure regulation. Under the influence of the sympathetic and parasympathetic nervous systems, they constrict and dilate to control the amount of blood that reaches the organs. Choice A is incorrect because arteries have less smooth muscle and are not able to constrict as much as arterioles. Choices C and D are incorrect because veins and venules are capacitance vessels: they act as a reservoir for blood.

603. D is correct. Pacemaker cells are found in the sinoatrial and atrioventricular nodes. Choice A is incorrect because while the vagus nerve modifies heart rate, it is not responsible for the automaticity of the heart. Choice B is incorrect because the bundle of His conducts the action potential but does not initiate it. Choice C is incorrect because papillary muscles are responsible for keeping the tricuspid and mitral valves closed during ventricular contraction.

Passage VI (Questions 604-609)

604. D is correct. Monocytes are the progenitor cells for macrophages.

605. B is correct. Uninhibited cell division is a factor common to many cancers. Cytotoxic T cells respond to and directly destroy infected and/or cancerous cells, whereas Helper T cells respond to pathogens circulating in the blood or lymph. Choices A, C, and D are part of the response to cellular infection. MHC molecules are only cell surface markers.

606. D is correct. Perforin is secreted by cytotoxic T cells. Cytotoxic T cells destroy infected Class I MHC cells.

607. A is correct. According to the passage, Class I MHC molecules are present on all <u>nucleated</u> cells. Mature red blood cells, or erythrocytes, do not have any membrane-bound organelles, including nuclei. Thus, erythrocytes have Class II MHC markers, and would not be affected by the disorder.

608. C is correct. The production of antibodies, according the passage, depends on (1) the antigen fragment forming a complex with the Class II MHC molecule at the cell surface; (2) Helper T cells recognizing the antigen and binding to the MHC molecule; (3) the Helper T cell stimulating B cells to differentiate into plasma cells, which release the antibodies. Cytotoxic T cells and perforin have nothing to do with antibody production.

609. B is correct. People with AB blood present both the A and B antigens on their cell surfaces, which means they must NOT produce antibodies against these antigens. Type O indicates the absence of A or B antigens.

Independent Questions (Questions 610-611)

610. C is correct. Memory B cells differentiate from B lymphocytes in response to a <u>specific</u> antigen. Phagocytosis, stomach acid, and the skin are all examples of nonspecific, or innate, immunity, whereas B lymphocytes are part of humoral, or acquired, immunity.

611. C is correct. Passive immunity refers to immunity in which memory B cells and antibodies are not produced by oneself, but are acquired from an external source. II and III are examples of passive immunity, whereas I is an example of active immunity. Vaccination would be another example of active immunity.

EXPLANATIONS 14

Answers to Questions 612–658

ANSWERS TO EXAMINATION 14

PHYSICAL SCIENCES	VERBAL REASONING	BIOLOGICAL SCIENCES
612. A	628. A	643. C
613. A	629. D	644. B
614. A	630. B	645. A
615. B	631. A	646. C
616. C	632. A	647. C
617. C	633. B	648. A
618. C	634. D	649. D
619. D	635. C	650. D
620. A	636. B	651. C
621. C	637. C	652. B
622. B	638. A	653. A
623. B	639. D	654. C
624. C	640. C	655. B
625. A	641. D	656. D
626. D	642. D	657. B
627. B		658. A

Passage I (Questions 612-616)

612. A is correct. Since input and output power is the same, $I_I V_I = I_O V_O$.

$$I_I(24,000) = (200)(120)$$

$$I_I = (200)(120)/(24,000) = 1 \text{ A}$$

613. A is correct. The relationship is as follows:

$$20,000V = \frac{5000}{3}(12)$$

$$\text{So } \frac{N_I}{N_O} = \frac{5000}{3}$$

614. A is correct. If the input voltage is constant, there is no magnetic field in the iron core, and thus no ouput voltage generated.

615. B is correct. The peak voltage may be found as such:

$$V_{MAX} = V_{RMS}\left(\sqrt{2}\right) = (120)(1.4) = 170 \text{ V}$$

616. C is correct. The changing current in the input loop has the shape of a sine wave, which will be reflected in the magnetic field. When the current reaches a peak or a trough, Lenz's law will force the magnetic field to change direction.

Passage II (Questions 617-624)

617. C is correct. The hydroxide ion accepts a proton in both reactions, which is the function of a Bronsted-Lowry base in both reactions.

618. C is correct. Use the dilution equation.

$$M_1 V_1 = M_2 V_2$$

$$(6\ M)(10 \text{ ml}) = (0.1\ M)V$$

$V = 600$ ml, however the student begins with 10 ml of solution, so the volume of water *added* was 590 ml.

619. D is correct. The pOH of the solution is 1 ($-\log 10^{-1} = 1$), so the pH must be $14 - 1 = 13$.

620. A is correct. Choice A shows the curve for the titration of a strong acid by a strong base. Choice B represents the titration of a weak acid with a strong base.

621. C is correct. A buret should always be rinsed with the titrating solution before starting. Rinsing the buret with anything else will change the concentration of the titrating solution.

622. B is correct. The carbonic acid from the carbon dioxide reaction will neutralize OH^- ions in the solution, so the actual hydroxide ion concentration will be lower than what is expected.

623. B is correct. The number of moles of H^+ must be equal to the number of moles of OH^- added at the equivalence point. Volume must be converted to liters to use the equation:

$$\text{Moles} = MV = (0.105 \text{ moles/L})(0.0244 \text{ L})$$

624. C is correct. The equivalence point for the titration of a strong acid with a strong base is 7. Bromthymol blue is the only choice that includes a pH of 7 in its range for color change.

Independent Questions (Questions 625-627)

625. A is correct. The more resistors added in parallel the smaller the total resistance of the circuit will be. If the total resistance decreases, then the total current must increase to maintain the same voltage.

626. D is correct. Magnetic fields do not exert force on a charged particle traveling parallel to the field lines.

627. B is correct. Using the formula for the energy stored in a capacitor: (the resistor and discharge time are not necessary)

$$E = (1/2) CV^2 = (0.5)(10 \times 10^{-6})(10)^2 = 5 \times 10^{-4} \text{ J}$$

Examination 14: Verbal Reasoning

Passage III (Questions 628-634)

628. Which of the following is the most significantly weakens in the validity of the paradigm expounded upon by the author?

A. The possibility that a bridge might not exist between chemistry and mathematics and between biology and physics was not discussed
CORRECT: The author made the connection between biology and mathematics but failed to demonstrate these other relationships. If a dependence and/or connection does not exist between the respective sciences listed, then the paradigm would be significantly weakened. Without addressing this possibility, there is a gap in the evidence proffered which weakens the credibility of the paradigm.

B. The paradigm does not take language into account
WRONG: Even though this statement is in itself correct, not taking language into account does not weaken the paradigm. Language is not a part of the

paradigm expounded upon in the first two paragraphs, so not taking it into account does not have any affect on the paradigm.

C. The paradigm only takes the hard sciences and mathematics into account

WRONG: This is a true statement, but the fact that only hard sciences and mathematics are taken into account does not weaken the paradigm. It can still be internally valid without taking into account the other sciences.

D. All paradigms must fall on the logical models expressed in lines 38-42

WRONG: This is not a reasonable choice. Nothing in the passage supports this statement. Also, the use of strong words such as, "all" and "must" warrant suspicion that this answer is incorrect.

629. Which of the following statements does NOT directly support the overall theme of the passage?

A. Mathematics is a fundamental way of characterizing reality

WRONG: This statement supports the overall theme of the passage, which is to expound on and support the validity of the paradigm in question. The author accomplishes this by showing how different levels of knowledge are reducible to more basic forms and also by showing the interrelation between the different sciences. This answer choice supports the above theme, as mathematics is referred to as the most fundamental form of knowledge. Mathematics is also seen as having the capacity to explain all the phenomena that exist the other sciences (lines 20-21).

B. Different sciences yield knowledge of reality at differing levels of perception and depth.

WRONG: This statement supports the overall theme of the passage, which is to expound on and support the validity of the paradigm. The author accomplishes this by showing how different levels of knowledge are reducible to more basic forms and also by showing the interrelation between the different sciences. This answer choice corroborates the above theme, as the paradigm would not exist if there were no difference in the levels of knowledge acquired through the different sciences. Without a differential, there can be no discussion of reducibility.

C. Despite possible shortcomings, the paradigm set out in the passage is reasonably valid.

WRONG: This statement supports the overall theme of the passage, which is to expound on and support the validity of the paradigm. The author accomplishes this by showing how different levels of knowledge are reducible to more basic forms and also by showing the interrelation between the

different sciences. This answer choice supports the above theme because it highlights the validity of the paradigm.

D. Chemistry characterizes the realm of elemental reactions and interactions.

CORRECT: This is an informational statement. It does not do anything to directly support or expound on the paradigm or support its validity.

630. In lines 73-75, the author implies that there is a need for further research. Which of the following would best address this need?

A. Explaining chemistry in terms of mathematics

WRONG: The need for further research is to see whether or not the forms of knowledge included in the western theory of knowledge but not included in the paradigm can be reduced and explained by more fundamental sciences. Chemistry and mathematics are already included in the paradigm.

B. Explaining psychology in terms of biology

CORRECT: The need for further research is to see whether or not the forms of knowledge included in the western theory of knowledge but not included in the paradigm can be reduced and explained by more fundamental sciences. Psychology is not included in the paradigm and biology, according the western theory of knowledge, is more fundamental than psychology. This would address the research need set out in lines 67-70.

C. Explaining language in terms of metaphor theory

WRONG: The need for further research is to see whether or not the forms of knowledge included in the western theory of knowledge but not included in the paradigm can be reduced and explained by more fundamental sciences. This would not address the research need because it does not explain language using a more fundamental science. Also, the passage never really discusses anything termed metaphor theory.

D. Explaining the hard sciences in terms of soft sciences.

WRONG: The need for further research is to see whether or not the forms of knowledge included in the western theory of knowledge but not included in the paradigm can be reduced and explained by more fundamental sciences. This does not address this need because it does not explain the hard sciences using a more fundamental science. In fact the soft sciences are, as per the western theory of knowledge, less precise than the hard sciences. Also, the hard sciences are already addressed by the paradigm so the research need set out in lines 65-68 would not be met by this choice.

631. The paradigm designated in the passage and the Western theory of knowledge are similar in that

    A.   Both place an emphasis on mathematics as a precise way of knowing
            CORRECT: Both models emphasize the primacy of mathematics (lines 28-29, 63-65)

    B.   Both acknowledge that there is ultimately no difference between the different sciences.
            WRONG: In fact, the opposite is true. Both models are predicated on the differential accuracies of various sciences as methods to know reality (lines 1-20, 44-49).

    C.   Both agree that language is more comprehensive in its scope than either chemistry or physics
            WRONG: Neither theory states that language is more comprehensive. In fact, language is not even included in the paradigm.

    D.   Both are diametrically opposed to the Eastern theory of knowledge.
            WRONG: The Eastern theory of knowledge is never discussed in the passage, so one cannot make any comparison between it on one side and the western theory of knowledge and paradigm on the other.

632. Removing which of the following statements would least affect the overall coherence and stability of the passage?

    A.   "the above paradigm cannot fall on the logical model: $A=B$, and $B=C$; therefore $A=C$. The equal signs in the previous paradigm are weak if not lacking (lines 38-40)
            CORRECT: The next part of the paragraph addresses a similar idea or concept. Therefore, if this section were removed there would be little effect on the passage as a whole.

    B.   "Biology involves the study of life. Life is, in turn, comprised of matter that must fundamentally be in some state of motion" (lines 47-49)
            WRONG: This statement is important. The author is able to explain biology in terms of mathematics by first simplifying all of biology to two entities (matter and motion) and then using mathematics to characterize those entities. If this statement were removed this whole argument would be undermined.

    C.   "such an approach obscures the possible lack of dependency between types of sciences …more than level removed"(lines 32-34)
            WRONG: This statement gives the main idea of the second paragraph. Removing it would have a significant effect on the passage as a whole.

    D.   "The paradigm concurs with the Western theory of knowledge" (line 59)

            WRONG: This is integral to the theme of the passage as it adds credibility and validation to the paradigm. Removing it would affect the passage as a whole.

633. Suppose that the author of the passage was hired as a curriculum director for a local high school. He would like the practically institute his paradigm in the curriculum. Which of the curriculum changes would be most closely be instituted?

    A.   Tripling class time given to the instruction of mathematics at the expense of other science classes
            WRONG: Even though the author sees mathematics as the most fundamental science, he never indicates the other sciences are completely unimportant. Such a curriculum would drastically devalue the other sciences. Also the first sentence stating that science is interrelated seems to show that in fact there is a need to study the other sciences (line 1).

    B.   Developing a more integrated scientific curriculum
            CORRECT: This underscores one of the major themes of the passage which is to show the interrelation between the different sciences. This is clearly expressed in line 1.

    C.   Halving class time devoted to the soft sciences
            WRONG: The soft sciences are not included in the paradigm.

    D.   Replacing biology and chemistry with physics
            WRONG: This move is too drastic. The author never mitigates or downplays the importance of any of the sciences in the course of the passage. He simply states that some sciences can be explained in terms of other more fundamental sciences. This choice is clearly NOT the best answer.

634. From the passage, we can most correctly infer that the author is

    A.   A theist arguing the existence of God based on the intelligent design of reality
            WRONG: Just because the author indicates that there is a mathematical order to reality does not make him a theist advancing arguments for the existence of God. This is too big a jump.

    B.   A PhD in mathematics from MIT
            WRONG: Just because the author places emphasis on mathematics does not imply that he is a mathematician. This is too distant of an inference to make.

    C.   A humanities professor at Columbia University
            WRONG: Nothing overtly indicates this in the passage.

D. There is insufficient textual evidence to make this determination

CORRECT: There were not enough clues in the passage to determine the identity of the author. The passage mostly concentrated on explaining and validating the paradigm set up in the first few lines.

Passage IV (Questions 635-642)

635. Which of the following statement would best support the central theme of the passage?

A. The complexities involved with the word 'until' are best illustration of certain modes of complex expression

WRONG: The whole discussion of the scholarly opinion concerning the interpretation of the word until was only an example. It is never stated as the best example of the sophistication involved in certain modes of complex expression such as formal argumentative writing. Therefore, this statement does not support the main idea.

B. Everyday talk may be loose but can become sophisticated if the mode of legal expression is used in conversation.

WRONG: Even though this is possible, it does not support the central theme of trying to get the reader to appreciate the subtle and complex issues involved in complex modes of expression.

C. Legal and formal argumentative modes of expression are inherently complex and highly sophisticated.

CORRECT: The passage is trying to get the reader to appreciate the subtle and complex issues involved in complex modes of expression. This choice is congruent with this purpose.

D. Agreement on the "rules" of establishing meaning adds to the complex subtleties of legal and formal argumentative expression

WRONG: This statement is not correct. In fact, the opposite is true (lines 31-34). If the statement is incorrect, it cannot support the central theme.

636. According the scholarly opinion given in the passage (lines 19-29), which answer choice would be most true regarding the statement: The book may be kept without a fine until tomorrow.

A. Tomorrow may or may not be included as a limit for keeping the book without a fine.

WRONG: This is incorrect because in the default situation (as applies to the given statement), the limit (tomorrow) is included in the scope of the primary statement/injunction (The book can be kept

without a fine). There is no ambiguity as to whether or not to include the limit.

B. The book may be kept until the end of tomorrow without having to give a fine.

CORRECT: This is correct because in the default situation (as applies to the given statement), the limit (tomorrow) is included in the scope of the primary statement/injunction (The book can be kept without a fine). We know that the default interpretation applies because both of the two conditions set out in lines 46-49 are met. Also there is no direct or indirect indication that the limit is not to be included.

C. The statement cannot be assessed according to the framework set up in the passage

WRONG: The passage gives ample information to make this determination. The book may be kept until the end of tomorrow without having to give a fine. This is because in the default situation (as applies to the given statement), the limit (tomorrow) is included in the scope of the primary statement/injunction (The book can be kept without a fine). See also b above.

D. Tomorrow is included in the period exempt from a fine, but the specific time tomorrow is unspecified

WRONG: The passage indicates that the entire limit (tomorrow in this case) is included in the scope of a primary statement/injunction (The book may be kept without a fine in this case) given that we are dealing with the default interpretive case (line 42).

637. Which of the following statements would not result in the default interpretation of the word 'until'?

A. Speak to the audience until nine o' clock

WRONG: This would result in the default interpretation. The limit is an appropriate time symbol and the primary statement/injunction (speaking) has the capacity to be extended. Also there is no direct or indirect indication that the limit is not to be included.

B. The house lease will continue until August 23

WRONG: This would result in the default interpretation. The limit is an appropriate time symbol and the primary statement/injunction (leasing a house) is an action that has the capacity to be extended. Also there is no direct or indirect indication that the limit is not to be included.

C. The money must be returned until the bank is satisfied*

CORRECT: This would not result in the default interpretation. The limit is not an appropriate time or space symbol. Rather it is a state. The primary statement/injunction does not have the capacity to be extended (returning in an instantaneous action). The two conditions are not met so the default interpretation will not apply. Instead, it will be read to mean that the money must be returned *in order that* the bank be satisfied.

D. The new property line continues until the red flag
WRONG: This would result in the default interpretation. The limit is an appropriate spatial marker and the primary statement/injunction (property line) has the capacity to be extended. Also there is no direct or indirect indication that the limit is not to be included.

638. If someone were to argue that the technicalities and rules mentioned in the passage are superfluous and merely an intellectual exercise, the author would most likely respond:

A. By stating that such a complex framework is necessary to resolve court cases
CORRECT: If there are no rules to establish meaning, almost anything can be twisted to mean something else. The author states that establishing meanings are necessary in order to be able to settle on a verdict or achieve closure in a debate (lines 30-33).

B. By agreeing with the objector
WRONG: The author would not agree with the objector because he feels that the rules are necessary to establish meanings for given utterances (lines 30-33).

C. By recapitulating the sophistication of legal and formal argumentative expression
WRONG: This would not convince the objector nor would it strengthen the author's stance.

D. Inventing a new and innovative argument to justify the convolution found in legal texts.
WRONG: The author would not need to advance new arguments since he already makes one in lines 30-33. Also, the author would not agree to the assertion that legal texts are convoluted given that he sees the necessity of sophistication in legal modes of expression.

639. If you were to discover that the "scholarly opinion" indicated in lines 36-51 was actually the result of a series of leisurely, philosophical discussions that the pharmacist author had with his programmer friend, how would the credibility of the passage's thesis be affected?

A. The credibility of the thesis would remain unchanged
WRONG: The credibility would be affected. See D below.

B. It would strengthen the credibility of the thesis because it shows the intellectual prowess of the author.
WRONG: The thesis of the passage is that legal and formal argumentative exposition is highly complex and sophisticated. The author's intellectual prowess has no bearing on this complexity and sophistication.

C. It would weaken the credibility of the thesis because it would show that the author was dishonest in stating the opinion was a scholarly one.
WRONG: The credibility of the thesis is not directly based, in this passage, on the credibility or trustworthiness of the author. Rather, its credibility is based on the ideas advanced to support it.

D. It would weaken the credibility of the thesis because there would be no expert evidence to show that legal and argumentative expression is a sophisticated process
CORRECT: The credibility of the thesis is directly based, in this passage, on the ideas advanced to support it. The whole 'until' discussion forms one of the major pieces of evidence to support the thesis that that legal and formal argumentative exposition is highly complex and sophisticated. If the "scholarly" opinion is in fact not scholarly, then this damages one of the main pieces of supporting evidences for the thesis and thus damages its credibility. This weakening of the thesis is due to the lack of scholarly evidence to support the thesis not the dishonesty involved in presenting unscholarly opinion as an academic one.

640. According to the passage, which of the following components usually found in legal documents might be lacking in casual conversation?

I. Careful word choice

II. Consideration of how the listener may understand what is being said

III. Circuitous word usage

A. I only
WRONG: Choice II is also correct.

B. II only
WRONG: Choice I is also correct.

C. I and II *
CORRECT: In the first paragraph, the author explains these factors as lacking in ordinary conversation. He then states that they are found in "legal writing and formal argumentation" (lines 4-9).

D. I, II, and III
WRONG: Choice III is incorrect. This is not supported by the passage.

641. If a grammarian were to offer an alternative framework for interpreting the word 'until' the author would likely react by:

A. Defending the framework given in the passage
WRONG: The author would only be driven to defend himself if a situation arose that was counter to his viewpoint. The offering of an alternative framework for interpreting the word 'until' does not create such a situation because the author acknowledges and accepts that one of the complexities of legal and argumentative modes of expression is that there is disagreement when it comes to setting rules for establishing meaning (lines 61-65).

B. Accepting the alternative framework in place of the framework expounded upon in the passage in lines 36-51
WRONG: The author acknowledges, accepts, and even asserts that there is a plurality of rule systems possible when it comes to legal and argumentative modes of expression (lines 61-65). Replacing one framework with another would negate this assertion and the author's appreciation of plurality.

C. Rejecting the alternative framework since there is a need to set an assigned meaning
WRONG: The author acknowledges, accepts, and even asserts that there is a plurality of rule systems possible when it comes to legal and argumentative modes of expression (lines 61-65). Rejecting one framework with another would negate this assertion and appreciation of plurality.

D. Regarding the alternative framework as a manifestation of the complexity involved in language expression
CORRECT: The author acknowledges, accepts, and even asserts that there is a plurality of rule systems possible when it comes to legal and argumentative modes of expression (lines 44-48). This plurality exemplifies the complexities of legal and argumentative modes of expression which is the major theme of the passage.

642. According to the passage, under which of the following conditions would the author most likely argue that a verbal agreement is unambiguous?

A. There is an audio recording of the agreement.
WRONG: Recording ambiguously worded speech will not reduce the ambiguity.

B. There is a video recording of the agreement.
WRONG: Video taping speakers of ambiguously worded speech will not reduce the ambiguity.

C. The exact words used by the agreeing parties is written down as they are spoken.
WRONG: Writing down ambiguously worded speech will not reduce the ambiguity.

D. The wording of the agreement was carefully prepared by both parties.
CORRECT: The whole point of the passage is about the ambiguity of speech because it not carefully crafted with precise meaning. Choice D addresses this problem.

Examination 14: Biological Sciences

Passage V (Questions 643-649)

643. **C is correct.** The acid chloride will work in place of the anhydride to provide the electrophile for the hydroxy nucleophile. It is the only reagent listed that has a carbonyl.

644. **B is correct.** Based on the chromatograms cholesterol has a smaller R_f value. As the reaction proceeds, the amount of reactant will decrease as the amount of product increases. This relationship will be demonstrated on the chromatograms. Cholesterol forms the lowermost spot on the chromatograms, and thus has a smaller R_f value.

645. **A is correct.** According to the passage, the chromatographic spots were demarcated under UV visualization. Cholesteryl acetate must absorb UV light in order to have been demarcated.

646. **C is correct.** Both cholesterol and cholesteryl acetate are more soluble in ether than water. The chromatograms contain two spots, indicating that both are present.

647. **C is correct.** Cholesterol and Cholesteryl acetate are not separated in the experiment. Both must be present in order to appear on the chromatograms. Acetic acid is produced from the anhydride as a byproduct of the reaction. A Sodium hydroxide wash is used to remove the acetic acid.

648. **A is correct.** Increasing the amount of the most polar solvent will increase the R_f value of both cholesterol and cholesteryl acetate. as ether is more polar than hexane, answer choic A is correct.

649. **D is correct.** Compounds that appear as separate spots on thin layer chromatography may also be separated by column chromatography. Distillation works for non-solid compoundts. Both compounds will extract in ether, as well as similar solvents. Recrystallization is not the best option as solubilites of the two compounds is quite similar.

650. **D is correct.** The Hydrogen atoms bonded to chemically equivalent Carbons will also be chemically equivalent, and thus have the same field strength (ppm) on NMR spectroscopy. Answer B is true, however, examination of peak integrations reveals that all hydrogens are accounted for.

651. **C is correct.** The integration of peak 5 indicates the presence of two hydrogens, while the splitting reveals 2 neighboring Hydrogens. The Carbons labeled *e* and *d* are the only Carbons with 2 Hydrogens, however, Carbon *d* has 3 neighboring Hydrogens. Furthermore, the chemical shift indicates that Carbon *e* is closer to an electronegative atom.

652. **B is correct.** Peak 4 is farther downfield, and thus less shielded.

653. **A is correct.** A peak at 0 ppm is TMS the reference.

654. **C is correct.** Peak 4 represents Carbon *g*, which is part of the methoxy group only present in the product.

655. **B is correct.** Isoamyl acetate's ester is the most feasible functional group to follow product formation. The carbonyl stretch for the ester group would be in the 1680 -1740 cm^{-1}.

656. **D is correct.** Peak 2 is a quartet, indicating the presence of 3 neighboring Hydrogens. Recall the "Splitting rule": the splitting of a peak is found by $n+1$, where n represents the number of neighboring hydrogens.

657. **B is correct.** IR spectroscopy is based on the vibration of polar covalent bonds only.

658. **A is correct.** 1,3-butadiene is a conjugated system while 1,4-butadiene is isolated. Thus 1,3-butadiene will absorb longer wavelengths of UV radiation.

EXPLANATIONS 15

Answers to Questions 659–705

ANSWERS TO EXAMINATION 15

Physical Sciences	Verbal Reasoning	Biological Sciences
659. B	675. D	690. B
660. D	676. B	691. C
661. A	677. A	692. B
662. C	678. D	693. D
663. B	679. A	694. D
664. D	680. B	695. D
665. B	681. A	696. C
666. C	682. A	697. B
667. D	683. A	698. D
668. D	684. C	699. B
669. A	685. D	700. B
670. D	686. B	701. C
671. C	687. A	702. B
672. D	688. B	703. C
673. A	689. D	704. A
674. D		705. A

Passage I (Questions 659-664)

659. B is correct. The passage states that a reflected wave has a phase change of 180°, as shown in choice B. Choice A does not demonstrate a phase change and choices C and D represent refracted waves, instead of reflected waves.

660. D is correct. The speed of light in the glass is equal to $c/n = (3 \times 10^8)/(1.5) = 2 \times 10^8$. Keep in mind that the light is traveling 1200 nm, not 600, since it passes back through the glass. Using the equation $t = d/v$:

$$t = d/v = (1200 \times 10^{-9})/(2 \times 10^8) =$$
$$600 \times 10^{-17} = 6 \times 10^{-15} \text{ sec.}$$

661. A is correct. Using the equation $2nd = m\lambda$, n = 1.5 and $\lambda = 750$ nm.

$$3d = 750m$$

None of the answer choices correspond to an m of 0 or 1. When $m = 2$, d can be equal to 500 nm.

662. C is correct. When light passes into a medium with a lower index of refraction, its speed decreases and its frequency remains the same. In order for the wave equation $v = \lambda f$, to be satisfied, λ must decrease when v decreases.

663. B is correct. The angle of reflection from a surface is equal to the angle of incidence. When moving into a medium with a greater index of refraction, light is bent towards the normal, so the angle of refraction must be less than 12°, and choice B is the only option available.

664. D is correct. Constructive interference occurs only when the peaks and troughs of the two waves line up perfectly. In other words, there can be no difference in the phases of the two waves.

Passage II (Questions 665-670)

665. B is correct. First, balance the electrons by multiplying the top equation by 3 and the bottom equation by 4. Then add them and cancel the electrons.

$$4 \text{ Al}^{3+} + 6 \text{ O}^{2-} + 3 \text{ C} \rightarrow 4 \text{ Al} + 3 \text{ CO}_2$$

$(4 \text{ Al}^{3+} + 6 \text{ O}^{2-})$ can be combined to form $2 \text{ Al}_2\text{O}_3$

666. C is correct. A reaction taking place in an electrolytic cell must be non-spontaneous as voltage is required to move the reaction forward. The free-energy change is always positive for a non-spontaneous reaction.

667. D is correct. Both Al^{3+} and Na^+ ions are present in the chamber. In order for Al^{3+} to be reduced to Al, it must have a greater reduction potential than Na^+. Otherwise, Na^+ would be reduced to Na instead.

668. D is correct. Al^{3+} gains electrons, so it is reduced (GER). C loses electrons, so it is oxidized (LEO). O^{2-} keeps the same oxidation state during the process, so it is neither oxidized nor reduced.

669. A is correct. Carbon dioxide gas bubbles appear when carbon combines with oxygen, Carbon changes its oxidation state from 0 to +4. Since it loses electrons, it is being oxidized. One may employ the mnemonic device, ANOX REDCAT, to associate oxidation with the anode.

670. D is correct. Use dimensional analysis.

$$\left(\frac{5 \text{ mol e}^-}{1}\right)\left(\frac{1 \text{ mol Al}}{3 \text{ mol e}^-}\right)\left(\frac{27 \text{ g Al}}{1 \text{ mol Al}}\right) = 45 \text{ g Al}$$

Independent Questions (Questions 671-674)

671. C is correct. An object placed outside the focal length of a concave mirror will form a real image. The lens equation yields:

$$\frac{1}{f} = \frac{1}{d_o} + \frac{1}{d_i}$$
$$\frac{1}{8} = \frac{1}{12} + \frac{1}{d_i}$$
$$d_i = 24 \text{ cm}$$

Since the image distance is larger than the object distance, the magnification will be greater than 1 and the image will be larger than the object.

672. D is correct. Lens B is more curved, so is has a smaller radius of curvature and a smaller focal length. As power is the reciprocal of focal length, smaller focal length indicates greater power.

673. A is correct. By reversing the sign of the potential for the silver half-reaction and then adding the two potentials together: $(-0.80 \text{ V}) + (-0.76 \text{ V}) = -1.56 \text{ V}$. Coefficients are not considered in the calculation of potentials for redox reactions.

674. D is correct. The equilibrium constant does not change when the concentrations of the reactants are changed. The increase in voltage is supported by the Nernst equation and LeChatelier' principle.

Passage III (Questions 675-681)

675. Which of the following statements would most completely depict the author's belief about the relationship between life and art?

A. social and historical context shape the art produced in that era

WRONG: Even though this statement in itself is true, it is not the most complete answer. It does not take into account the effect that art has on society.

B. Art influences the social environment in which it exists

WRONG: Even though this statement in itself is true, it is not the most complete answer. It does not take into account the effect that the societal milieu in which a work is produced has on that work.

C. There is no interaction between life and art

WRONG: This is not correct. The author does believe that there is an interaction between life and art. This is the main idea behind the first paragraph of the passage (lines 19-22).

D. Life and art influence each other

CORRECT: This is the most complete answer. It takes into account how the socio-historic context in which a piece of art is produced is influenced by its context, as well as, how the piece of art influences and shapes that same context. This answer choice is most consistent with the passage (lines 19-22), which indicates that a two-way interaction exists.

676. The criticism published in the *Endinburgh Magazine and Literary Miscellany is* most likely dated:

A. 1859

WRONG: This was never stated in the passage.

B. 1818

CORRECT: It is stated in line 20 that this criticism was penned in the same year that *Frankenstein* was written. In line 1, the author reveals that Frankenstein was written in the year 1818.

C. Late nineteenth century

WRONG: This was never stated in the passage.

D. There is not enough information to ascertain the date

WRONG: There is enough information. See B above.

677. Which of the following types of thematic literature would be most readily accepted, and thus most popular, if published in 1820?

A. A controversial horror novel

CORRECT: This is the best answer. We are told in the passage that the readership at this time was "demanding more and more exciting material in the fictional pieces that they read" (lines 33-34). This answer is the most "exciting" of the answer choices given. To answer this question, one needs to keep in mind that the first criticism was written in the same year that Frankenstein was published, 1818. THe second paragraph reveals the nature of the readership during this time period.

B. An analysis of the Industrial Revolution

WRONG: This would likely not be the most popular book during this time period. The readership during this time period was looking for more and more exciting material. This genre would not fit this profile.

C. A run-of-the-mill romantic love story

WRONG: One might be tempted to choose this answer. However, one should make careful note of the modifier "run-of-the-mill" in the answer choice. A mundane novel would probably not appeal to the readership as much as a something that is controversial (choice A), since the readership was looking for something different and exciting (lines 33-34).

D. A novel promoting atheism

WRONG: Even though a piece like this would be highly controversial, on the basis of the passage, it is too controversial. The author states that the social milieu at the time is more religious and orthodox than it is in contemporary society. God as a controversial topic is mentioned again in the first criticism (lines 29-31). It follows that a novel regarding complete rejection of God would not be so readily accepted.

678. Which of the following INCORRECTLY pairs a criticism with its perspective on Frankenstein

A. *Endinburgh Magazine and Literary Miscellany-* marginally heretic

WRONG: Marginally heretic is an accurate representation of the stance that *Endinburgh Magazine and Literary Miscellany* took toward Frankenstein. In lines 30-31, the author states that the "attribution of the ability to create to anyone other than God did in fact border on impiety" during this era. We would say that the criticism only considered it marginally heretic because it excused some of the controversial nature of the book in light of the changing perceptions and demands of the readership (lines 35-37).

B. Elizabeth Nitche- overly expressive syntax
WRONG: This is an accurate pairing. Nitche sees Shelly writing style as "grandiloquent" (line 40).

C. Goldberg- social commentary
WRONG: This is a correct pairing. Goldberg sees the theme of isolation in Frankenstein as Shelly's commentary on society as oppose to an expression of her own personal isolation (lines 50-52).

D. Kingsley Amis- futuristic science fiction
CORRECT: This is an inaccurate pairing. Amis simply studies the way that ideas expressed in Frankenstein have impacted and influenced future works (lines 56-58). There is no indication that Shelly wrote the novel as a prediction of the future.

679. Given only the information in the passage, the first two criticisms are most alike in that they :

A. Give attention to the style in which Frankenstein was written
CORRECT: Both criticisms do this. The first criticism "acknowledges the "beauty and power" of Shelly's writing" (line 26). The second criticism criticizes Mary Shelly for her "grandiloquent style" (lines 39-40).

B. Analyze the future ramifications Frankenstein on other literature
WRONG: Only the last criticism does this (lines 58-61).

C. Critique Shelly for her shortcomings as a writer
WRONG: Only the second criticism critiques Shelly for her shortcomings as a writer. The first criticism rather applauds Shelly as a writer by acknowledging the "beauty and power" of Shelly's writing" (line 26).

D. Analyze the coherence of Shelly's ideas expressed in Frankenstein.
WRONG: Neither of the criticisms looks at the coherence of Shelly's ideas in Frankenstein. This is simply not stated or implied in the passage.

680. The criticism written by Elizabeth Nitche was most likely published during which time period?

A. 1800-1815
WRONG: This cannot be the correct answer because it would require that the criticism be written even before Frankenstein was published in 1818.

B. 1945-1960
CORRECT: The author presents us with criticisms in chronological order. We are given time periods for all the criticisms except for the second. The first criticism was done in 1818 (line 1). The third criticism was done in 1959 (line 46). The last one, even though we are not given a specific date, is the more recent than any of the other criticisms. This indicates that we are being chronologically presented with different criticisms of Frankenstein, perhaps to have the reader appreciate the changing responses to *Frankenstein* over time. In any case, we can infer that the second criticism was written between the first and third criticisms in the passage roughly placing it in the time period of 1819 to 1959. This makes B the only consistent answer choice.

C. 1970-1985
WRONG: This would be too recent, as it would likely post-date even the third criticism.

D. The time period cannot be inferred from the given information
WRONG: We can infer the time period from the passage because, as the criticisms are presented in chronological order. See B above.

681. In the above passage, the word "criticism" most closely refers to which of the following?

A. Scholarly Analysis and study
CORRECT: Criticism is not being used in the literal sense. This is best exemplified by the last criticism that does not extend any criticism or reproach to Shelly herself or *Frankenstein*. All the criticisms have in common the fact that they all analyze various aspects of Frankenstein academically.

B. Effort to uncover the shortcomings in Shelly's Frankenstein
WRONG: This is not the best answer. Even though some of the criticism may uncover some of Shelly's shortcomings, "criticism" is not being used in the literal sense in this passage. This is best exemplified by the last criticism that does not extend any criticism or reproach to Shelly herself or Frankenstein.

C. Thematic commentary
WRONG: This is not the best answer. Though some criticisms, such as the third, do examine the themes in Frankenstein, it is not necessary that a "criticism," as used in the passage, is limited to thematic analysis.

D. Disapproval and disparagement of Shelly for her inclusion of "impious" content
WRONG: This is not the sense in which the word is being used in the passage. This answer choice is only characteristic of the first criticism.

682. Suppose Shelly had written another book about a scientist cloning a human being. Based upon the passage, which of the following might object to this book on moral grounds?

I. Endinburgh Magazine and Literary Miscellany

II. Elizabeth Nitche

III. M.A. Goldberg

IV. Kingsley Amis

A. I only
   CORRECT: The passage says that they criticism of Frankenstein for impious material mentioning specifically the attribution of the ability to create life to someone other than God.

B. IV only
   WRONG: The Kingsley discussion doesn't present Kingley's opinion on artificial creation or the need to take moral responsibility. It only says that Frankenstein brings those topics up as issues.

C. I and IV only
   WRONG see choice B

D. I, II, III, and IV
   WRONG see choice B

Passage IV (Questions 683-689)

683. Given the information in the passage, which of the following would be most plausible to infer about *The Issa Valley*?

A. It is loaded with bright, colorful, and detailed imagery of lakes and forests
   CORRECT: This is best answer. In lines 66-67, the author of the passage states that *The Issa Valley* is "filled with rich, beautiful descriptions of nature."

B. It is loaded with crass, obscene anathemas hurled at Christendom
   WRONG: There is nothing to indicate this in the passage. Milosz's approach involves a sophisticated commentary on Christianity and what he views as its discrepancies (lines 39-41). His approach seems analytical (lines 3-7) as oppose to crassly deprecatory and disparaging.

C. It is filled with praise and justification for pagan practices
   WRONG: The passage indicates that Milosz's view of paganism is, if anything, neutral (lines 56-59)

D. It includes themes of coming to terms with the unpredictable nature of the world
   WRONG: This answer is unrelated to the passage. The unpredictability of the natural world is not an issue that is stated or implied in the passage.

684. According to the passage, which of the following locales would Czeslaw Milosz most prefer?

A. The capital city of Lithuania
   WRONG: Just because the story takes place in Lithuania does not provide sufficient support for this answer. Also, the capital city would be very urban and this is diametrically opposed to the rural life of nature that the author clearly prefers (lines 67-69).

B. Vatican City
   WRONG: Both the urban nature and the Christian association of this city would point one away from this answer as both are entities that the author does not prefer (lines 29-31, 68-69)

C. Walden Pond
   CORRECT: Even though one may not be familiar with Thoreau and his retreat to Walden Pond, the word "Pond" should indicate a natural setting. Given Milosz's preference for nature, this is the best choice (line 67-69).

D. The comfort of his own home
   WRONG: This answer choice is too vague. We are never told where Milosz's home is nor are we ever given enough information such that would strongly imply that he has a preference to stay home.

685. According to the passage, Christianity and paganism are most similar in that

A. Their constituents are hypocrites
   WRONG: Pagans are never labeled as hypocrites in the passage.

B. They give birth to many legends and myths
   WRONG: According to the passage, this would only true of pagan religion (lines 54-56).

C. They make superordinary the mundane existence of everyday Lithuanian life
   WRONG: According to the passage, this would only true of pagan religion (line 59-60).

D. They offer their constituents a way to make sense of and/or deal with the world
   CORRECT: This is the best answer. Paganism, as stated in the passage, is "just one mode amongst many in which man tries to make sense of the world around him" (lines 61-63). This understanding would provide a framework for them as to how to act and deal with the world. The purposes that Christianity serves, as outlined in lines 36-38 indicate that Christianity is largely a theoretical framework that allows individuals to react to different life situations and "deal" with the world.

686. If one had to predict based on the information given in the passage, Thomas might most likely grow up to be a:

A. Political revolutionary
   WRONG: Even though Thomas grew up in the

tutelage of Joseph the Black, a nationalist revolutionary, this exposure lead, according to the passage, to an enduring hate for hypocrisy (lines 14-16). There is nothing in the passage to indicate Thomas's revolutionary leanings.

B. Recluse in the forest
CORRECT: This would be consistent with the main theme in the book which emphasizes most the importance of nature (line 67-69). Also, we are told that Nature is Thomas's reprieve (lines 72-73)

C. Protestant priest
WRONG: With the book's critical view of Christianity and Thomas's scorn for the religion's constituents, this would not be a likely choice. Inferring that Milosz's criticism is confined to Catholicism is not indicated in the passage and would require reading too far into the question and the passage.

D. Painter
WRONG: There is no evidence in the passage to point the reader toward this choice. Thomas's artistic abilities are never discussed in the passage.

687. If Milosz were to discover that he had erred in his perception of the hypocrisy of Christians, how might his view change?

A. His antagonistic views would only be slightly softened
CORRECT: Milosz's antagonism toward Christianity is based not only on what he views as the hypocrisy of its constituents but also what he deems as the "many failings, shortcomings, and discrepancies <u>in the religion itself</u>" (lines 40-41). Thus, his stance is not likely to change that drastically.

B. He would hold a neutral view of Christianity
WRONG: Milosz would still likely hold an antagonistic stance toward Christianity. This is because Milosz's antagonism toward Christianity is based not only on what he views as the hypocrisy of its constituents but also what he deems as the "many failings, shortcomings, and discrepancies <u>in the religion itself</u>" (lines 40-41).

C. He would become a weak proponent of the Christian faith
WRONG: The passage would indicate otherwise. Milosz's antagonism toward Christianity is based not only on what he views as the hypocrisy of its constituents but also what he deems as the "many failings, shortcomings, and discrepancies <u>in the religion itself</u>" (lines 40-41). With this view, he would be unlikely to be a proponent of the Christian faith.

D. His views would remain unchanged

WRONG: This is not the correct answer because Milosz's antagonistic stance toward Christianity is based on two premises: 1. the hypocrisy of its constituents and 2. the shortcomings of the religion itself (lines 40-41). If one of these premises were proved false, then it is unlikely that his stance would remain entirely unchanged.

688. In which way does Thomas feel that accepting Christ as his savior is hypocritical ?

A. It is tantamount to not taking responsibility for one's actions
WRONG: This is not the reasoning given in the passage. Thomas does feel that he is responsible for his own actions, but denying this responsibility could hardly be characterized as hypocrisy. What Thomas views as hypocritical is not being true to his own belief (lines 21-23). It is hypocritical to him to believe one thing and live otherwise.

B. It goes against his personal belief system
CORRECT: This is the best answer. Thomas views not being true to his own beliefs as being hypocritical. Hypocrisy to him is to believe one thing and live otherwise (lines 21-23).

C. It requires that one place less emphasis on the natural world
WRONG: It is never indicated or implied in the passage that accepting Christ as one's savior and interacting with Nature are mutually exclusive. From the passage, it is clear that the author prefers Nature to Christianity and paganism.

D. It creates a dichotomy within him consisting of both pagan and Christian values
WRONG:The Christian concept of absolution by accepting Christ and paganism are not looked upon as mutually exclusive entities in the passage (lines 19-21, 33-34). Furthermore, it is not stated in the passage that Thomas has any strong beliefs or affiliation with Christianity and paganism as would be required for such a dichotomy to exist.

689. According to the passage, what approach does Milosz take in exploring issues of Christianity, paganism, and Nature?

I. He analyzes the basics tenets and workings of all three

II. He sees how individuals existentially experience all three

III. He makes implicit judgments on the inherent worth of all three

A. I only
WRONG: II and III are also correct.

B. II only
WRONG: I and III are also correct.

C. I and II only

WRONG: III is also correct.

D. I, II, and III

CORRECT: I is correct because Milosz "questioning the premises on which they [Christianity, paganism, and Nature] are based" (lines 7-8). II is correct because Milosz "explores how they are interwoven with both human emotions and cognitions" (lines 9-10). III is correct because Milosz makes makes implicit value judgments on all three entities in the passage. He takes an antagonistic stance towards Christianity, a neutral stance toward paganism, and a positive stance toward Nature (lines 33-34, 37-38, and 68-69, respectively).

Examination 15: Biological Sciences

Passage V (Questions 690- 697)

690. **B is correct.** As stated in the question stem, slow twitch fibers depend more on aerobic processes (i.e. Krebs cycle) for energy. Figure 2 in the passage shows that maximal intake (and therefore consumption) of oxygen *decreases while in flight*. Due to the decreased availability of oxygen, slow twitch fibers will be forced to use anaerobic processes (i.e., glycolysis) for energy, which would decrease their overall efficiency.

691. **C is correct.** In order for a muscle to contract, myosin (thick) and actin (thin) myofilaments must bind to each other and undergo a power stroke that is powered by ATP. Maximal muscle contraction is accomplished when there is maximal overlap between these thick and thin myofilaments, allowing for the biggest power stroke of them all. Potassium is not directly involved with powering muscle contraction. The length of a sarcomere has nothing to do with the number of myofibrils recruited; this answer is also nonsensical in that a myofibril is made up of many sarcomeres.

692. **B is correct.** By definition, voluntary muscles such as the semitendinous are skeletal muscles. Smooth and cardiac muscle, on the other hand, are involuntary muscles. Skeletal muscle is striated and *multinucleated*, forming syncytia that function as a singular unit. Cardiac muscle, on the other hand, is also striated but mononucleated. Both skeletal and cardiac muscle is imbedded with T-tubule networks, which help transmit action potentials to the interior of the muscle cell.

693. **D is correct.** Muscle contraction is directly dependent on the presence of calcium, which is stored and released from the sarcoplasmic reticulum. The surge of calcium release causes a change in troponin-tropomyosin conformation. This conformational change allows for myosin-actin binding, which then leads to the power

stroke involved in contraction. Calcium levels in the blood are tightly controlled by *calcitonin*, a hormone produced by the *thyroid gland.*

694. **D is correct.** The passage states that the primary anti-gravity muscles include the gastrocnemius, quadriceps, and the musculature of the back and neck. In the absence of gravity, it can be assumed that these muscles would atrophy mostly readily and quickly. While biceps are not stated to be a specific anti-gravity muscle, it can be assumed that they will still atrophy more than the heart. The heart, albeit a muscle, ought not to atrophy as it continues to pump blood regardless of the absence of gravity.

695. **D is correct.** Unlike the heart, which is a free-floating muscle within the thoracic cavity, skeletal muscle is attached at each end to bones. Therefore, the maximal length of skeletal muscle is fixed with very little room for excess stretch. The hypertrophy (increase in cell size) of muscles seen with weightlifting or moderate exercise is a result of repeated muscle *contraction*, not expansion or stretching. Muscles cannot expand with force, but only contract. Hyperplasia is the increase in the number of cells.

696. **C is correct.** Cardiac muscle differs from skeletal muscle in several ways: unlike skeletal muscle, which is multinucleated, cardiac muscle is mononucleated. Although cardiac muscle does not form synticia, since it is mononucleated, it behaves like a synticium through the connections of intercalated disks, which allow for action potentials to be propagated from one cardiac cell to another instantaneously. Intercalated disks are not seen in skeletal muscle. While the action potential (AP) in skeletal muscles is generated solely through the influx of sodium through sodium-gated channels, the AP in cardiac cells is prolonged through the use sodium-calcium channels as well. However, both cardiac and skeletal muscle is microscopically striated.

697. **B is correct.** The firing of an action potential is an "all or none" process that, once fired, serves only to propagate itself, NOT to increase the force of a contraction. Recruitment of additional fibers, increasing the amount of calcium released from the sarcoplasmic reticulum, and muscle hypertrophy (such as seen with weight lifting) can all increase the force of muscle contraction.

Passage VI (Questions 698- 703)

698. **D is correct.** The fact that the disorder is only seen in males points toward sex-linked inheritance. Since the parents are both unaffected, the disorder must be recessive.

699. **B is correct.** If the child died, he must have been homozygous for achondroplasia. As the father is

heterozygous, the mother must have an allele for achondroplasia as well. Thus the mother is also a heterozygote, or dwarf.

700. B is correct. The genes for colorblindness and Huntington's are on different chromosomes (sex-linked vs autosomal, respectively) and thus they assort independently. Since Huntington's is dominant and both parents are heterozygotes, there is a 75% chance of having children with the disorder. There is a 50% chance of having a colorblind child (whether they are a boy or a girl). The chances of them having BOTH are simply (75%)(50%) = 37.5%

701. C is correct. The fact that Bob's daughters are all affected while both of his sons are normal strongly implicates the X-chromosome. If the disorder was sex-linked recessive, then Jane's genotype would be homozygous for the affected X chromosome. This would result in all of her sons being affected. Since there is a normal son, the disorder must be sex-linked dominant, and Jane must be heterozygous. Furthermore, the fact that all of Jane's children are affected even though the father is normal implies that the disease allele is dominant.

702. B is correct. Bob passes a Y chromosome to all of his sons. The boys have a 50% chance of receiving either the normal or defective X chromosome from their heterozygous mother.

703. C is correct. According to the passage, dominant lethal disorders can only exist if they cause death after reproductive maturity. As the number of individuals whom survive until reproductive age decreases, the defective alleles are slowly removed from the gene pool vial natural selection.

Independent Questions (Questions 704-705)

704. A is correct. Any sex-linked recessive disorder will be far more common in males since they only have one X chromosome. Menstruation is only the shedding of the uterine lining. Although female hemophiliacs would exhibit significantly greater bleeding, similar to fibroid menorrhagia, mentstruation can be very easily prevented with hormonal treatment. Choice III is the reasoning behind the contraindication of estrogen and progesterone-containing oral contraceptives for women with increased clotting, however, this is not the reason why the incidence of female hemophilia is low.

705. A is correct. Mitochondrial DNA is inherited solely from the mother.

428

EXPLANATIONS 16

Answers to Questions 706–751

ANSWERS TO EXAMINATION 16

PHYSICAL SCIENCES	VERBAL REASONING	BIOLOGICAL SCIENCES
706. C	722. B	736. B
707. B	723. D	737. A
708. A	724. B	738. D
709. C	725. C	739. C
710. C	726. D	740. A
711. B	727. D	741. D
712. A	728. D	742. C
713. D	729. D	743. B
714. C	730. A	744. B
715. C	731. B	745. D
716. D	732. C	746. D
717. A	733. B	747. D
718. A	734. C	748. A
719. A	735. A	749. D
720. D	689. D	750. D
721. D		751. B
		752. A

Passage I (Questions 706-710)

706. C is correct. Use the lens equation. The focal length is one-half of the radius of curvature, so $f = 6.25$ cm. Keep in mind that the image distance is negative.

$$\frac{1}{f} = \frac{1}{d_o} + \frac{1}{d_i}$$

$$\frac{1}{6.25} = \frac{1}{d_o} + \frac{1}{-25}$$

$$d_o = 5 \text{ cm}$$

707. B is correct. According to the passage, the eye cannot clearly perceive an object that is closer than 25 cm. The passage also states that the maximum magnification occurs when the image is at a distance of 25 cm.

708. A is correct. The image appears on the same side of the lens as the object, so it is a virtual image. All virtual images are upright.

709. C is correct. The angular size is equal to the ratio $\frac{h}{d}$, which is $\frac{1}{3}$ for the object. The passage states that when an object is placed at the focal point, the angular size of the image is the same as the angular size of the object.

710. C is correct. The largest visible image occurs when

$$M = 1 + \frac{25}{f} = 6.$$

The smallest visible image occurs when $M = \frac{25}{f} = 5$.

711. B is correct. Set up a ratio using angular size.

$$(2)/(100) = (30)/d$$

$d = 1500$ cm $= 15$ m. Meters do not have to be converted to centimeters, as long as the units remain consistent across the ratio.

Passage II (Questions 712-717)

712. A is correct. In the reaction ,the oxidation state of Fe^{2+} is increased to 3+, so it lost electrons and was oxidized (LEO). The oxidation state of O_2 went from 0 to 2–, so it gained electrons and was reduced (GER).

713. D is correct. Use the coefficient on the reactant side and solve for x.

$$x + 1 = 4$$

$$x = 3$$

714. C is correct. The voltages given are for the oxidation taking place in Reaction 1 and the reduction taking place in Reaction 2, so neither sign has to be switched when the two are combined to form a redox reaction. Adding the voltages together reveals the standard emf: 1.23 V + 0.44 V = 1.67 V.

715. C is correct. Salt water contains more ions than fresh water, so it is a better conductor. The passage states that mobile ions in the water are a necessary part of the rusting process.

716. D is correct. According to Reactions 1 and 2, hydrogen ions are necessary for the oxidation of iron, so a solution with a high pH and thus, a low concentration of hydrogen ions, will not be conducive to rust formation.

717. A is correct. The oxidation potentials for Sn and Zn can be found by changing the signs of the reduction potentials shown in the passage. The oxidation potentials for the three metals are: Sn (0.14 V), Fe (0.44 V), Zn (0.76 V). The higher the oxidation potential, the more reactive the metal.

Independent Questions (Questions 718-721)

718. A is correct. When the source and observer are moving apart, the Doppler shift will cause the wave to have lower frequency and larger wavelength. Speed is the same for both.

719. A is correct. Dispersion occurs when white light is broken up into its component frequencies. Choice B is an example of diffraction. Choice C is an example of total internal reflection. Choice D is an example of interference.

720. D is correct. K has an oxidation state of +1 and the four oxygens each have an oxidation state of –2, so Cl must have an oxidation state of +7 for the molecule to remain neutral.

721. D is correct. If $\Delta G°$ is negative, then the reaction is spontaneous under standard conditions. If the reaction is spontaneous under standard conditions, then the voltage must be positive and the equilibrium constant must favor the products by having a value greater than 1.

Passage III (Questions 722-728)

722. Bandura's theory of social learning can be best categorized as:

A. A theory that emphasizes the role of society on the way one learns
WRONG: This is not indicated in the passage. It would be incorrect to infer this statement from the name (social learning) of the theory. One must look to see what the second set of approaches, which includes Bandura's social learning theory, have in common.

B. A theory that interprets human behavior in terms of the learned social consequences of one's behavior in given situations
CORRECT: This is the most consistent choice with the information in the passage. The second set of approaches, which includes Bandura's social learning theory, put an emphasis on behavior (line 21). This choice states that social learning theory looks at how societal consequences in given situations (environmental conditions/circumstances) effects human behavior. This falls in the purview of the second set of approaches as outlined in lines 22-24.

C. A theory that is fundamentally different from the Big 5 traits theory
WRONG: It cannot be fundamentally different because both theories belong to the same set of approaches (lines 29-30).

D. A theory that looks at how past social interactions influence the way one perceives the world
WRONG: This would better define or characterize the final set of approaches (lines 41-43) and would not apply to Bandura's theory of social learning.

723. The attempt understand the person in terms of a human story is most consistent with which category of approaches?

A. The first category
WRONG: The first category looks at the human in terms of the unconscious (line 15).

B. The second category
WRONG: The second theory concentrates interaction between the environment and behavior (lines 26-27).

C. The third category
WRONG: This category concentrates on understanding man in terms of his conscious self (line 32).

D. The fourth category
CORRECT: This category of approaches studies man as an ongoing narrative of experiences (lines 44-46).

724. According to the passage, there is most probably a diverse range of methods to understand humans because:

A. Humans have unconscious, conscious, behavioral, and social aspects
WRONG: These are the different aspects of the human that various approaches address in order to understand personality. However, the passage does not state that the difficulty in studying personality arises from this multi-faceted nature of humans. These are just various ways in which researchers have approached the study of personality.

B. Human are inherently complex
CORRECT: This idea is expressed in lines 6-7. The passage is stating the inherent intricacy of man makes understanding him "no simple task" (lines 6-7). The passage further states that due to this intricacy multitudinous formulations have been designed to understand man (lines 7-8).

C. Our methods of scientifically studying personality are not yet mature
WRONG: The author does imply that the field of personology may not be linear in its progression toward understanding man (lines 1-4). However, it is not stated that this has lead to the diversity of theories produced to understand man.

D. Man is the product of his social context, a context that has too many variables to ever be fully understood
WRONG: This reasoning is not supported by the passage.

725. Which of the following assertions would most weaken the main idea of this passage

A. Ultimately, we can achieve a reasonable understanding of personality
WRONG: The author does state that the field of personology may not be linear in its progression toward understanding man, that the field may not mature, so to speak, over time (lines 1-4). However, this is not the main idea of the passage.

B. Existentialism is not appropriately classified in this scheme because there are significant differences between it and the other approaches of the third category
WRONG: This statement does threaten the validity of the passage in that it suggests existentialism has been misclassified. However, existentialism was only offered as an illustrative example of the third category of approaches and its classification does not comprise the main idea of the passage

C. There are many theories whose approach to understanding man does not fall into any of the four categories listed.
CORRECT: The main idea of the passage is that the multitudinous conception about personality can be seemingly comprehensively compartmentalized into four broad categories (lines 11-12). If numerous theories do not fall into this scheme, then the main idea is threatened.

D. McAdams created this classification during a time of great turmoil
WRONG: This does not threaten the main idea directly. The main idea of the passage is that the multitudinous conception about personality can be comprehensively compartmentalized into four broad categories (lines 11-12). We cannot assume that McAdams construction of this scheme in a time of person turmoil is a threat to it validity.

726. According to the author, in which following ways are all the modern approaches of personology most similar?

A. Each of the modern approaches looks at multiple aspects of the person
WRONG: We cannot make this conclusion from the passage. Actually, it would seem from the passage that each set of approaches concentrate on one specific aspect of human nature (the unconscious, behavior, intellect, and socio-historical context) rather than multiple aspects.

B. Modern approaches all address the central role of the intellect in understanding man
WRONG: According to the passage, only the third category fits this description.

C. Modern approaches all agree that man is a complex entity that is difficult to study
WRONG: This is tricky: The fact that man is a complex entity is the author's interpretation. This is not necessarily the view promulgated by specific approaches or theories.

D. Modern approaches may not be more accurate in understanding man than earlier approaches
CORRECT: The authors states that, as time passes, personology unlike other scientific fields may not mature in terms of its understanding of personality (lines 2-4). This would mean that modern theories are not necessarily more insightful than older ones.

727. A man goes to work and is reprimanded by his boss for a mistake that he did not commit. He keeps quiet, but feels perturbed and uneasy the rest of the day. When he gets home, he kicks the dog and yells at his wife for not having supper ready. He has a short fuse for the rest of the evening but cannot seem to understand why he is act-

ing as such. Which of the following approaches would be the most appropriate to study and explain this man's behavior?

A. Bandura's social learning theory
WRONG: This is not the best answer because it does not take into account the fact that the individual is not fully aware of what is driving his actions.

B. Maslow's theory of self actualization
WRONG: This is not the best answer because it does not take into account the fact that the individual is not fully aware of what is driving his actions.

C. Erik Erickson's theory of life stages
WRONG: This theory is not mentioned in the passage.

D. Freudian theory of conflict sublimation
CORRECT: Even if one is not familiar with the concept of sublimation, the fact that Freud is mentioned leads one to understand that the first category of approaches is being referred to in this answer choice. This category focuses on unconscious drives, desires, and conflicts in understanding the individual (lines 13-16). This approach would be the most appropriate to analyze this person's behavior because it takes into consideration that the individual in the vignette is not cognizant of what is driving this behavior.

728. A young college student falls passionately in love with a colleague and they marry. Growing up, the student's parents had been exacting and very strict. The student is now in a stage in his life where people generally feel the need to belong. The young bride finds her new husband very clingy and controlling. Which of the following theories stated in the passage would take all these factors into account when analyzing the student's personality?

A. Big 5 traits theory
WRONG: This theory would not take into account the various life experiences of the individual over time. It would concentrate more on how a certain person would act in a given situation in set point in time.

B. Behaviorist theory
WRONG: This theory is not discussed in the passage.

C. Existentialism
WRONG: This theory would focus on the person's conception of the world around himself and how that conception would drive behavior (lines 36-37). It would not take into account the various life experiences of the individual over time nor would it take into account the person's life stage.

D. No such theory was mentioned in the passage
CORRECT: This is the best answer. The fourth

433

category of approaches looks at the individual in terms of his previous experiences. These approaches also would likely take into account the individual's life stage as this may be understood to be a part of the individual's social context at the time (lines 42-46). There are no examples given from this category in the passage.

Passage IV (Questions 729-736)

729. The term *Congressional staff* most accurately refers to:

A. Senators and Congressmen
WRONG: Senators are Congressmen. This fact should call into question the validity of this answer choice. Congressmen consist of members of the House of Representatives and the Senate. Congressional staff consists of outside personnel whose job it is to aid Congress members in various capacities (lines 54-55). These Congressional staff are not however Congress members themselves.

B. Members of congressional committees and sub-committees
WRONG: Congressional committees consist of Democratic and Republican Congress members (lines 8-9). Congressional staff is not synonymous with Congress members themselves. Rather Congressional staff aid Congress members in various capacities (lines 54-55).

C. The president's cabinet
WRONG: This is never stated in the passage.

D. L.A.'s, fellows, and press secretaries
CORRECT: This is the best answer. Even though press secretaries are never mentioned in the passage, we do know that Congressional staff consists of personnel that "educate, brief, and advice Congress members on the scores of issues they are required to debate and adjudicate on" (lines 53-55). L.A.'s and fellows are mentioned verbatim (lines 53-55).

730. Consider a case in which a group of Senators are in almost complete agreement on a bill that has come out of conference. However, they would like to make some slight changes to the bill. Which of the following courses of action are at their disposal?

A. Start all the way at the beginning of the legislative process by introducing their desired changes in the form of a new bill.
CORRECT: The passage indicates that once a bill comes out of conference, no further amendments are allowed (lines 34-35). The only choice left would then be to reintroduce the changes in the form of a new bill.

B. Filibuster to prevent the passage of the bill in vote unless their changes are incorporated into the bill
WRONG: First, filibustering is not discussed in this particular passage. Second, The passage indicates that once a bill comes out of conference, no further amendments are allowed (lines 34-35). If the bill out of conference is final then this option (making slight changes to a bill that has come out of conference) is not at the disposal of the Senators, via filibustering or any other means.

C. Make the changes to the bill and resubmit the bill to the conference committee
WRONG: The passage indicates that once a bill comes out of conference, no further amendments are allowed (lines 34-35). The Senators would not be able to make amendments to the bill at this juncture be it by resubmitting the bill to a committee.

D. Use lobbying power to convince Congressmen of the importance to incorporate the desired changes into the bill
WRONG: This is not stated in the passage. Furthermore, The passage indicates that once a bill comes out of conference, it is final and no further amendments are allowed (lines 34-35).

731. The president's party holds majority in both the House and the Senate. Consider the situation in which a bill has gone out of Congress to the president. For political reasons, the president would like the bill to die without issuing a formal veto. Which of the following actions might the President take to achieve this end?

A. Wait for the ten-day presidential review period to pass
WRONG: If the president were to wait for the ten-day presidential review period to pass, then the bill would not die. In fact, the bill would automatically be passed (lines 38-39).

B. Ask party members in Congress to create a movement to have Congress adjourn
CORRECT: If Congress adjourns during the ten-day presidential review period, then the bill will die. This is called a pocket veto (lines 40-42)

C. The president has no options. He must issue a formal veto to stifle the passage of the bill into law.
WRONG: This is not true. Theoretically, the president can create a motion in Congress to adjourn during the ten-day presidential review period and thereby effect a pocket veto (lines 43-44).

D. The president will put pressure on the minority leader in Congress to get a 2/3 consensus for a veto
WRONG: The Congress cannot veto a bill by 2/3 majority while it is undergoing presidential review.

732. Some Congressmen want to ensure that the president does not veto a health care reform bill. They forward the president the bill, so that he may review it ahead of time, while the bill is still in consideration at the congressional level. With this goal in mind, the most appropriate stage to forward the bill would be:

A. As soon as the bill is introduced
WRONG: The bill will go through multiple debates and amendments in Congress after its introduction. For example, it must still be submitted for committee review and debated on the floor. By the time, the bill finally makes it to presidential review it is likely to have been altered. There is no guarantee then that the president will sign this altered bill into law. It would be best to forward the bill when it is in its last stage of debate in Congress, so that whatever changes the president would like to make can be incorporated into the final version of the bill that will be submitted for presidential review.

B. During committee action
WRONG: The bill has yet to go through multiple debates and possible revisions in Congress after committee review. By the time, the bill is submitted for presidential review it is likely to have been altered. There is no guarantee then that the president will sign this altered bill into law. Also, at this stage, there is ample opportunity for the bill to be placed out of consideration. It would be best to forward the bill when it is in its last stage of debate in Congress, so that whatever changes the president would like to make may be incorporated into the final version of the bill that will be submitted for presidential review.

C. During conference committee
CORRECT: This is the best time to forward the bill. Forwarding the bill during conference will allow Congress to incorporate any amendments that the president would prefer just before the bill becomes final (lines 30-31). This final bill would face little alteration as it would contain all the changes that the president desired without much further alterations.

D. Soon after a pocket veto
WRONG: Once a pocket veto has been issued the bill is dead (lines 40-42).

733. What the term "reported favorably" in line 13 most likely refer to?

A. The complete consensus of both chambers
WRONG: The bill will be reported favorably by committee in the chamber in which the bill was introduced. The other chamber has not become involved yet. The second chamber will become involved later (lines 23-25), and thus there cannot be a consensus.

B. That the bill is mostly agreed upon by committee but may be subsequently modified
CORRECT: This answer is the most consistent with the information in the passage (lines 15-20). The committee agrees and passes the bill by voting. Then a committee report is written. This report is then debated and appropriate modifications are made (lines 15-20).

C. That the bill was passed into law by majority vote
WRONG: The bill will not be passed into law until much later. The bill still has to go through various stages in Congress and presidential review (lines 25-34).

D. The media presents the bill positively during reporting
WRONG: This is not indicated in the passage.

734. A tobacco company spent millions of dollars lobbying over the past six fiscal years. This year they decide to evaluate the efficacy of their lobbying efforts. Based on the passage, which of the following is most likely the biggest obstacle to the tobacco company's lobbying platform?

A. Financial constraints due to new tax laws concerning the sale of tobacco
WRONG: Financial constraints are not discussed in the passage as concerns lobbying (lines 58-59).

B. Changing constituency of Congress members
WRONG: Even though lobbyists do meet with Congress members, we are told that these meetings are less rare than those with Congressional staff. According to the passage, lobbyist influence changes mostly at the level of Congressional staff (lines 58-59).

C. Changing constituency of Congress staff members
CORRECT: According to the passage, lobbyists work mostly at the level of Congressional staff (lines 58-59). If this staff were to change, then the tobacco company would have to form new contacts. We can infer, based on the passage, that this is the biggest difficulty in the company's efforts to lobby.

D. Inability to find enough time to convince Congress
WRONG: This is not discussed in the passage.

735. Which of the following statements is TRUE?

A. A bill is first deliberated upon by committee before is debated on the floor
CORRECT: This is true. First the committee will review the bill. If it is reported favorably, a committee report will be drafted. Later, the bill is debated on the House or Senate floor (lines 10-15).

B. Anyone can introduce a bill to Congress but only a Congressman can draft a bill

WRONG: It is actually the other way around. Only a Congressman can introduce a bill, but anyone can draft one (lines 5-6).

C. A bill will be considered "enrolled" so long as it is passed by one chamber of Congress

WRONG: Both chambers need to pass the bill for it to be considered "enrolled" (lines 26-27).

D. A three-fifths vote is required to override a presidential veto.

WRONG: A two-thirds vote is required, not a three-fifths vote, to override a presidential veto (lines 44-45).

Examination 16: Biological Sciences

Passage V (Questions 736-743)

736. B is correct. According to the passage, "Osteoid primarily contains proteoglycans and collagen". Vitamin C is necessary for collagen formation and maintenance; vitamin C deficiency causes scurvy. The symptoms of scurvy include skin lesions, poor wound healing, blood vessel fragility, and softening of bones leading to spontaneous bone breakage. Vitamin A is important for the visual cycle. Vitamin B12 is important for the maintenance of red blood cells and nervous system. Vitamin E is an important antioxidant and membrane component.

737. A is correct. PTH and calcitonin act in opposition to each other, and thus both would not be elevated or decreased at the same time. This rules out answer choices C and D. According to the passage, "Osteoblasts and osteocytes maintain and form bone…" When Osteoblasts are inactive, osteoid production would be minimal and they would be flat in appearance. Increased PTH and/or decreased calcitonin would favor the dissolution of bone by osteoblast inhibition and osteoclast stimulation.

738. D is correct. Estrogen is a sterol and is most closely related to Vitamin D. Thus, estrogen can be expected to mimic or enhance the action of vitamin D, which increases Ca^{2+} and PO_4^{3-} reabsorption in the kidney. By this logic, answer choice A is incorrect. Stimulating osteoclast activity would exacerbate the symptoms of osteoporosis, ruling it out as an effective therapy. According to the passage, answer choice C characterizes osteomalacia.

739. C is correct. Vitamin D increases Ca^{2+} and PO_4^{3-} reabsorption in the kidney, and thus would favor hydroxyapatite deposition. Collagen and proteoglycans are components of osteoid synthesized by osteoblasts and should not accumulate in kidney; answer choices A

and D are eliminated. While vitamin D can be expected to accumulate in most soft tissue membranes due to its lipidic nature, it will not harden into kidney stones.

740. A is correct. PTH increases the rate of bone resorption by stimulating osteoclast activity. Calcitonin is an effective treatment for the early stage of Paget's disease to slow the initial bone resorption. In late stage Paget's disease, calcitonin or Vitamin D would only exacerbate bone formation; answer choices B and D are incorrect. PTH and calcitonin act in opposition to one another so coadministration would not be effective.

741. D is correct. Osteoblasts synthesize osteoid; an excessive number and activity of osteoblasts in osteosarcoma results in increased osteoid synthesis. This mimics rickets (osteomalacia) where the ratio of mineral to organic bone material is lower than normal. Sickle cell anemia is a disease of the blood; answer choice C is incorrect. According to the passage, osteoporosis is characterized by "equal loss of both organic and inorganic bone matrix", and thus the ratio of osteoid to mineral does not change. Scurvy would inhibit collagen synthesis, and thus increase the ratio of mineral to organic bone material.

742. C is correct. According to the passage, osteoporosis is characterized by "equal loss of both organic and inorganic bone matrix". The question states that protein synthesis by osteoblasts is decreased upon glucocorticoid administration; this accounts for decreased osteoid production in the resulting osteoporosis. Increased bone resorption must also take place to account for the loss of inorganic bone matrix. PTH is the only hormone in the answer choices that increases bone resorption. Calcitonin decreases bone resorption and vitamin D is not a hormone; answer choices A and D are eliminated. PTH and calcitonin act in opposition to one another.

743. B is correct. Calcitonin is a peptide hormone produced by parafollicular cells of the thyroid gland. PTH (parathyroid hormone) is a polypeptide hormone produced by the parathyroid glands. Vitamin D is not a hormone, and is obtained from the diet and/or formed in the skin by exposure to UV light.

Passage VI (Questions 744-750)

744. B is correct. For a gene pool to be stable, there must be no *net* migration in or out of the population, but there can be some migration.

745. D is correct. Genetic drift describes any change in allelic frequency which occurs as a result of small sample size. These changes may be attributed to statistical fluctuations, founder effects, or bottlenecks.

746. D is correct. The summed frequencies for all alleles must equal 1. If 9% of the population is homogenous A, then the frequency of A is 30% (square root of .09). If 16% of the population is homogenous B, then the frequency of B is 40% (square root of 0.16). A + B + C = 1; 0.3 + 0.4 + C = 1; The frequency of C is 30%.

747. D is correct. If 1 in 100 lizards had scaly skin, then the frequency for allele a would be 0.1 (square root of 0.01). The frequency for allele A would thus be $1 - 0.1 = 0.9$. The frequency of heterozygotes would be $0.1 \times 0.9 \times 2 = 0.18$.

748. A is correct. If the frequency of s is 0.4, then the frequency of S is 0.6. The lizards with phenotypically smooth skin are either homozygous dominant or heterozygous. The frequency is $0.6 \times 0.6 = 0.36$ for homozygous dominant and $2 \times 0.6 \times 0.4 = 0.48$ for heterozygous. The sum of these is 84% and, in a population of 10,000, you would get 8,400.

749. D is correct. All of these factors may contribute to the increased prevalence of an allele on one of the two islands. Choice A and B suggest that scales present an evolutionary advantage to lizards on Island 1. Choice C exemplifies a *founder effect*.

750. D is correct. One may only use Hardy-Weinburg calculations to predict the characteristics of a population; population statistics cannot be applied to single births.

Independent Question (Question 751)

751. A is correct. 'Bottlenecking' occurs when the population size is severely reduced and the group of those left behind has a different gene pool than the original.
